T0226797

Implant Procedures for the General Dentist

Editor

HARRY DYM

DENTAL CLINICS OF NORTH AMERICA

www.dental.theclinics.com

April 2015 • Volume 59 • Number 2

ELSEVIER

1600 John F. Kennedy Boulevard • Suite 1800 • Philadelphia, Pennsylvania, 19103-2899

http://www.dental.theclinics.com

DENTAL CLINICS OF NORTH AMERICA Volume 59, Number 2
April 2015 ISSN 0011-8532, ISBN: 978-0-323-35972-6

Editor: John Vassallo; j.vassallo@elsevier.com
Developmental Editor: Stephanie Wissler

Dental Clinics of North America (ISSN 0011-8532) is published quarterly by Elsevier Inc., 360 Park Avenue South, New York, NY 10010-1710. Months of issue are January, April, July, and October. Business and Editorial Offices: 1600 John F. Kennedy Boulevard, Suite 1800, Philadelphia, PA 19103-2899. Periodicals postage paid at New York, NY and additional mailing offices. Subscription prices are $280.00 per year (domestic individuals), $485.00 per year (domestic institutions), $135.00 per year (domestic students/residents), $340.00 per year (Canadian individuals), $628.00 per year (Canadian institutions), $410.00 per year (international individuals), $628.00 per year (international institutions), and $200.00 per year (international and Canadian students/residents). International air speed delivery is included in all *Clinics* subscription prices. All prices are subject to change without notice. **POSTMASTER:** Send address changes to *Dental Clinics of North America*, Elsevier Health Sciences Division, Subscription Customer Service, 3251 Riverport Lane, Maryland Heights, MO 63043. **Customer Service (orders, claims, online, change of address): Elsevier Health Sciences Division, Subscription Customer Service, 3251 Riverport Lane, Maryland Heights, MO 63043. Tel: 1-800-654-2452 (U.S. and Canada). Fax: 314-447-8029. E-mail: journalscustomer service-usa@elsevier.com (for print support); journalsonlinesupport-usa@elsevier.com (for online support).**

Reprints. For copies of 100 or more, of articles in this publication, please contact the Commercial Reprints Department, Elsevier Inc., 360 Park Avenue South, New York, NY 10010-1710. Tel.: 212-633-3874; Fax: 212-633-3820; E-mail: reprints@elsevier.com.

The *Dental Clinics of North America* is covered in *MEDLINE/PubMed (Index Medicus), Current Contents/Clinical Medicine, ISI/BIOMED* and *Clinahl.*

Contributors

EDITOR

HARRY DYM, DDS
Chairman, Department of Dentistry/Oral and Maxillofacial Surgery; Program Director Oral and Maxillofacial Surgery, Residency Training Program, The Brooklyn Hospital Center, Brooklyn; Clinical Professor, Oral and Maxillofacial Surgery, Columbia University College of Dental Medicine, New York, New York; Senior Attending, Woodhull Hospital, Brooklyn; Attending, New York Harbor Healthcare System, Brooklyn, New York

AUTHORS

SHELLY ABRAMOWICZ, DMD, MPH
Assistant Professor in Oral and Maxillofacial Surgery and Pediatrics, Division of Oral and Maxillofacial Surgery, Department of Surgery, Emory University, Atlanta, Georgia

ARVIND BABU RS, BDS, MDS, DFO
Oral and Maxillofacial Pathologist; Lecturer and Research Coordinator, Dentistry Programme, Faculty of Medical Sciences, The University of the West Indies, Mona, Kingston, Jamaica, West Indies

GOLALEH BARZANI, DMD
Resident, Oral and Maxillofacial Surgery Training Program, The Brooklyn Hospital Center, Brooklyn, New York

HUSSAM BATAL, DMD
Assistant Professor, Oral and Maxillofacial Surgery, Boston University, Boston, Massachusetts

DUSTIN BOWLER, DDS
Oral and Maxillofacial Surgery Training Program, The Brooklyn Hospital Center, Brooklyn, New York

RICARDO A. BOYCE, DDS, FICD
Assistant Clinical Professor with Columbia University SDM and NYU College of Dentistry; Full-time Attending and the Director of the General Practice Residency Program, Department of Dentistry, The Brooklyn Hospital Center, New York, New York

MICHAEL H. CHAN, DDS
Director of Oral and Maxillofacial Surgery, Oral and Maxillofacial Surgery/Dental Service, Department of Veterans Affairs, New York Harbor Healthcare System (Brooklyn Campus); Attending, Department Dentistry/Oral and Maxillofacial Surgery, The Brooklyn Hospital Center, Brooklyn, New York

EARL CLARKSON, DDS
Program Director, Department of Oral and Maxillofacial Surgery, Woodhull Hospital; Attending Physician, The Brooklyn Hospital Center, Brooklyn, New York

LADI DOONQUAH, MD, DDS
Consultant Surgeon, Department of Surgery; Associate Lecturer, Faculty of Medical Sciences, University Hospital of the West Indies, University of the West Indies, Kingston, Jamaica

HARRY DYM, DDS
Chairman, Department of Dentistry/Oral and Maxillofacial Surgery; Program Director Oral and Maxillofacial Surgery, Residency Training Program, The Brooklyn Hospital Center, Brooklyn; Clinical Professor, Oral and Maxillofacial Surgery, Columbia University College of Dental Medicine, New York, New York; Senior Attending, Woodhull Hospital, Brooklyn; Attending, New York Harbor Healthcare System, Brooklyn, New York

SCOTT D. GANZ, DMD
Maxillofacial Prosthodontist Private Practice, Fort Lee; Attending, Hackensack University Medical Center, Hackensack; Attending, Rutgers School of Dental Medicine, Newark, New Jersey

CURTIS HOLMES, DDS
Resident, Department Dentistry/Oral and Maxillofacial Surgery, The Brooklyn Hospital Center, Brooklyn, New York

PATRICK D. KELLY, DDS
Resident, Division of Oral and Maxillofacial Surgery, Loyola University Stritch School of Medicine, Loyola University Medical Center, Maywood, Illinois

GARY KLEMONS, DDS
Department of Dentistry, Attending for Restorative Implantology and Cosmetic Dentistry, The Brooklyn Hospital Center, New York, New York; Private Practice, Brooklyn, New York

RYAN LODENQUAI, BSc, MBBS
Resident, Department of Surgery, Faculty of Medical Sciences, University of the West Indies, Kingston, Jamaica

STEPHEN MACLEOD, BDS, MD, FACS
Division of Oral and Maxillofacial Surgery and Dental Medicine, Department of Surgery, Loyola University Medical center, Maywood, Illinois

PUSHKAR MEHRA, BDS, DMD
Chairman, Oral and Maxillofacial Surgery, Boston University, Boston, Massachusetts

ANIKA D. MITCHELL, BSc, MBBS
Resident, Department of Surgery, Faculty of Medical Sciences, University of the West Indies, Kingston, Jamaica

NAVEEN MOHAN, DDS
Resident, Department of Dentistry/Oral and Maxillofacial Surgery, The Brooklyn Hospital Center, Brooklyn, New York

ORRETT OGLE, DDS
Lecturer, Mona Dental Program, Faculty of Medical Sciences, University of the West Indies, Kingston, Jamaica; Attending, The Brooklyn Hospital Center, Brooklyn, New York; Former Chief, Oral and Maxillofacial Surgery, Woodhull Hospital, Brooklyn, New York

JAMES PARELLI, DMD, MD, MS.Ed
Division of Oral and Maxillofacial Surgery, Department of Surgery, Emory University, Atlanta, Georgia

KEVIN ROBERTSON, DDS
Division of Oral and Maxillofacial Surgery and Dental Medicine, Department of Surgery, Loyola University Medical Center, Maywood, Illinois

STEVEN RICHARD SCHWARTZ, DDS
Diplomate, American Board of Oral and Maxillofacial Surgery; Private Practice, Oral and Maxillofacial Surgery, Brooklyn; Director of Surgical Implantology, Woodhull Medical and Mental Health Center, Division of Oral and Maxillofacial Surgery, Department of Dentistry; Senior Attending, Division of Oral and Maxillofacial Surgery, Department of Dentistry, The Brooklyn Hospital Center; Private Practice, New York Oral and Maxillofacial Surgeon, Brooklyn, New York

TIMOTHY SHAHBAZIAN, DDS
Division of Oral and Maxillofacial Surgery and Dental Medicine, Department of Surgery, Loyola University Medical Center, Maywood, Illinois

MARK J. STEINBERG, DDS, MD, FACS
Clinical Professor of Surgery, Division of Oral and Maxillofacial Surgery, Loyola University Stritch School of Medicine, Maywood, Illinois; Private Practice, Northbrook, Illinois

AVICHAI STERN, DDS
Attending and Clinical Coordinator, Oral and Maxillofacial Surgery Training Program, The Brooklyn Hospital Center, Brooklyn, New York

JONATHAN M. TAGLIARENI, DDS
Chief Resident, Department of Oral and Maxillofacial Surgery, The Brooklyn Hospital Center, Brooklyn, New York

JOSHUA WOLF, DDS
Attending, Department of Dentistry/Oral and Maxillofacial Surgery, The Brooklyn Hospital Center, Brooklyn, New York

AMIR YAVARI, DDS
Private Practice, Boston, Massachusetts

Contents

Dental implants provide completely edentulous and partial edentulous patients the function and esthetics they had with natural dentition. It is critical to understand and apply predictable surgical principles when treatment planning and surgically restoring edentulous spaces with implants. This article defines basic implant concepts that should be meticulously followed for predictable results when treating patients and restoring dental implants. Topics include biological and functional considerations, biomechanical considerations, preoperative assessments, medical history and risk assessments, oral examinations, radiographic examinations, contraindications, and general treatment planning options.

Clinicians worldwide are increasingly adopting guided surgical applications for dental implants. Clinicians are becoming more aware of the benefits of proper planning through advanced imaging modalities and interactive treatment planning applications. All aspects of the planning phase are based on sound surgical and restorative fundamentals. As an integral part of the implant team, dental laboratories have now moved from analog to the digital world, providing the necessary support to the new digital workflow.

In this article, current literature on fixed and removable prosthodontics is reviewed along with evidence-based systematic reviews, including advice from those in the dental profession with years of experience, which help restorative dentists manage and treat their cases successfully. Treatment planning for restorative implantology should be looked at in 4 sections: (1) review of past medical history, (2) oral examination and occlusion, (3) dental imaging (ie, cone-beam computed tomography), and (4) fixed versus removable prosthodontics. These 4 concepts of treatment planning, along with proper surgical placements of the implant(s), result in successful cases.

Tissue response represents an important feature in biocompatibility in implant procedures. This review article highlights the fundamental characteristics of tissue response after the implant procedure. This article also highlights the tissue response in compromised osseous conditions. Understanding the histologic events after dental implants in normal and abnormal bone reinforces the concept of case selection in dental implants.

Short-length implants (<10 mm) can be used effectively in atrophic maxillae or mandibles even with crown/implant ratios that previously would have been considered excessive. Short implants can support either single or multiple units and can be used for fixed prostheses or overdentures. The use of short-length implants may avoid the need for complicated bone augmentation procedures, thus allowing patients who were either unwilling or unable for financial or medical reasons to undergo these advanced grafting techniques to be adequately treated.

Appropriate treatment of implants is becoming increasingly important for the general dentist as the number of implants placed per year continues to increase. Early diagnosis of peri-implantitis is imperative; initiating the correct treatment protocol depends on a proper diagnosis. Several risk factors exist for the development of peri-implantitis, which can guide patient selection and treatment planning. Treatment of peri-implantitis should be tailored to the severity of the lesion (as outlined by the cumulative interceptive supportive treatment protocol), ranging from mechanical debridement to explantation. Several surgical and nonsurgical treatment alternatives exist. There is little consensus on superior treatment methods.

Dental implants have had tremendous improvement since their initial introduction into clinical practice. With ongoing advances in implant technology and materials, better data emerge to allow shorter time between placement and restoration. This allows the restorative dentist and surgeon to provide improved treatment options to patients. Most evidence that exists supports the practice of immediately placed (after extraction) and immediately loaded implants. Additional high-quality studies are still needed to develop specific guidelines for a standardized approach to immediate rehabilitation.

Injuries to branches of the trigeminal nerves are a known complication during dental implant placement. These injuries tend to be more severe than those experienced during other dentoalveolar procedures. This article reviews the types of nerve injuries and areas and situations of which clinicians should be cognizant when placing dental implants. Strategies to avoid injuries, and a management algorithm for suspected nerve injuries, are also discussed.

Naveen Mohan, Joshua Wolf, and Harry Dym

Pneumatization of the maxillary sinus secondary to posterior maxillary tooth loss is an extremely common finding. Significant atrophy of the maxilla prevents implant placement in this region. For several decades, sinus augmentation has been used to develop these sites for dental implant placement. The main techniques for increasing the vertical bone height of the posterior maxilla are the transalveolar and lateral antrostomy approaches. The clinical and radiographic examinations dictate the appropriate method for each clinical situation. Both techniques have been shown to have high success rates. However, practitioners must be aware of potential complications and how to address them.

Ladi Doonquah, Ryan Lodenquai, and Anika D. Mitchell

The deficient alveolar ridge has been an impediment to the placement of dental implants in the past. A greater comprehension of bone biophysiology and biotechnology has greatly increased the surgical options available to rehabilitate these patients. Technology and regenerative science has also allowed clinicians to simplify some of the approaches to these patients. This article presents the authors' perspective on the current surgical treatment methodologies that have been most beneficial in reconstructing atrophic alveolar bone.

Avichai Stern and Golaleh Barzani

Autogenous bone harvest is the gold standard for restoring deficiencies of the recipient site. A deficient site requires adequate grafting before placement of implants; therefore, proper understanding of the wide variety of grafting options is the key to successfully planned implant dentistry. This provides general dentists with a better understanding of autogenous bone harvest and the variety of techniques available to provide the best outcomes for the patient.

Michael H. Chan and Curtis Holmes

Restoration of the atrophic edentulous maxilla and mandible with implant retained prostheses has involved the use of axially placed implants in regions of the maxilla and mandible based on the adequate availability of bone, often using a staged surgical approaches. Anatomic limitations including pneumatized maxillary sinus, proximity of the inferior alveolar nerve and lack of available native bone have many clinicians performing traditional grafting procedure prior to implant placement. Utilization of the "All-on-4" concept has overcome these anatomic restrictions by allowing placement of 2 vertical and 2 angled implants in the premaxilla and anterior mandible. This technique has enabled immediate placement of full arch fixed restoration at the time of implant surgery if sufficient torque is achieved. It has biomechanical advantages including increasing in A-P spread, enhancing load distribution with cross arch stabilization, shorten cantilever, longer implants to be placed by titling them posteriorly, and maintenance of marginal bone height. High implant survival rates of in the maxilla (92.5–100%), in the mandible (93–100%) and restoration (99.2–100%) prove that the "All-on-4" concept is a viable treatment option for edentulous patients with atrophic alveolar ridges circumventing these traditional grafting procedures.

Adequate quality and quantity of soft tissue plays an integral part in the esthetic outcome of dental implants. Adequate band of attached tissue decreases the incidence of mucositis and improves hygiene around implants. This article discusses a variety of techniques for soft tissue augmentation. Soft tissue grafting can be achieved at various stages of implant therapy. Epithelial connective tissue grafts are commonly used to increase the band of attached tissue. Subepithelial connective tissue grafts are great for increasing soft tissue thickness and improving the gingival biotype.

Alveolar bone that is insufficient to support implant placement due to lack of height or width may be augmented with grafting materials including bone morphogenic protein to create sites that are adequate for implant place-ment and long-term stability of implant-supported prosthesis. Bone morphogenic protein can be used alone or in concert with other bone graft materials as an alternative to invasive allograft bone harvesting procedures.

The structural and functional union of the implant with living bone is greatly influenced by the surface properties of the implant. The success of a dental implant depends on the chemical, physical, mechanical, and topographic characteristics of its surface. The influence of surface topography on osseointegration has translated to shorter healing times from implant placement to restoration. This article presents a discussion of surface characteristics and design of implants, which should allow the clinician to better understand osseointegration and information coming from implant manufacturers, allowing for better implant selection.

DENTAL CLINICS OF NORTH AMERICA

ISSUE OF RELATED INTEREST

Oral and Maxillofacial Surgery Clinics February 2015 (Vol. 27, No. 1)
Contemporary Management of Temporomandibular Joint Disorders
Daniel E. Perez, and Larry M. Wolford, *Editors*
Available at: www.oralmaxsurgery.theclinics.com

NOW AVAILABLE FOR YOUR iPhone and iPad

DENTAL CLINICS OF NORTH AMERICA

Preface

Implant Procedures for the General Dentist

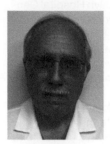

Harry Dym, DDS
Editor

I am very pleased to once again have the privilege of being part of the *Dental Clinics of North America* and working with such talented editors as Mr. John Vassallo and Ms. Stephanie Carter. This is a wonderful scholarly series dedicated to bringing new, relevant and evidence based scientific information to a readership committed to providing quality dental/oral care to their patients.

Implant surgery is a vital service that we as dentists can offer our patients and it is an area of practice that is growing by leaps and bounds. I have been involved in dental and oral surgical resident education for over thirty years and am a firm believer that general dentists have the ability, skill and knowledge to practice and master many different areas in the field of dentistry, based on their education, training and experience. General dentists, as the clinical gate keepers, have the initial opportunity to engage their patients in the discussion of implants. A more complete background in this subject will allow them to grow their clinical practice and meet the needs of their patients.

I am grateful to my esteemed colleagues who have so capably contributed to this text and I am confident that it will be a resource that will be of great help to those practitioners interested in introducing implant surgery into their practice as well as to those already offering implant surgical services to their patients.

As I have done in the past, I would like to take this opportunity to thank certain individuals who I have been fortunate enough to have worked with or interacted with these past many years (and in some cases decades) and without whose guidance, wisdom and loyalty, my professional and personal life would surely have diminished.

1. Dr Peter M. Sherman, Chairman of Dentistry and Oral and Maxillofacial Surgery at Woodhull Hospital, mentor, colleague and most trusted and loyal friend for 35 years.

Dent Clin N Am 59 (2015) xiii–xiv
http://dx.doi.org/10.1016/j.cden.2014.12.002
0011-8532/15/$ – see front matter © 2015 Published by Elsevier Inc.

2. Dr Earl Clarkson and Dr Orrett Ogle, loyal friends and colleagues for over three decades.
3. Dr Richard Becker, MD, CEO and President of The Brooklyn Hospital Center, a forward thinking leader who has always appreciated the critical and vital importance of dental and oral surgery to the overall health of our community patients, and enthusiastically supports our program's initiatives.
4. Dr Benson Yeh, Vice President for Academic Affairs at The Brooklyn Hospital Center and Dr Gary Stephens, Chief Medical Office at The Brooklyn Hospital Center.
5. Mr. Carlos Naudon, Chairman of the Board of Trustees at The Brooklyn Hospital Center and Mr. George Harris, Trustee of The Brooklyn Hospital Center and dear friends, for their commitment and dedication to The Brooklyn Hospital Center.
6. Dr Ricardo Boyce, general dentistry residency program director at The Brooklyn Hospital Center, committed educator and dedicated clinician.
7. Ms. Melissa Molina, Executive Assistant and Oral and Maxillofacial Residency Coordinator who was directly involved in helping me coordinate this issue.
8. Rabbi Isaac B. Sadowsky, a Talmudic scholar who has devoted his entire life to the dissemination and teaching of Torah.
9. Dr Stan Bodner, a dedicated friend, for his counsel and good cheer.
10. My wife Freidy and children Yehoshua, Chani, Hindy, Daniel, Michal, Akiva and Stephanie and my grandchildren Noach, Shira, Malka, Shoshana and Menachem, for their love, sense of humor, and constant caring and Mrs. Hedy Rosner, my devoted mother in law, for her continual interest, caring and love.

Harry Dym, DDS
Chairman, Dentistry and Oral Surgery
The Brooklyn Hospital Center
121 Dekalb Avenue
Brooklyn, NY 11205, USA

Clinical Professor of Oral and Maxillofacial Surgery
Columbia University College of Dental Medicine
630 West 168th street
NY 10032, USA

Program Director, Oral and Maxillofacial Surgery
Residency Training Program
The Brooklyn Hospital Center
121 Dekalb Avenue
Brooklyn, NY 11205, USA

Senior attending, Woodhull Hospital
760 Broadway, Brooklyn
NY 11206, USA

Attending, New York Harbor Healthcare System
423 East 23rd street, New York
NY 10010, USA

E-mail address:
hdymdds@yahoo.com

Basic Concepts and Techniques of Dental Implants

Jonathan M. Tagliareni, DDS[a],*, Earl Clarkson, DDS[a,b]

KEYWORDS

- Implants • Implant surgery • Patient assessment • Basic implant concepts

KEY POINTS

- Dental implants provide a predictable, effective, and reliable means to replace dentition.
- Dental implants provide completely edentulous and partial edentulous patients the function and esthetics they had with natural dentition.
- It is critical to understand and apply predictable surgical principles when treatment planning and surgically restoring edentulous spaces with implants.
- Basic implant concepts should be meticulously followed for predictable results when treating patients and restoring dental implants.

IMPLANT BASIC CONCEPTS

Dental implants provide a predictable, effective, and reliable means for tooth replacements. Additionally, dental implants provide completely edentulous and partial edentulous patients the function and esthetics they had with natural dentition. It enables patients to regain normal masticatory function, esthetics, speech, smile, and deglutition. In patients with orofacial pain, it may resolve painful symptoms as well as improve facial esthetics and appearance. Edentulous patients gain a feeling of higher self-esteem and well-being. In patients with craniomaxillofacial defects, implants can be used to replace ears, noses, eyes, and other maxillofacial defects. Moreover, congenital, traumatic, and developmental oral defects can be treated with implants.

BIOLOGICAL AND FUNCTIONAL CONSIDERATIONS

Osseointegration is the primary goal of implant placement. In 1952, Brånemark began extensive studies on the microscopic circulation of bone marrow healing. These

The authors have nothing to disclose.
[a] Department of Oral and Maxillofacial Surgery, The Brooklyn Hospital Center, Brooklyn, NY 11201, USA; [b] Department of Oral and Maxillofacial Surgery, Woodhull Hospital, Brooklyn, NY 11206, USA
* Corresponding author.
E-mail address: JTagliareni.dds@gmail.com

studies led to a dental implant application in the early 1960s in which a 10-year implant integration was established in dogs without significant adverse reactions in the soft and hard tissues. Osseoeintegration can be defined as the direct structural and functional connection between organized, living bone and the surface of a load-bearing implant without intervening soft tissue between the implant and bone.[1] Clinically, osseoeintegration can be defined as the asymptomatic rigid fixation of an implant in bone with the ability to withstand occlusal forces.[2] Rigid fixation is a clinical term that implies no observable movement of the implant when a force of 1 to 500 g is applied (**Fig. 1**).

Advancements in biomaterials, implant science, and nanotechnology; improved biotechnology; and an understanding of the bone–implant interface have resulted in improved outcomes and an expanded utilization of implants. Improved imaging techniques help aid in diagnosis; a varied availability of implant geometries, surfaces, and refined surgical techniques has made it possible for most healthy patients to receive implants. Numerous materials are available to aid in bone regeneration in the maxillofacial region, including bone substitute composite grafts and autogenous bone. These tissue types involve the key concepts of osteogenisis, osteoinduction, osteoconduction, and osteopromotion (**Boxes 1** and **2**).

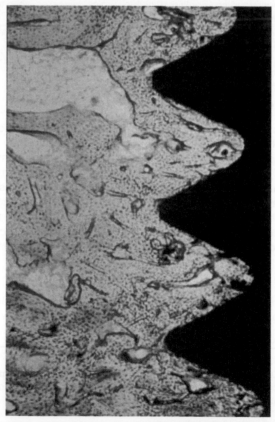

Fig. 1. Osseointegration, as coined by Brånemark, describes a direct bone–implant interface under the power of a light microscope. (*From* Misch CE. Generic root form component terminology. In: Misch CE, editor. Dental implant prosthetics. St Louis (MO): Elsevier Mosby; 2015; with permission.)

Box 1
General considerations
• Informed consent
• Perioperative antibiotics
• Imaging modalities
• Documentation

Surgical preparation in a standard sterile fashion is recommended for all implant procedures. The goal is to minimize mechanical and thermal injuries to the bone. Osteotomies should be completed under copious irrigation using sharp osteotomy drills at high torque and slow speed. It is critical to maintain bone temperatures under 47°C. Bone necrosis and failure of integration can occur when temperatures exceed 47°C.

The material of choice for implants needs to be biocompatible with bone and biologically inert. Titanium is an optimal material that encompasses both of these required qualities.

Volume and quality of bone that contacts the implant determine its initial stability. This stability must be maintained in order for bone to form at the implant surface. Immobility of the implant is imperative for successful osseointegration. Implants can be placed using a staged surgical plan depending on the initial stability and quality of bone available. A single-stage surgery requires adequate primary stability and can be loaded immediately. A 2-staged approach requires submerging the implant when initial stability is less than adequate. A surgical uncovering and placement of healing abutment is required in 3 to 4 months (**Figs. 2** and **3**).

SOFT TISSUE

Understanding and managing the peri-implant soft tissue are critical to long-term success clinically and esthetically. The soft tissue consists of connective tissue covered by epithelium, extending into an epithelial lined sulcus. Junctional epitheliam lines the most apical portion, which forms an attachment. Soft tissue thickness should be assessed prior to surgery, noting that soft tissue thickness affects the vertical edentulous space. The minimum vertical space needed for a cemented crown is 9 mm; however, the tissue thickness is as much as 3 mm in the posterior mandible, affecting the depth of implant placement.

BIOMECHANICAL CONSIDERATIONS

Long-term success of properly placed implants depends heavily on restorative biomechanical factors. The load-bearing capacity of the integrated implant has to be greater

Box 2
Predictable osseoeintegration factors
• Atraumatic surgery
• Biocompatible material
• Placement of implant with initial stability
• Immobility of implant

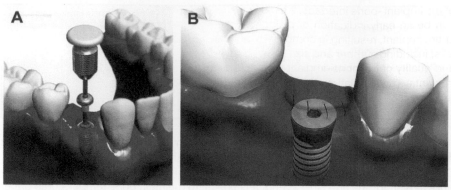

Fig. 2. (*A*) A first-stage cover screw is inserted into the implant body before obtaining primary closure of the soft tissue at stage I surgery. (*B*) The tissue covers the first-stage cover screw during bone integration of the implant. (*From* Misch CE. Generic root form component terminology. In: Misch CE, editor. Dental implant prosthetics. St Louis (MO): Elsevier Mosby; 2015; with permission.)

than the anticipated load during function.[3] When loads exceed the load-bearing capacity, biological failure and mechanical failure can occur. Mechanical failure may present as a complete fracture through implant fixture or porcelain splinting from restorative prosthesis. When the functional load exceeds the load-bearing capacity

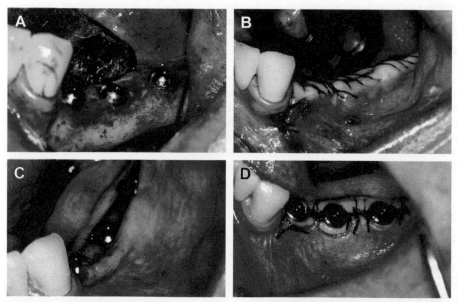

Fig. 3. (*A*) A posterior mandible with 3 implants and first-stage cover screws inserted. (*B*) Primary closure of the soft tissue at implant stage I surgery decreases the risk of postoperative infection and implant movement during initial healing. (*C*) A second-stage surgery uncovers the implants after initial integration. (*D*) A permucosal extension is inserted into the implant body and the sutures sutured around them. (*From* Misch CE. Generic root form component terminology. In: Misch CE, editor. Dental implant prosthetics. St Louis (MO): Elsevier Mosby; 2015; with permission.)

of the implant–bone interface, a biological failure occurs. Bone loss around the implant can be an early indication of biological failure. Bone loss may progress around the entire implant, resulting in complete biological failure and loss of implant. Several factors, including number and size of implants, arrangement and angulation, and volume and quality of the bone–implant interface, determine the load-bearing capacity of the implants. The angulation of the implants as it relates to the occlusal plane and the direction of the occlusal forces is an important determinate in optimizing the translation of the forces to the implants and surrounding bone.[3] Prosthetics should direct loads through the long axis of the implant. Ideally, loads applied should be less than 20°, minimizing load magnification, which initiates bone loss at the bone–implant junction (**Box 3**).

CHIEF COMPLAINT

Patients convey their problems in their own words to a health care provider. A clinician explores conversationally the details of a patient's concerns, apprehensions, and goals of committing to treatment. Expectations of the patient must be managed into realistic goals for both clinician and patient.

MEDICAL HISTORY AND RISK ASSESSMENT

A comprehensive medical history must be documented thoroughly and is required for every patient evaluated (**Box 4**). The surgeon is responsible for reviewing the obtained data and discussing pertinent findings through an insightful interview with the surgical candidate. A full understanding of a patient's health status is critical to evaluate a patient's ability to tolerate the procedure and recover with a favorable prognosis.

With any surgical procedure, the absolute and relative contraindications need to be evaluated. When discussing surgical implant therapy, there are only few medical absolute contraindications, including patients who are acutely ill and those with uncontrolled metabolic disease.[4] Patients may become candidates once the illness is resolved and the metabolic disease is under control. Relative contraindications include bone metabolism disorders and issues with patient healing ability. These conditions may include immunpcompromised patients, diabetes, osteoporosis, bisphosphonate usage, and medical treatment, including chemotherapy and irradiation of the head and neck.[5]

DENTAL HISTORY

A comprehensive examination, including history of patients with all dental specialties, should be obtained. Information regarding patients' past history with an oral and

---

Box 3
Preoperative assessment

- Chief complaint
- Medical history and risk assessment
- Dental history
- Intraoral evaluation
- Diagnostic casts and photographs
- Radiographic examination

Box 4
Contraindications

Absolute contraindications to implant placement

- Acute illness
- Magnitude of defect/anomaly
- Uncontrolled metabolic disease
- Bone and/or soft tissue pathology/infection

Relative contraindications

- Diabetes
- Osteoporosis
- Parafunctional habits
- HIV
- AIDS
- Bisphosphonate usage—oral and intravenous
- Chemotherapy
- Irradiation of head and neck
- Behavioral, neurologic, psychosocial, psychiatric disorders

---

maxillofacial surgeon, general dentist, prosthodontist, and endodontist can yield insight into patient motivation and candidacy for implant therapy.

ORAL EXAMINATION

An oral examination evaluating hard and soft tissue relevant to implant placement is imperative. A clinician should examine existing teeth and prosthetics, periodontal health, oral hygiene, vestibular depths, jaw relationships, interarch spaces, and maximum incisal opening. Additionally, the clinician should examine for parafunctional habits, including clenching and grinding, observing for wear facets on the occlusal surfaces. Height and width of edentulous ridges should be visualized and palpated. The soft tissue should be scrutinized meticulously, documenting clinical biotype and zones of keratinization, areas of redundancy, mobility, and possible pathology.

RADIOGRAPHIC EXAMINATION

The radiographic examination can include traditional projections, such as standard periapical, occlusal, and panoramic films (**Box 5**). More comprehensive treatment planning can be completed using complex cross-sectional imaging, including CT and cone-beam CT. Three classifications for radiographic imaging techniques can be considered. Phase 1, or presurgical implant imaging, involves past radiographs and new radiologic examinations to assist in finalizing a comprehensive treatment plan. Presurgical imaging allows clinicians to determine the quality and quantity of bone available, vital structure identification, evaluation of implant sites, and presence or absence of pathology. Phase 2, or the surgical and intraoperative imaging phase, is used to assist the surgical intervention of patients. Phase 3, or postprosthetic implant imaging, gives access to maintenance plans, information regarding function, and integration of the implant (**Fig. 4, Table 1**).

Box 5
Types of imaging modalities

- Periapical radiography
- Panoramic radiography
- Occlusal radiography
- Cephalometric radiography
- Conventional tomographic radiography
- CT (3-D)
- CBCT
- Medical CT
- MRI (3-D)
- Interactive CT (3-D)

Abbreviation: CBCT, cone-beam CT.
From Resnik RR, Misch CE. Radiographic imaging in implant dentistry. In: Misch CE, editor. Dental implant prosthetics. St Louis (MO): Elsevier Mosby; 2015; with permission.

Quantifying measurements from radiographs needs to account for magnification. Traditional panoramic images magnify up to 25%. The magnification factor can be calculated at the given site by dividing the actual diameter of the object by the diameter measured on the on the radiographic image (**Fig. 5**). Patients may wear a diagnostic template containing 5-mm ball bearings during the panoramic radiograph, allowing surgeons to quantify the magnification in the radiograph (see **Fig. 5**).

When the 25% average magnification is accounted for, it categorizes patients into 3 different groups: (1) there is obviously enough vertical bone to place an implant; (2) there is obviously not enough vertical bone to place an implant; and (3) the amount of bone is not obvious (**Boxes 6–8**).[6]

Critical to implant placement is a comprehensive treatment plan and the ability to identify preoperative conditions that may lead to complications. Measuring vertical restorative space or crown height space is paramount in the successful placement

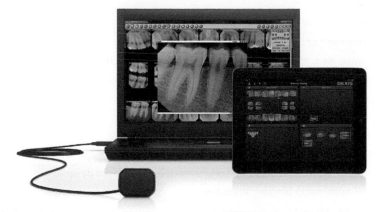

Fig. 4. Digital radiographic system that includes a digital sensor and computer. (*Courtesy of Dexis, LLC.*)

Table 1
Comparison of film versus digital-based images

	Film	Digital
Image	Analog	Analog or digital
Cost	Film, chemicals	Up front
Radiation	High	50%–90% Less
Viewing	Delayed	Immediate
Resolution	14–18 Lines/mm	12–20 Lines/mm
Gray scale	16 Shades	256 Shades
Film	Thin, flexible	Thin, cord
Enhancement	Unchangeable	Wide range
Storage	Chart	Computer

Data from Park ET, Williamson GF. Digital radiography: an overview. J Contemp Dent Pract 2002;3:1–13.

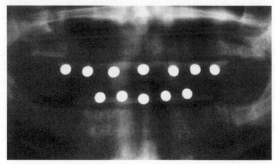

Fig. 5. Panoramic radiograph with 5-mm ball bearings on the crest of a mandible.

Box 6
Panoramic radiographic images

Advantages

• Easy identification of opposing landmarks

• Initial assessment of vertical height of bone

• Convenience, ease, and speed in performance in most dental offices

• Evaluation of gross anatomy of the jaws and any related pathologic findings

Limitations

• Distortions inherent in the panoramic system

• Errors in patient positioning

• Do not demonstrate bone quality

• Misleading measurements because of magnification and no third dimension

• No spatial relationship between structures

From Resnik RR, Misch CE. Radiographic imaging in implant dentistry. In: Misch CE, editor. Dental implant prosthetics. St Louis (MO): Elsevier Mosby; 2015; with permission.

Box 7
Radiographic evaluations—structures

- Incisive foramen
- Maxillary sinus
- Nasal cavity
- Mental foramen
- Mandibular canal
- Anterior loop of the mandibular canal
- Cortical bone
- Bone trabeculation
- Sinus health
- Pathology

Box 8
Measurements specific to implant placement

- 5 mm anterior to mental foramen
- 2 mm superior to mandibular canal
- 3 mm from adjacent implants
- 1.5 mm from adjacent teeth
- 1 mm inferior to maxillary and nasal sinus

Box 9
Solutions for deficient vertical space

- Alveoloplasty/alveolectomy
- Soft tissue augmentation
- Abutment type selection
- Selection of different prosthesis
- Orthodontic intrusion
- Fabrication of traditional fixed or partial prosthesis

Box 10
Solutions for excessive vertical space

- Block grafting
- Guided bone regeneration
- Distraction osteogenesis
- Placement of traditional partial or complete removable dentures

and restoration of endosseous implants. Vertical restorative space can be identified as the distance from the crest of the residual alveolar ridge to the occlusal plane of the planned restoration in the opposite dentition[7]; 9 mm is the minimum vertical space needed for a posterior single-unit fixed restoration, measured from the crestal bone to the occlusal plane of the opposing dentition, or 6 mm from the soft tissue to occlusal plane. Implants should be placed at least 3 mm below the most apical point of the free gingival margin, maintaining the peri-implant biological width (**Boxes 9** and **10**).[7]

REFERENCES

1. Branemark PI. The osseointegration book: from Calvarium to Calcaneus. Berlin (Germany); Chicago: Quitessenz Verlags; 2005.
2. Zarb G, Albrektsson T. Osseointegration – a requiem for the periodontal ligament? Int J Periodontics Restorative Dent 1991;14:251–62.
3. Chapter 14. In: Hupp J, Ellis E, tucker M, editors. Contemporary oral and maxillofacial surgery. 6th edition. St. Louis (MO): Mosby; 2014. p. 234–63.
4. Esposito M, Hirsch JM, Lekholm U, et al. Biological factors contributing to failures of osseointegrated oral implants. (II). Etiopathogenesis. Eur J Oral Sci 1998;106: 721–64.
5. Shin EY, Kwon YH, Herr Y, et al. Implant failure associated with oral bisphosphonate – related osteonecrosis of the jaw. J Periodont Implant Sci 2010;40:90–5.
6. Misch CE. Dental Implant Prosthetics. Chapter 7 Radiographic imaging in Implant dentistry. 2nd edition. St. Louis (MO): Mosby; 2015.
7. Al-Faraje L. Surgical complications in oral implantology: etiology, prevention, and management. Hanover Park (IL): Quintessence Publishing; 2011.

Three-Dimensional Imaging and Guided Surgery for Dental Implants

 CrossMark

Scott D. Ganz, DMD[a,b,c,*]

KEYWORDS

- Computed tomography/cone beam computed tomography • Dental implants
- Computer-aided design • Computer-aided manufacturing
- Guided Surgery Applications

KEY POINTS

- As technology continues to improve, and imaging modalities become widely available, clinicians worldwide are increasingly adopting guided surgical applications for dental implants.
- All aspects of the 3-D Interactive treatment planning phase are based on sound surgical and restorative fundamentals.
- As an integral part of the implant team, dental laboratories have now moved from analog to the digital world, providing the necessary support to the new digital workflow.
- Guided surgery applications are dependent on careful diagnosis using the advanced tools that 3-dimensional imaging offers in combination with advanced interactive treatment planning software.
- Clinicians who wish to achieve true restoratively driven implant dentistry must be aware that the diagnostic phase often begins before the scan is taken.
- The use of diagnostic wax-ups, radiopaque scanning appliances, and the incorporation of intraoral optical scanners can significantly enhance the process and improve accuracy.
- The digital workflow is here to stay, providing clinicians with enhanced diagnostic tools for enhanced implant planning, surgical intervention, and links to computer-aided design software and computer-aided manufacturing process, and will continue to evolve over the next decade.

A 2-dimensional periapical radiograph has been the standard in dentistry for aiding clinicians in the diagnosis and treatment planning for various procedures including, but not limited to, the detection of dental caries, identifying pathology, periodontal disease, endodontic treatment, need for tooth extraction, and locating receptor sites for dental implants (**Fig. 1**). However, periapical radiographs and panoramic radiology are

The author has nothing to disclose.
[a] Maxillofacial Prosthodontist Private Practice, Fort Lee, NJ 07024, USA; [b] Hackensack University Medical Center, Hackensack, NJ 07601, USA; [c] Rutgers School of Dental Medicine, Newark, NJ 07103, USA
* Maxillofacial Prosthodontist Private Practice, Fort Lee, NJ 07024, USA.
E-mail address: drganz@drganz.com

Dent Clin N Am 59 (2015) 265–290
http://dx.doi.org/10.1016/j.cden.2014.11.001
0011-8532/15/$ – see front matter © 2015 Elsevier Inc. All rights reserved.

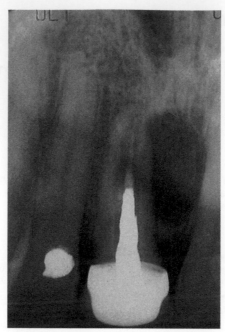

Fig. 1. A 2-dimensional periapical radiograph may not be sufficient to diagnose 3-dimensional anatomy or pathology.

inherently limited in the ability to accurately represent maxillomandibular structures. Two-dimensional radiography can only relate information about height or mesial-distal width but can not describe bone density, thickness of the cortical plates, or the true relationship of the natural tooth to the alveolar housing. When planning for dental implants, and especially when guided surgical applications are considered, it is essential that the true 3-dimensional anatomic presentation is understood and that all adjacent vital structures be accurately visualized.

The advent and acceptance of 3-dimensional computed tomography (CT), and newer-generation lower-dose cone beam CT scan devices (CBCT) in combination with interactive treatment planning software provides the clinicians with the ability to truly appreciate each patient's anatomic reality. Regardless of the device used to acquire the dataset (CT vs CBCT), it is imperative that there is an understanding of how each image can provide important undistorted information that can be used for diagnosis and treatment planning for a variety of surgical and prosthetic interventions to improve accuracy and limit complications. Generally, the 3-dimensional dataset consists of 4 basic views: (1) the axial, (2) the cross-sections, (3) the panoramic reconstructed view, and the 3-dimensional reconstructed volume. Each of these views is important, as no one view alone should determine the ultimate desired treatment.

The cross-sectional view is important to help determine the quality of the bone, the thickness of the cortical plates, sinus pathology, periapical pathology, and the trajectory of the tooth within the alveolus. Often the natural tooth is positioned far to the facial or buccal of the alveolar bone (**Fig. 2**). Therefore, when considering dental implant placement, clinicians can mistakenly try to position the implant within an extraction socket, which can result in less than satisfactory results. An appreciation

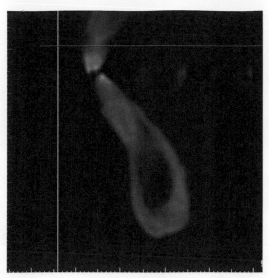

Fig. 2. The labial position of the mandibular tooth in relationship to the trajectory of the anterior mandibular bone as depicted in a cross-sectional view.

of the cross-sectional image can aid clinicians in determining the topography of the alveolus, root morphology, and extent of any facial/buccal concavities (**Fig. 3**A). If the site is critical for the planned reconstruction, then bone grafting procedures may need to be considered if there are bony defects present, often not detected by 2-dimensional imaging modalities. The posterior maxillary arch is another region in which cross-sectional imaging can provide anatomic details not visualized by any other means. The facial-palatal dimensions of the maxillary sinus can be fully appreciated, as can any sinus pathology or thickening of the Schneiderian membrane as seen in **Fig. 3**B (red arrow). The thickness of the lateral sinus wall, and often vessels present within the lateral wall, can also be seen, in anticipation of a planned sinus augmentation procedure (yellow arrow). The placement of a simple cotton roll in the vestibule can add significantly to the diagnostic potential by lifting the lip from the alveolus ("lip-lift technique"), aiding in the appreciation of the bone, the vestibule, and the soft tissue, which is especially significant for the aesthetic zone of the maxillary sinus (red arrow in **Fig. 4**). The yellow arrow points to the thickness of the soft tissue covering the cortical bone (green arrows), and the cross-sectional view shows the path of the incisal nerve (magenta arrows). This diagnostic information is invaluable, improves accuracy of planning, and aids in the prevention of surgical and restorative complications.

Before the acquisition of a CT or CBCT scan, it is often desirable to complete a diagnostic wax-up or a duplicate of the patient's existing well-fitting denture to aid in restoratively driven planning. If a radiopaque material is used (Bariopaque, Salvin Dental Charlotte, NC), it will be visible on the scan, providing a link between the desired tooth position as it relates to the underlying bone (**Fig. 5**A). The ability to visualize the tooth position greatly enhances treatment planning. Using an interactive treatment planning software application, a realistic implant can be virtually positioned within the cross-sectional alveolar bone (see **Fig. 5**B). The yellow projection represents the path of the abutment, which, in this example, travels through the facial aspect of the tooth. This relationship would require an abutment to receive a

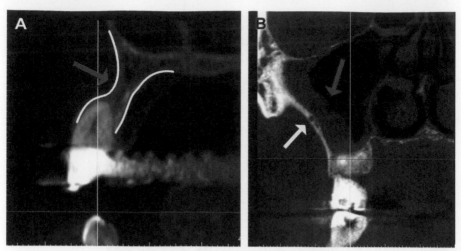

Fig. 3. (*A*) The cross-sectional image can aid clinicians in determining the topography of the alveolus, root morphology, and the extent of any facial/buccal concavities (*red arrow*). (*B*) In the posterior maxilla, the facial-palatal dimensions of the maxillary sinus can be fully appreciated as well as any sinus pathology or thickening of the Schneiderian membrane (*red arrow*) and the presence of intraosseous vessels (*yellow arrow*).

cement-retained restoration. If a screw-retained restoration is desired, the apical end (arrow) of the implant must be rotated toward the facial cortical plate so that the abutment projection can emerge from the palatal or cingulum aspect of the tooth (see **Fig. 5**C). This may result in a compromised volume of bone surrounding the implant and grafting may be required for long-term success. If the implant is placed so that the most volume of bone will surround the implant, an angulated abutment can be

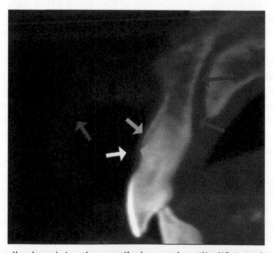

Fig. 4. A cotton roll placed in the vestibule or the "lip-lift" technique provides an unobstructed view to the facial soft tissue and cortical plate of bone (*red arrow*). The path of the incisal canal (*magenta arrows*), thin facial cortical plate (*green arrow*), and gingival tissue (*yellow arrow*) is clearly visible in the cross-sectional slice.

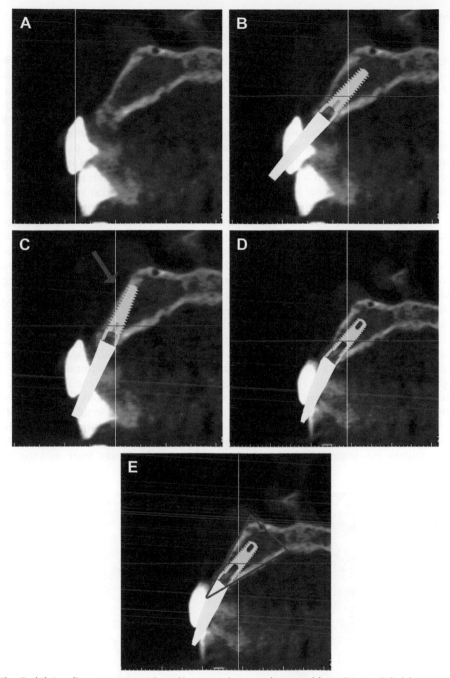

Fig. 5. (*A*) A radiopaque material used in a scanning template provides a diagnostic link between the desired tooth position as it relates to the underlying bone (Bariopaque; Salvin Dental, Charlotte, NC). (*B*) A realistic implant can be virtually positioned within the cross-sectional alveolar bone using an interactive treatment planning software application to plan for a cement-retained restoration. (*C*) The apical end (*arrow*) of the implant must be rotated toward the facial cortical plate so that the abutment projection can emerge from the palatal or cingulum aspect of the tooth for a screw-retained restoration. (*D*) An angulated abutment can be simulated for either a cement-retained or screw-retained restoration. (*E*) The Triangle of Bone defines an area allowing clinicians to analyze the bone within the zone of the triangle (*in red*) as a determinant for placement of an implant.

placed for either a cement-retained or screw-retained restoration (see **Fig. 5D**). The author has designated this zone the "Triangle of Bone" as seen in **Fig. 5E**. The Triangle of Bone defines an area allowing clinicians to analyze the bone within the triangle as a determinant for placement of an implant. To further appreciate the power of the diagnostic software, a slice through the 3-dimensional reconstructed volume illustrates a realistic implant with an abutment projection piercing through the desired tooth position as represented by the barium sulfate scanning template (**Fig. 6**). If a screw-retained restoration will be the treatment plan of choice, an angled hex-engaging screw-receiving abutment must be used and can be simulated with a realistic abutment in the cross-sectional view and 3-dimensional reconstruction volumetric view (**Fig. 7**).

To facilitate the diagnosis process for guided surgery applications, and to maximize accuracy of the planning and template design, it is often desirable to have a diagnostic wax-up fabricated by the dental laboratory. This can be accomplished for a single tooth replacement, a full arch, or full mouth reconstruction. Alginate impressions are poured in stone, and delivered to the dental laboratory with a bite, for mounting with or without a facebow, depending on the needs of the case. The diagnostic wax-up is then fabricated to achieve the desired prosthetic outcome and can be used as a presentation/communication aid for the patient to gain case acceptance. This Master Diagnostic Model (MDM; Valley Dental Arts, Stillwater, MN) is examined for accuracy and bite relationship in all views (**Fig. 8A**). The MDM is then placed into a desktop optical scanner to be digitized for use with the computer software applications (see **Fig. 8B**). The software can also allow for virtual articulation similar to what has been used for conventional crown and bridge restorative dentistry in the fabrication of computer-aided design and computer-aided manufacturing (CAD CAM)–milled restorations. Advances in CT and CBCT interactive diagnostic software can provide additional links to further improve diagnostic accuracy, making it possible to integrate the standard triangulation language (STL) dataset from desktop or

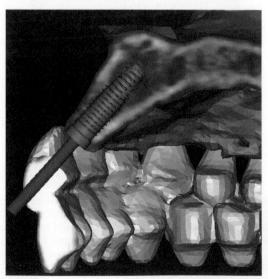

Fig. 6. A realistic manufacturer-specific implant with an abutment projection (*in red*) can pierce through the desired tooth position as represented by the barium sulfate scanning template, seen in the 3-dimensional volumetric clipping view.

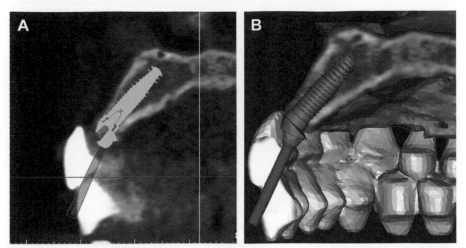

Fig. 7. (A, B) An angled hex-engaging, screw-receiving abutment can be simulated with a realistic abutment in both the cross-sectional view, and 3-dimensional reconstruction volumetric view for a planned screw-retained restoration.

intraoral optical scanner devices. The models are imported into the software where they will be registered or "married" to the anatomic representations of the CT or CBCT axial and coronal slices. The models can then be further verified with the 3-dimensional volumetric views and the final positioning of the maxillary and mandibular STL models confirmed as superimposed to the CBCT dataset (**Fig. 9**). The importance of merging these datasets can not be underestimated when planning dental implant surgery and is essential for certain template-guided surgical applications.

The 3-dimensional volumetric reconstructions of the mandibular arch (**Fig. 10**) can aid in the visualization of the existing anterior teeth (blue), and an assessment of the posterior distal edentulous bony anatomy. The bilateral mental foramen and nerves can also be seen (orange). Implants can be planned for the posterior mandible, with yellow abutment projections showing the relative parallelism but without appreciation of where they will emerge within the desired occlusal scheme (**Fig. 11**A). Once the

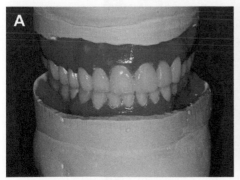
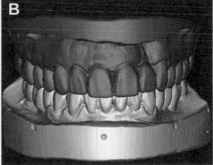

Fig. 8. (A) A maxillary and mandibular diagnostic wax-up fabricated by the dental laboratory can be used to enhance the planning process. (B) The wax-up on the stone cast is placed into a high-resolution desktop scanner to be digitized, creating a virtual model (STL).

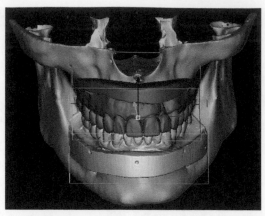

Fig. 9. The maxillary and mandibular STL models were superimposed onto the CBCT dataset and the final position confirmed for accuracy using x, y, z axis reference lines (*red, green, blue markings*).

MDM STL model was superimposed, the direction of the implants can be modified to fit within the envelope of the tooth position (see **Fig. 11**B). The implant positions can be confirmed in all views, specifically within the alveolar bone of the cross-sectional image as related to the outline of the MDM STL model (**Fig. 12**A). Further inspection using the clipping function of the interactive treatment planning software, provides state-of-the-art views of how the implant is represented within the bone and how the abutment projection (yellow) emerges from the occlusal aspect of the superimposed diagnostic model (see **Fig. 12**B).

CASE PRESENTATION

A 62-year-old man presented with a preexisting maxillary reconstruction and a lower failing reconstruction (**Fig. 13**). The maxillary reconstruction needed replacement, as the vertical dimension of occlusion was compromised (overopened by 5.5 mm),

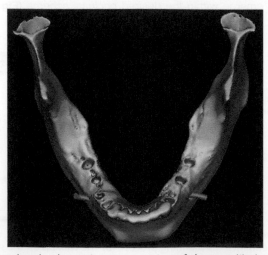

Fig. 10. The 3-dimensional volumetric reconstruction of the mandibular arch.

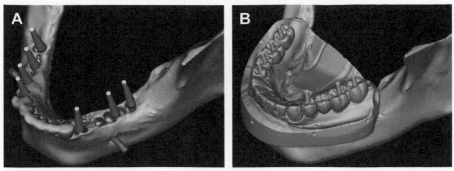

Fig. 11. (*A*) Implants planned for the posterior mandible, with yellow abutment projections show the relative parallelism but without appreciation of the desired tooth position. (*B*) Once the STL model of the wax-up is superimposed, the direction of the implants can be modified to fit within the envelope of the tooth position.

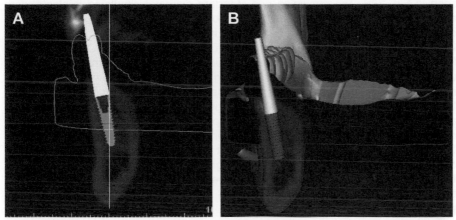

Fig. 12. (*A*) The simulated implant positions can be confirmed specifically within the alveolar bone of the cross-sectional image as related to the outline STL model. (*B*) The clipping function of the planning software provides state-of-the-art views of how the abutment projection (*yellow*) emerges from the occlusal aspect of the superimposed diagnostic model.

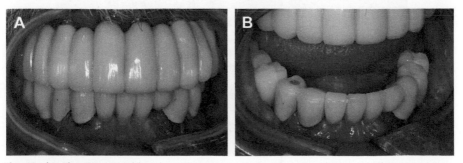

Fig. 13. (*A, B*) A 62-year-old male patient presented with a preexisting maxillary reconstruction and a mandibular failing fixed reconstruction.

making it difficult for the patient to function or speak properly. The panoramic view as reconstructed from the CBCT dataset shows the existing implants in the maxilla, and failing teeth supporting a fixed bridge in the anterior mandible, 3 existing posterior right mandibular implants supporting a separate fixed bridge, and a single implant located on the mandibular left side (**Fig. 14**). The cross-sectional images representing the 3 mandible right implants were evaluated (**Fig. 15**). Proximity of the existing implant to the mental foramen is seen in **Fig. 15**C. The cross-sectional images of 2 of the remaining natural teeth confirm the circumferential bone loss around the roots (**Fig. 16**A, B) and the proximity to the mental foramen on the left distal wide-diameter implant (see **Fig. 16**C).

The axial view shows the right posterior implants and the left single implant with circumferential bone loss around the existing anterior natural teeth with the parallel positioning of 6 simulated implants for an implant-supported restoration (**Fig. 17**). The existing bridgework did not allow for a diagnostic wax-up for this case. Therefore, the positioning of the 3 standard-diameter (4.0) implants was achieved within the framework of the preexisting restorations in the cross-sectional images (**Fig. 18**). The prognathic chin area and the favorable density of the bone can be seen in **Fig. 18**B. The remaining one-standard diameter simulated implants were also verified in relation to the surrounding bone volume and the 2 wider (4.5 mm diameter) implants close to the path of the inferior alveolar nerve (orange) as seen in (**Fig. 19**). The 3-dimensional reconstructed volume from the CBCT scan data allows for inspection of the anatomical structures and bone loss surrounding the natural tooth roots (**Fig. 20**A) and the preexisting anterior fixed bridgework. The existing implants are illustrated in blue (**Fig. 20**B). Using a software segmentation process, the bridge was virtually removed, aiding in the implant planning process. The yellow abutment projections helped in the spatial positioning of the implants in a parallel orientation for ease of prosthesis fabrication (**Fig. 21**A). The complex relationship between the mandibular bone, the inferior alveolar nerves, the existing bridge, and proposed implants can be seen through use of "selective transparency" (see **Fig. 21**B). Once all implant positions have been verified and confirmed by all members of the implant team, a template can be fabricated for the guided surgical procedure.

The tooth-supported, stereolithographic surgical template was fabricated to sit on the restorations and left single implant that would remain (**Fig. 22**). The fit of the template was confirmed on the working stone cast through the inspection windows.

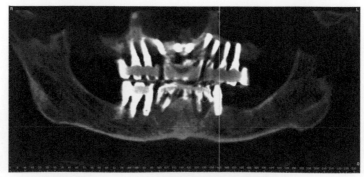

Fig. 14. Preoperative panoramic reconstruction shows preexisting implants and failing anterior mandibular bridge on natural teeth.

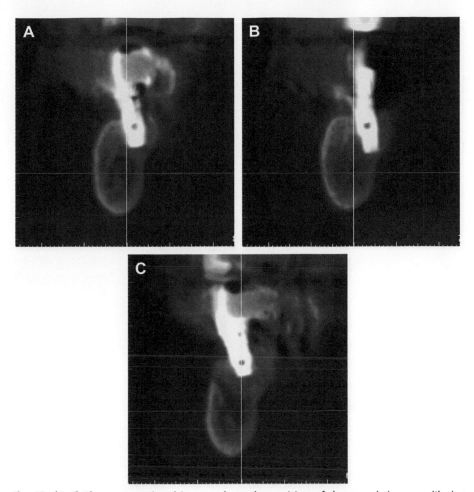

Fig. 15. (*A–C*) The cross-sectional images show the position of the preexisting mandibular right posterior implants.

To facilitate the immediate extraction, immediate implant placement, and transitional restoration, a resin stereolithographic model was fabricated (**Fig. 23**). The model had preprocessed holes for implant replicas (analogs) to be placed. The surgical guide was verified on the model and assessed for accuracy. Temporary titanium abutments were positioned on the model for the fabrication of a screw-retained transitional restoration (**Fig. 24**). The implants were planned to be parallel to facilitate the laboratory phase and to enhance the passive fit of the CAD CAM framework. The surgical template can provide for control of direction and depth, which is necessary to fabricate an immediate or delayed restoration based on the plan. To achieve the most accurate result, additional instrumentation is required from the implant manufacturer to allow for full template guidance as described by the author (**Fig. 25**A).

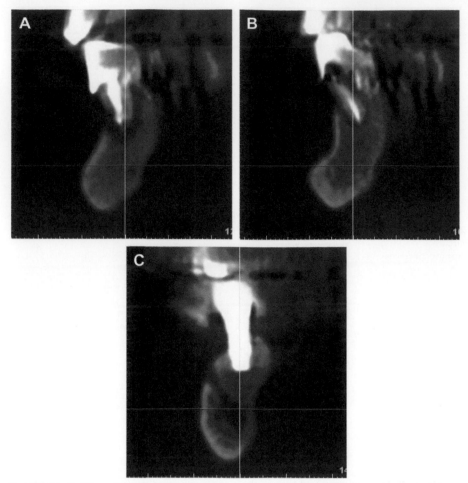

Fig. 16. (*A–C*) Circumferential bone loss around the roots of 2 remaining natural teeth were confirmed in the cross-sectional view (*A, B*) and the proximity of the wide-diameter implant to the mental foramen (*C*).

Three classifications of surgical guidance are proposed by the author, which are based on 3-dimensional CT/CBCT scan imaging. The proposed Ganz-Rinaldi Classification divides guided implant surgery into 3 specific types: (1) diagnostic freehand guidance; (2) template-assisted guidance; and (3) full template guidance.

Diagnostic Freehand Guidance

A CT or CBCT scan is acquired for the purpose of dental implant placement. The dataset as seen on the device's native software allows inspection of the essential views: axial, cross-sectional, coronal, sagittal, panoramic, and 3-dimensional reconstructed views to assess anatomic landmarks for the purposes of dental implant or bone grafting surgical procedures. The information will be assimilated, measurements made with the software, and the surgical intervention will be performed using freehand drilling without templates for either implant placement or for bone grafting.

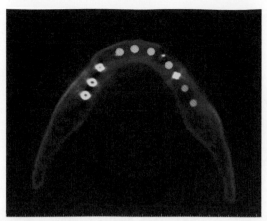

Fig. 17. The axial view shows the right posterior implants, the left single implant with circumferential bone loss around the existing anterior natural teeth, and the parallel positioning of 6 simulated implants to support an implant-supported restoration.

Template-Assisted Guidance

The Digital Imaging and Communications in Medicine (DICOM) data from the CT or CBCT device is exported into a third-party interactive treatment planning software application, which has the appropriate tools to simulate implant placement. It should also have the ability to export the data for the fabrication of surgical guides or templates. Templates that can be fabricated are categorized as tooth-supported, mucosal-supported, or bone-supported templates. Template-assisted protocols provide for limited control implant angulation and depth of the osteotomy.

Full Template Guidance

Similar to template-assisted, full-template guidance takes the additional step of using implant-specific and manufacturer-specific drills and implant mounts to direct the implant through the embedded cylinders within the template once the osteotomy has been prepared. The implant mounts or carriers should match the implant connection and diameter of the implant utilized (see **Fig. 25**A). The osteotomy will be prepared through the template with specific drills to control diameter and depth, and then the implants will be accurately placed through the same cylinders with manufacturer-specific implant mounts that deliver the implant to the specific depth required (see **Fig. 25**B).

SURGICAL INTERVENTION

Using local anesthetic agents, the anterior mandibular fixed bridge and teeth were removed (**Fig. 26**). A full-thickness mucoperiosteal flap was performed to debride the tooth sockets and decorticate for subsequent bone grafts. The tooth borne template was placed over the existing crowns, and the fit verified through the inspection windows (**Fig. 27**A). The sequential drilling was performed through the proper-diameter guide keys, which fit into the cylinders embedded in the surgical guide (see **Fig. 27**B). Once the drilling was completed, the appropriate fixture mount was attached to the implant, and the implant was delivered to the site through the template (**Fig. 28**). As 3 of the 4 initial fixtures were finally seated, the template achieved even more stability (**Fig. 29**).

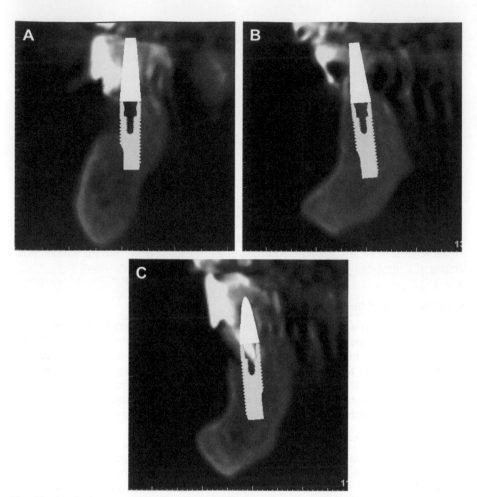

Fig. 18. (*A–C*) Three standard-diameter (4.0) implants were simulated within the envelope of the preexisting restorations as seen in the cross-sectional images.

The fixtures were torqued into the osteotomy site until flush with the top of the surgical guide. The temporary titanium cylinders were attached, the bone grafts placed, membrane positioned over the graft, and the soft tissue approximated for closure with sutures. An immediate transitional restoration was delivered, and the occlusion was checked. Postoperative instructions were provided to the patient.

RESTORATIVE PHASE

The patient was monitored for the 8-week period before impressions were taken to complete the restoration (**Fig. 30**). The newly placed implants exhibit parallelism, which aides in the laboratory phase of prosthesis construction and passivity of fit. A stone cast, which incorporated implant analogs, was fabricated and verified with a rigid intraoral verification index. CAD CAM software was used to design the framework for the definitive restoration. The diagnostic wax-up was scanned and imported

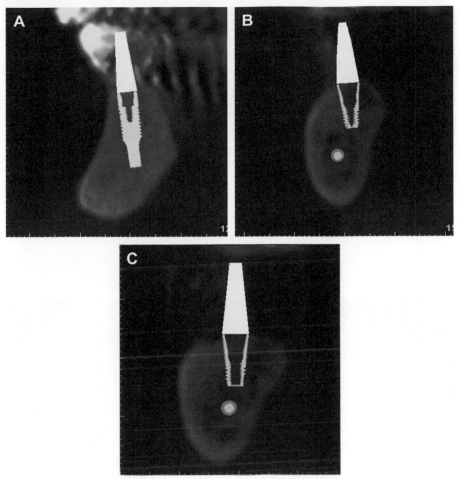

Fig. 19. (A–C) The remaining one-standard diameter implant was verified in relation to the surrounding bone volume (A) with 2 wider (4.5 mm diameter) implants that were in close proximity to the inferior alveolar nerve (*orange*).

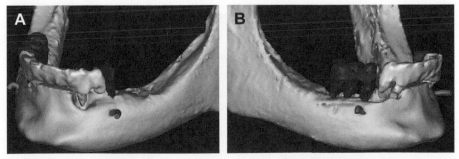

Fig. 20. (A, B) The 3-dimensional reconstructed volume from the CBCT scan data allows for inspection of the preexisting structures and bone loss around the natural tooth roots (existing implants illustrated in *blue*).

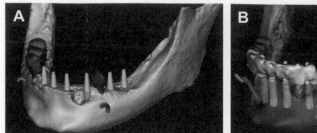
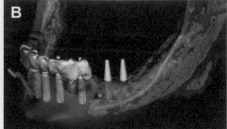

Fig. 21. (*A*) The abutment projections (*yellow*) helped in the spatial positioning of the implants in a parallel orientation to aid in prosthesis fabrication. (*B*) The complex relationship between the bone, the inferior alveolar nerves, the existing bridge, and simulated implants can be visualized through use of selective transparency.

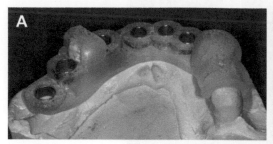
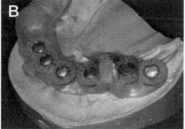

Fig. 22. (*A*, *B*) The tooth-supported, stereolithographic surgical template seated on the stone cast.

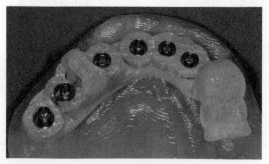

Fig. 23. A stereolithographic resin model was fabricated to facilitate the immediate implant placement and transitional screw-retained restoration.

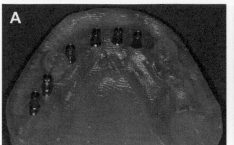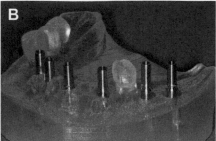

Fig. 24. (A, B) The stereolithographic model had preprocessed holes for implant replicas (analogs) to be placed with titanium screw–receiving abutments positioned to aid in the fabrication of a screw-retained transitional restoration.

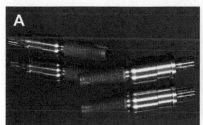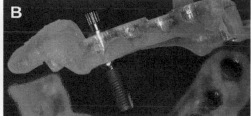

Fig. 25. (A, B) To achieve full template guidance, additional instrumentation is required from the implant manufacturer to allow implants to be delivered through the template.

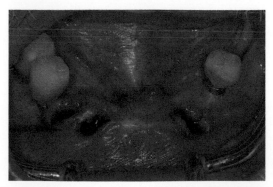

Fig. 26. The anterior mandibular fixed bridge with the natural tooth roots was carefully removed.

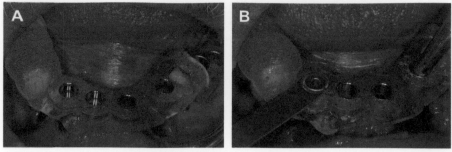

Fig. 27. (*A*) The tooth-borne surgical template was placed over the existing crowns and the seating verified through the inspection windows. (*B*) The sequential drilling was performed through the proper-diameter guide keys, which fit into the cylinders embedded in the surgical guide.

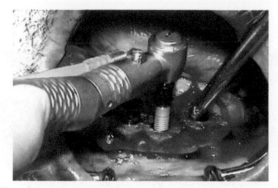

Fig. 28. Once drilling for each osteotomy was completed, the appropriate fixture mount was attached to the implant, and the implant was delivered through the template into the bone.

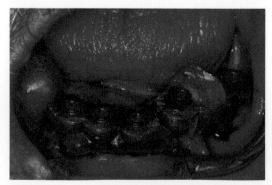

Fig. 29. Three of 4 initial fixtures were seated to depth, providing increased stability of the template.

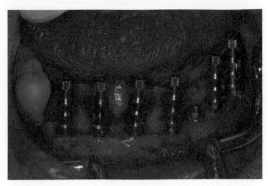

Fig. 30. After monitoring the patient for 8 weeks, fixture-level impressions were taken.

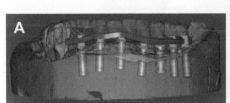

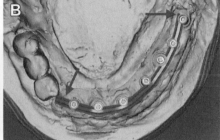

Fig. 31. (*A*) The diagnostic wax-up was scanned and imported into the CAD design software, for the design of the virtual restoration. (*B*) A titanium-milled, hybrid-type screw-retained CAD CAM bar was designed on the computer workstation, and red arrows indicated areas to discuss with the laboratory.

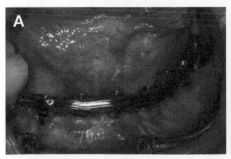

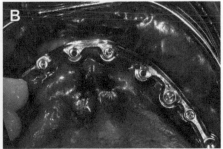

Fig. 32. (*A*) The titanium screw–retained bar was inspected in the mouth for accuracy and passive fit. (*B*) The occlusal view of the CAD CAM bar framework with favorable soft tissue response.

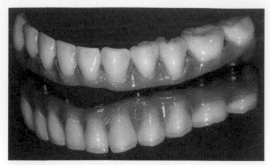

Fig. 33. The final hybrid screw-retained mandibular restoration fabricated with denture teeth and pink composite processed to the framework.

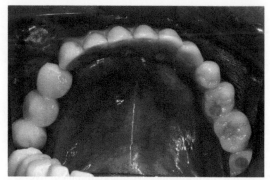

Fig. 34. The occlusal view of the definitive prosthesis representing normal tooth morphology and arch form.

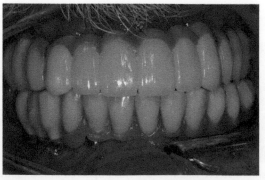

Fig. 35. The retracted view of the maxillary and mandibular prostheses at the correct vertical dimension.

into the CAD design software, and the virtual tooth set-up completed (**Fig. 31**A). The concept of selective transparency is also used to link the implant positions to the tooth positions, which determine the framework design of the screw-retained prosthesis. It was planned for a titanium-milled bar, hybrid-type, screw-retained restoration. The CAD CAM bar design is illustrated in **Fig. 31**B. Once the virtual wax-up was confirmed, the framework was milled. The titanium screw–retained bar was inspected on the working cast for accuracy and passive fit and then delivered to the mouth (**Fig. 32**A). The bar framework was checked intraorally for fit, and soft tissue response (see **Fig. 32**B). A resin base was then attached to the frame to complete the tooth set up for try-in. The occlusion and phonetics were verified intraorally. The maxillary reconstruction was also remade simultaneous to the mandible on the preexisting implants, correcting the occlusal discrepancy in conjunction with new implants placed for the mandibular arch. The patient accepted the esthetics for the maxillary and mandibular restorations. The final hybrid screw-retained mandibular restoration contained denture teeth and pink composite processed to the framework (**Fig. 33**). The occlusal view of the definitive prosthesis is seen in **Fig. 34** representing normal tooth morphology and arch form. The retracted view reveals the maxillary and mandibular prostheses at the correct vertical dimension (**Fig. 35**).

SUMMARY

As the technology continues to improve, and imaging modalities become widely available, clinicians worldwide are increasingly adopting guided surgical applications for dental implants. Although CT/CBCT diagnosis and treatment planning are still not universally taught in dental schools at either the undergraduate or postgraduate levels, clinicians are becoming more aware of the benefits of proper planning through advanced imaging modalities and interactive treatment planning applications. It should be emphasized that all aspects of the planning phase are based on sound surgical and restorative fundamentals. There is one other catalyst that is important for the continued expansion and adoption of the technology—the fact that dental laboratory technicians are becoming entirely fluent in the use of virtual CAD design software and CAM, and have invested in the necessary equipment to provide these services as the technology continues to evolve. As an integral part of the implant team, dental laboratories have now moved from analog to the digital world, providing the necessary support to the new digital workflow.

However, it must also be stated that "It's not the Scan, it's the PLAN," meaning that guided surgery applications are dependent on careful diagnosis using the advanced tools that 3-dimensional imaging offers in combination with advanced interactive treatment planning software. Yet this alone is not sufficient. Clinicians who wish to achieve true restoratively driven implant dentistry must be aware that the diagnostic phase often begins before the scan is taken. The use of diagnostic wax-ups, radiopaque scanning appliances, and the incorporation of intraoral optical scanners can significantly enhance the process and improve accuracy. Perhaps the most exciting aspect about the new digital workflow is the ability to take the information from the diagnostic wax-up as confirmed by the 3-dimensional planning and combine this with CAD CAM software to design first a transitional restoration and then the final restoration. The digital workflow is here to stay, providing clinicians with enhanced diagnostic tools for enhanced implant planning, surgical intervention, and links to the CAD CAM process and will continue to evolve over the next decade.

FURTHER READINGS

Abduo J, Lyons K, Bennani V, et al. Fit of screw-retained fixed implant frameworks fabricated by different methods: a systematic review [review]. Int J Prosthodont 2011;24(3):207–20.

Alqerban A, Jacobs R, Souza PC, et al. In-vitro comparison of 2 cone-beam computed tomography systems and panoramic imaging for detecting simulated canine impaction-induced external root resorption in maxillary lateral incisors. Am J Orthod Dentofacial Orthop 2009;136(6):764.e1–11 [discussion: 764–5].

Amet EM, Ganz SD. Functional and aesthetic acceptance prior to computerized tomography or implant placement. Implant Dent 1997;6(3):193–7.

Angelopoulos C, Aghaloo T. Imaging technology in implant diagnosis. Dent Clin North Am 2011;55(1):141–58.

Araryarachkul P, Caruso J, Gantes B, et al. Bone density assessments of dental implant sites: 2. Quantitative cone-beam computerized tomography. Int J Oral Maxillofac Implants 2005;20:416–24.

Arisan V, Karabuda ZC, Ozdemir T. Accuracy of two stereolithographic guide systems for computer-aided implant placement: a computed tomography-based clinical comparative study. J Periodontol 2010;81(1):43–51.

Basten CH. The use of radiopaque templates for predictable implant placement. Quintessence Int 1995;26:609–12.

Bavitz BJ, Harn SD, Hansen CA, et al. An anatomical study of mental neurovascular bundle-Implant relationships. Int J Oral Maxillofac Implants 1993;8:563–7.

Behneke A, Burwinkel M, Behneke N. Factors influencing transfer accuracy of cone beam CT-derived template-based implant placement. Clin Oral Implants Res 2012;23(4):416–23.

Benavides E, Rios HF, Ganz SD, et al. Use of cone beam computed tomography in implant dentistry: the International Congress of Oral Implantologists consensus report. Implant Dent 2012;21(2):78–86.

Benington PC, Khambay BS, Ayoub AF. An overview of three-dimensional imaging in dentistry. Dent Update 2010;37(8):494–6, 499–500, 503–4.

Berco M, Rigali PH Jr, Miner RM, et al. Accuracy and reliability of linear cephalometric measurements from cone-beam computed tomography scans of a dry human skull. Am J Orthod Dentofacial Orthop 2009;136(1):17.e1–9 [discussion: 17–8].

Berdougo M, Fortin T, Basten CH, et al. The use of barium sulfate for implant templates. J Prosthet Dent 1996;76:451–4.

Borrow W, Smith JP. Stent marker materials for computerized tomograph-assisted implant planning. Int J Periodontics Restorative Dent 1996;16:61–7.

Chan HL, Misch K, Wang HL. Dental imaging in implant treatment planning. Implant Dent 2010;19(4):288–98.

Cordaro L, Torsello F, Roccuzzo M. Implant loading protocols for the partially edentulous posterior mandible [review]. Int J Oral Maxillofac Implants 2009;24(Suppl):158–68.

Danza M, Zollino I, Carinci F. Comparison between implants inserted with and without computer planning and custom model coordination. J Craniofac Surg 2009;20(4):1086–92.

De Vos W, Casselman J, Swennen GR. Cone-beam computerized tomography (CBCT) imaging of the oral and maxillofacial region: a systematic review of the literature [review]. Int J Oral Maxillofac Surg 2009;38(6):609–25.

Di Giacomo GA, Cury PR, de Araujo NS, et al. Clinical application of stereolithographic surgical guides for implant placement: preliminary results. J Periodontol 2005;76(4):503–7.

Drago C, Saldarriaga RL, Domagala D, et al. Volumetric determination of the amount of misfit in CAD/CAM and cast implant frameworks: a multicenter laboratory study. Int J Oral Maxillofac Implants 2010;25(5):920–9.

Dreiseidler T, Mischkowski RA, Neugebauer J, et al. Comparison of cone-beam imaging with orthopantomography and computerized tomography for assessment in presurgical implant dentistry. Int J Oral Maxillofac Implants 2009;24(2):216–25.

Dula K, Mini R, van der Stelt PF, et al. The radiographic assessment of implant patients: decision-making criteria. Int J Oral Maxillofac Implants 2001;16(1):80–9.

Eggers G, Patellis E, Mühling J. Accuracy of template-based dental implant placement. Int J Oral Maxillofac Implants 2009;24(3):447–54.

Ersoy AE, Turkyilmaz I, Ozan O, et al. Reliability of implant placement with stereolithographic surgical guides generated from computed tomography: clinical data from 94 implants. J Periodontol 2008;79(8):1339–45.

Farley NE, Kennedy K, McGlumphy EA, et al. Split-mouth comparison of the accuracy of computer-generated and conventional surgical guides. Int J Oral Maxillofac Implants 2013;28(2):563–72.

Fortin T, Champleboux G, Bianchi S, et al. Precision of transfer of preoperative planning for oral implants based on cone-beam CT-scan images through a robotic drilling machine. Clin Oral Implants Res 2002;13(6):651–6.

Fortin T, Isidori M, Blanchet E, et al. An image-guided system-drilled surgical template and trephine guide pin to make treatment of completely edentulous patients easier: a clinical report on immediate loading. Clin Implant Dent Relat Res 2004;6(2):111–9.

Ganz SD. CT scan technology - an evolving tool for predictable implant placement and restoration. International Magazine of Oral Implantology 2001;1:6–13.

Ganz SD. Use Of stereolithographic models as diagnostic and restorative aids for predictable immediate loading of implants. Pract Proced Aesthet Dent 2003;15(10):763–71.

Ganz SD. Presurgical planning with CT-derived fabrication of surgical guides. J Oral Maxillofac Surg 2005;63(9 Suppl 2):59–71.

Ganz SD. Use of Conventional CT and cone Beam for improved dental diagnostics and implant Planning. AADMRT Newsletter, Spring Issue 2005. (AADMRT).

Ganz SD. Conventional CT and cone beam CT for improved dental diagnostics and implant planning. Dent Implantol Update 2005;16(12).

Ganz SD. Techniques for the use of CT imaging for the fabrication of surgical guides. Atlas Oral Maxillofac Surg Clin North Am 2006;14:75–97 Elsevier Saunders.

Ganz SD. The reality of anatomy and the triangle of bone. Inside Dent 2006;2(5):72–7.

Ganz SD. The reality of anatomy and the triangle of bone. Inside Dent. Proceedings of ICOI World Congress XXIV. Supplement Implant Dentistry;14:182–91. 2006.

Ganz SD. 3-D imaging and cone beam CT is "Where the action is!". Inside Dent 2007;102–3.

Ganz SD. CT-derived model-based surgery for immediate loading of maxillary anterior implants. Pract Proced Aesthet Dent 2007;19(5):311–8.

Ganz SD. Restoratively driven implant dentistry utilizing advanced software and CBCT: realistic abutments and virtual teeth. Dent Today 2008;27(7):122, 124, 126–7.

Ganz SD. Using interactive technology: "in the zone with the triangle of bone". Dent Implantol Update 2008;19(5):33–8 [quiz: p1].

Ganz SD. Computer-aided design/computer-aided manufacturing applications using CT and cone beam CT scanning technology. Dent Clin North Am 2008;52(4):777–808.

Ganz SD. Defining new paradigms for assessment of implant receptor sites - the use of CT/CBCT and interactive virtual treatment planning for congenitally missing lateral incisors. Compend Contin Educ Dent 2008;29(5):256–67.

Ganz SD. Advanced case planning with SimPlant. In: Tardieu P, Rosenfeld A, editors. The art of computer-guided implantology. Chicago, Illinois: Quintessence Publishing; 2009. p. 193–210.

Ganz SD. Advances in diagnosis and treatment planning utilizing CT scan technology for improving surgical and restorative implant reconstruction: tools of empowerment. In: Jokstad A, editor. Osseointegration and dental implants. Iowa, Ames: Wiley-Blackwell; 2009. p. 88–116.

Ganz SD. Bone grafting assessment: focus on the anterior and posterior maxilla utilizing advanced 3-d imaging technologies. Dent Implantol Update 2009; 20(6):41–8.

Ganz SD. Implant complications associated with two- and three dimensional diagnostic imaging technologies. In: Froum SJ, editor. Dental implant complications - etiology, prevention, and treatment. West Sussex (United Kingdom): Wiley-Blackwell; 2010. p. 71–99.

Ganz SD. The use of CT/CBCT and interactive virtual treatment planning and the triangle of bone: defining new paradigms for assessment of implant receptor sites. In: Babbush C, Hahn J, Krauser J, et al, editors. Dental implants - the art and science. (MO): Saunders Maryland Heights; 2010. p. 146–66.

Guerrero ME, Jacobs R, Loubele M, et al. State-of-the-art on cone beam CT imaging for preoperative planning of implant placement. Clin Oral Investig 2006;10: 1–7.

Haney E, Gansky SA, Lee JS, et al. Comparative analysis of traditional radiographs and cone-beam computed tomography volumetric images in the diagnosis and treatment planning of maxillary impacted canines. Am J Orthod Dentofacial Orthop 2010;137(5):590–7.

Harris D, Buser D, Dula K, et al. E.A.O. guidelines for the use of diagnostic imaging in implant dentistry. A consensus work-shop organized by the European Association for Osseointegration in Trinity College Dublin. Clin Oral Implants Res 2002; 13:566–70.

Horwitz J, Zuabi O, Machtei EE. Accuracy of a computerized tomography-guided template-assisted implant placement system: an in vitro study. Clin Oral Implants Res 2009;20(10):1156–62.

Israelson H, Plemons JM, Watkins P, et al. Barium-coated surgical stents and computer-assisted tomography in the preoperative assessment of dental implant patients. Int J Periodontics Restorative Dent 1992;12:52–61.

Jabero M, Sarment DP. Advanced surgical guidance technology: a review [review]. Implant Dent 2006;15(2):135–42.

Jacobs R, Mraiwa N, Van Steenberghe D, et al. Appearance of the mandibular incisive canal on panoramic radiographs. Surg Radiol Anat 2004;26:329–33.

Katsoulis J, Pazera P, Mericske-Stern R. Prosthetically driven, computer-guided implant planning for the edentulous maxilla: a model study. Clin Implant Dent Relat Res 2009;11(3):238–45.

Kim KD, Park CS. Effect of variable scanning protocols on the pre-implant site evaluation of the mandible in reformatted computed tomography. Korean J Oral Maxillofac Radiol 1999;29:21–32.

Kim KD, Jeong HG, Choi SH, et al. Effect of mandibular positioning on preimplant site measurement of the mandible in reformatted CT. Int J Periodontics Restorative Dent 2003;23(2):177–83.

Klein M, Abrams M. Computer-guided surgery utilizing a computer-milled surgical template. Pract Proced Aesthet Dent 2001;13(2):165–9 [quiz: 170].

Klein M, Cranin AN, Sirakian A. A computerized tomographic (CT) scan appliance for optimal presurgical and pre-prosthetic planning of the implant patient. Pract Periodontics Aesthet Dent 1993;5:33–9.

Lal K, White GS, Morea DN, et al. Use of stereolithographic templates for surgical and prosthodontic implant planning and placement. Part I. The concept. J Prosthodont 2006;15(1):51–8.

Lam EW, Ruprecht A, Yang J. Comparison of two-dimensional orthoradially reformatted computed tomography and panoramic radiography for dental implant treatment planning. J Prosthet Dent 1995;74:42–6.

Laster WS, Ludlow JB, Bailey LJ, et al. Accuracy of measurements of mandibular anatomy and prediction of asymmetry in panoramic radiographic images. Dentomaxillofac Radiol 2005;34(6):343–9.

Lin MH, Mau LP, Cochran DL, et al. Risk assessment of inferior alveolar nerve injury for immediate implant placement in the posterior mandible: a virtual implant placement study. J Dent 2014;42(3):263–70. http://dx.doi.org/10.1016/j.jdent.2013.12.014.

Mischkowski RA, Ritter L, Neugebauer J, et al. Diagnostic quality of panoramic views obtained by a newly developed digital volume tomography device for maxillofacial imaging. Quintessence Int 2007;38(9):763–72.

Mol A, Balasundaram A. In vitro cone beam computed tomography imaging of periodontal bone. Dentomaxillofac Radiol 2008;37(6):319–24.

Moreira CR, Sales MA, Lopes PM, et al. Assessment of linear and angular measurements on three-dimensional cone-beam computed tomographic images. Oral Surg Oral Med Oral Pathol Oral Radiol Endod 2009;108(3):430–6.

Mraiwa N, Jacobs R, van Steenberghe D, et al. Clinical assessment and surgical implications of anatomic challenges in the anterior mandible. Clin Implant Dent Relat Res 2003;5(4):219–25.

Naini RB, Nokar S, Borghei H, et al. Tilted or parallel implant placement in the completely edentulous mandible? a three-dimensional finite elementanalysis. Int J Oral Maxillofac Implants 2011;26(4):776–81.

Nickenig HJ, Eitner S. Reliability of implant placement after virtual planning of implant positions using cone beam CT data and surgical (guide) templates. J Craniomaxillofac Surg 2007;35(4–5):207–11.

Norton MR, Ganeles J, Ganz SD, et al. 2010 Guidelines of the Academy of Osseointegration for the provision of dental implants and associated patient care. Int J Oral Maxillofac Implants 2010;25(3):620–7.

Orentlicher G, Goldsmith D, Horowitz A. Computer-generated implant planning and surgery: case select. Compend Contin Educ Dent 2009;30(3):162–6, 168–73.

Orentlicher G, Goldsmith D, Horowitz A. Applications of 3-dimensional virtual computerized tomography technology in oral and maxillofacial surgery: current therapy. J Oral Maxillofac Surg 2010;68(8):1933–59.

Ozan O, Turkyilmaz I, Ersoy AE, et al. Clinical accuracy of 3 different types of computed tomography-derived stereolithographic surgical guides in implant placement. J Oral Maxillofac Surg 2009;67(2):394–401.

Peñarrocha M, Boronat A, Garcia B. Immediate loading of immediate mandibular implants with a full-arch fixed prosthesis: a preliminary study. J Oral Maxillofac Surg 2009;67(6):1286–93.

Rinaldi M, Ganz SD, Mottola A. Computer-guided applications for dental implants, bone grafting, and reconstructive surgery. Elsevier, in press.

Rodriguez-Recio O, Rodriguez-Recio C, Gallego L, et al. Computed tomography and computer-aided design for locating available palatal bone for grafting: two case reports. Int J Oral Maxillofac Implants 2010;25(1):197–200.

Rosenfeld AL, Mecall RA. Use of interactive computed tomography to predict the esthetic and functional demands of implant-supported prostheses. Compend Contin Educ Dent 1996;17:1125–46.

Rosenfeld AL, Mecall RA. Use of prosthesis-generated computed tomographic information for diagnostic and surgical treatment planning. J Esthet Dent 1998;10: 132–48.

Rosenfeld A, Mandelaris G, Tardieu P. Prosthetically directed placement using computer software to insure precise placement and predictable prosthetic outcomes. Part1: diagnostics, imaging, and collaborative accountability. Int J Periodontics Restorative Dent 2006;26:215–21.

Rothman, Stephen LG. Computerized Tomography of the enhanced alveolar ridge. In: Rothman, editor. Dental applications of computerized tomography. Chicago: Quintessence Publishing Co, Inc; 1998. p. 87–112.

Rugani P, Kirnbauer B, Arnetzl GV, et al. Cone beam computerized tomography: basics for digital planning in oral surgery and implantology. Int J Comput Dent 2009;12(2):131–45.

Sakakura CE, Morais JA, Loffredo LC, et al. A survey of radiographic prescription in dental implant assessment. Dentomaxillofac Radiol 2003;32:397–400.

Sarment DP, Shammari K, Kazor CE. Stereolithographic surgical templates for placement of dental implants in complex cases. Int J Periodontics Restorative Dent 2003;23:287–95.

Sonick M. A Comparison of the accuracy of periapical, panoramic, and computed tomographic radiographs in locating the Mandibular Canal. Int J Oral Maxillofac Implants 1994;9:455–60.

Spyropoulou PE, Razzoog ME, Duff RE, et al. Maxillary implant-supported bar overdenture and mandibular implant-retained fixed denture using CAD/CAM technology and 3-D design software: a clinical report. J Prosthet Dent 2011;105(6):356–62.

Tahmaseb A, De Clerck R, Wismeijer D. Computer-guided implant placement: 3D planning software, fixed intraoral reference points, and CAD/CAM technology. A case report. Int J Oral Maxillofac Implants 2009;24(3):541–6.

Tahmaseb A, Wismeijer D, Coucke W, et al. Computer technology applications in surgical implant dentistry: a systematic review. Int J Oral Maxillofac Implants 2014; 29(Suppl):25–42.

Terzioğlu H, Akkaya M, Ozan O. The use of a computerized tomography-based software program with a flapless surgical technique in implant dentistry: a case report. Int J Oral Maxillofac Implants 2009;24(1):137–42.

Testori T, Robiony M, Parenti A, et al. Evaluation of accuracy and precision of a new guided surgery system: a multicenter clinical study. Int J Periodontics Restorative Dent 2014;34(Suppl 3):s59–69.

Tyndall DA, Price JB, Tetradis S, et al, American Academy of Oral and Maxillofacial Radiology. Position statement of the American Academy of Oral and Maxillofacial Radiology on selection criteria for the use of radiology in dental implantology with emphasis on cone beam computed tomography. Oral Surg Oral Med Oral Pathol Oral Radiol 2012;113(6):817–26.

Valente F, Schiroli G, Sbrenna A. Accuracy of computer-aided oral implant surgery: a clinical and radiographic study. Int J Oral Maxillofac Implants 2009;24(2):234–42.

Treatment Planning for Restorative Implantology

Ricardo A. Boyce, DDS, FICD[a],*, Gary Klemons, DDS[a,b]

KEYWORDS

- Past medical history • Examination and occlusion • Dental imaging
- Fixed and removable prosthodontics • Dental implant success

KEY POINTS

- More than 30 million Americans are missing all of their teeth, according to the American Academy of Implant Dentistry.
- More than 5 million implants are inserted annually in the United States.
- Patients are demanding fixed prosthodontics as opposed to removable prosthodontics.
- In the completely edentulous patient and some partially edentulous patients, implants have become the treatment of choice. To meet these demands, the restorative dentist should have a good foundation in fixed and removable prosthodontics, to have continued success in restorative implantology.
- The goal is to deliver the best implant crown or prosthesis for the patient.
- If problems occur along with increased office visits, patients can become frustrated and discouraged.
- Treatment planning for restorative implantology should be looked at in 4 sections: (1) review of past medical history, (2) oral examination and occlusion, (3) dental imaging (ie, cone-beam computed tomography), and (4) fixed versus removable prosthodontics. These 4 concepts of treatment planning, along with proper surgical placements of the implant(s), result in successful cases.

More than 30 million people Americans are missing their teeth, according to the American Academy of Implant Dentistry. Misch[1] commented that "more than 5 million dental implants are inserted each year in the United States" and "more than $1 billion in implant products was sold in the United States in 2010." Implantology (surgical or restorative) is practiced by general dentists, prosthodontists, oral surgeons, periodontists, and endodontists. The restorative dentist should have a good foundation in fixed and removable prosthodontics to have continued success in restorative implantology.

The authors have nothing to disclose.
^a Department of Dentistry, The Brooklyn Hospital Center, New York, NY, USA; ^b Private Practice, Brooklyn, NY, USA
* Corresponding author.
E-mail address: raboycedds@yahoo.com

Dent Clin N Am 59 (2015) 291–304
http://dx.doi.org/10.1016/j.cden.2014.10.009
0011-8532/15/$ – see front matter © 2015 Elsevier Inc. All rights reserved.

dental.theclinics.com

Wood and Vermilyea[2] stated "it is imperative that the dentist restoring the implants, after consultation with appropriate specialists, be responsible for the treatment planning."

The restorative dentist should discuss the case with the surgeon (by telephone, in person, or via written form). There should not be any confusion regarding the implant system being used and the parts needed. Before consents are signed, the restorative dentist should make sure that they have the tools needed to restore the case. The surgeon and clinician should maximize the exchange of information regarding the surgery. The restorative dentist should inquire about (1) if there were any surgical complications, (2) insertion torque, (3) if there was a need for bone grafting or sinus lift, (4) the size/diameter of the platform and length of the implant, (5) the implant manufacturer, (6) the estimated time of placement of the healing cap, and (7) the clearance from the surgeon to begin the restorative treatment. When there is teamwork between the surgeon, restorative dentist, and the laboratory technician, the result can be a masterful replica of a normal oral cavity. The untrained eye simply does not know the difference.

All responsibilities fall in the lap of the surgeon and restorative dentist. All discussions should be finalized with the patient so that they understand the risks, benefits, and options/alternatives from a surgical and restorative standpoint. Lewis and Klineberg[3] stated that "patients should be informed of the spectrum of potential complications and maintenance issues that can occur with implant-borne prostheses, and informed of the biological consequences and associated future costs." Klein[4] went further in saying "Patient expectations of treatment time, provisional prosthesis requirements, and esthetic demands should be discussed." Dentistry's covenant of trust[5] begins by stating "The dental profession holds a special position of trust with society... the profession makes a commitment to society that its members will adhere to high ethical standards of conduct." The patient's health, well-being, comfort, and peace of mind should always be at the forefront of any dental services rendered.

Patients should know in advance approximately how many office visits are involved and should be given a cost for the restoration(s), including parts. A frustrated patient does not refer others and could seek legal action if they are stuck with a bill and the final outcome was not delivered as promised. The restorative dentist should be careful about what they say or promise to a patient; it is best not to promise anything. In this chapter, treatment planning for restorative implantology there will be four sections: (1) review past medical history, (2) oral examination and occlusion, (3) dental imaging (ie, cone-beam computed tomography [CBCT]), and (4) fixed versus removable prosthodontics. These 4 concepts of treatment planning, along with proper surgical placements of the implant(s), result in a successful implant cases (**Fig. 1**). The fifth concept, dental implant surgery will be discussed in the other chapters of this book.

There are many philosophies that differ and create debates among the groups of specialists mentioned earlier. Quality dentistry should be documented daily and incorporated into the practice of implant dentistry to provide successful cases and patient satisfaction. In this article, current literature is reviewed, along with evidence-based systematic reviews (to eliminate bias views), including advice from those in the dental profession with years of experience, which helps the restorative dentist manage and treat their cases successfully.

REVIEW OF PAST MEDICAL HISTORY

It is prudent for the clinician to review each patient's medical history, which often sets the stage for the treatment to be delivered. The dentist who chooses not to treat those

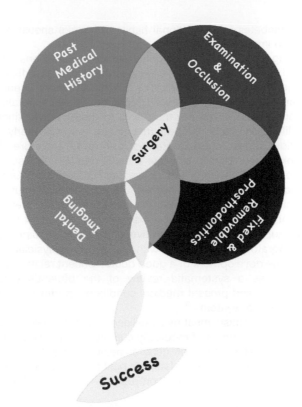

Fig. 1. The five concepts for dental implant success. (*Courtesy of* R. Boyce, DDS, Brooklyn, NY.)

patients who are medically complex or compromised should consider referring them to those in the profession who believe that they have sufficient training in management of their conditions. Lengthy and complex implant cases may not be suited for patients with multiple medical disorders in the ambulatory setting, so good judgment is needed with these patients. This group of patients may be better managed in a hospital setting, particularly in the operating room (OR). This is not difficult for oral surgeons and hospital dentists who place implants and who have OR privileges. An anesthesiologist can properly induce general anesthesia, monitor the patient's vital signs, and administer several medications intravenously (for the benefit of the induced patient), which allows the surgeon to focus on the precise details of preprosthetic surgery or implant placement. Most preprosthetic procedures (soft tissue, some bony) can be performed in the ambulatory setting, whereas more complex procedures (ie, vestibuloplasty, floor-of-the-mouth lowering, skin/mucosal/bone grafts, and multistage reconstructive surgery) require treatment in the OR, with overnight observation in a hospital.[6]

A similar concept applies to patients seeking the restoration of implants. If the general dentist does not feel confident that they can restore the implants, they have the ethical responsibility to refer the patient to someone in the profession who can properly manage the case (ie, a prosthodontist). The reasons include the length of chair time, the cost of the restoration(s), and the number of visits involved. Henry and Liddelow[7] recommended that inexperienced operators should use conventional loading protocols (instead of immediate loading) and that patient-mediated factors (eg, uncontrolled diabetes, parafunctional habits, smoking) should be regarded as contraindications to immediate loading, and so forth.

Patients are living longer, and many taking multiple medications for chronic conditions are in need of dental care. Some of these patients demand fixed prosthodontics as opposed to removable prosthodontics. Such demands present challenges to the dentist, regardless of the specialty. The patient who can obtain rehabilitative restorations or prostheses of greater than 60% of there lost dentition can have a good quality of life. The ability to chew (masticate) foods properly means that a patient can swallow, digest, and excrete foods normally, therefore eliminating the possibility of choking by trying to swallow a bolus, which can also lead to a host of digestive problems. Greenberg and colleagues[8] stated that "Oral health is an integral part of total health, and oral health care professionals must meet the advances in medicine, in order to be at the forefront of the overall health care team." The patient interview of the history is the most important part of the diagnostic patient workup, because it is imperative for the clinician to properly diagnose, collect data (ie, laboratory tests), consult with primary care physician/MD or specialists, and allow for the development of a good doctor-patient relationship.[9] The medical history comprises a systematic review of the patient's chief complaint, information about past and present medical conditions, pertinent social and family histories, and a review of systems.[8]

Marder[10] stated that dentists must use intelligence, common sense, and physician consent for the proper treatment of medically compromised patients. He also added that when there is "deterioration of general health, increased risk of infection, prolonged bleeding, or even demise exists, it is best to defer treatment until systemic stability or disease remission has been accomplished – and never without consultation with a physician."

Several studies[11–14] have established the negative effect of tobacco use on implant success and the likelihood of failure after second-stage surgery. Every clinician should be knowledgeable about different risk factors that can undermine the success of the implant. **Table 1** includes a list of notable medical conditions that should raise warning flags or caution before implant placement.

The term cluster phenomenon was used to describe a group of patients with implant failures with multiple systemic disorders and medications that include but are not limited to osteoporosis, diabetes, mental depression, heavy smoking habits, and parafunctional mandibular movements.[15] Parafunctional habits include tooth clenching, grinding, biting on pencils, chewing on ice, or bruxism. Balshi[16] reported that "overload caused by improper prosthesis design or parafunctional habits is considered to be one of the primary causes of late-stage implant failure."

Table 1 Risk factors for implant placement	
Moderate to severe neutropenia	Psychological instability
Patients on corticosteroids	Radiation therapy
Chemotherapy	Coronary artery disease (ie, myocardial infarction within 6 mo)
Osteoporosis (patients on intravenous bisphosphonates)	Gravid patient
Poorly controlled diabetes	Heavy smoking habits
Malignancy/terminal illness	Cluster phenomenon

DENTAL IMAGING: RADIOGRAPHS/CONE-BEAM COMPUTED TOMOGRAPHY

Oral rehabilitation is a term that takes on different circumstances and meanings to specialists in the dental profession. The responsibility for implantology is shared by the surgeon (ie, oral surgeon, prosthodontist, periodontist, perioprosthetic specialist, endodontist, and general dentist/implantologist) and restorative dentist (ie, prosthodontist, periodontist, and general dentist/implantologist). Traditionally, the restorative dentist initiated the consultation and recommended the region for the implant, then referred the patient to the oral surgeon, who then placed the implant(s). There are more dentists and specialists who are placing and restoring the implant(s). If the traditional planning for implant placement is used, then, there must be excellent communication between both doctors. As mentioned earlier, it is important that the same implant system is used and agreed, to eliminate any problems.

The oral and maxillofacial radiologist is often forgotten but has been instrumental in the transition from conventional radiology to CBCT. Preoperative consultation with an oral and maxillofacial radiologist can be helpful especially when there is a need to rule out and interpret disease (especially intraosseous disease). The surgeon must be cautious of certain anatomic structures in the maxilla and mandible before implant placement, such as the inferior alveolar nerve (IAN), mental nerve, nasopalatine canal, bony defects found on the facial surface of maxillary anteriors, the lingual concavity of the mandible, and pneumatization of the maxillary sinus.[17] These common findings in the human anatomy can place the surgeon at risk of injuring the lingual nerve or IAN, resulting in neuropraxia, axonotmesis, or neurotmesis, and leading to neuropathy, paresthesia, or anesthesia, respectively. Soderstrom and colleagues[18] stated that "the type, orientation, and amount of available bone and its orientation are crucial in treatment planning for implant location"; therefore, a variety of radiographic techniques may be implemented to obtain the best placement. Many dentist or oral surgeons in private practice may not have CBCT, because of cost; therefore, they have to depend on panoramic and periapical radiograph(s). Mupparapu and Beideman[19] made an important note that "panoramic radiographs are not to be used for specific anatomic measurements because of uneven (10% to 30%) magnifications within different regions of the image." The anatomic findings must be well understood before implant placement to prevent errors. The use of CBCT may be overemphasized, because there are times when patients seem to have sufficient bone (mesiodistally) with conventional film; however, after the use of CBCT, the patient may not have adequate bone for an implant buccolingually, which can lead to perforations or fenestrations, which can result in failure (see **Figs. 2–4**). In cases similar to this, patients may opt to have adjunctive surgical procedures or settle for fixed bridge or a removable appliance. Adjunctive treatments, such as onlay bone grafting/guided tissue regeneration, sinus lift, distraction osteogenesis, and ridge splitting, can be performed by the surgeon to overcome anatomic challenges.[20–22] The following adjunctive procedures can bring additional costs to the patient. Every treatment plan should be made according to the patient's budget; therefore, all fees should be discussed in advance, so that the patient can decide if they can afford the package. It is imperative that all risks, benefits, and options/alternatives are discussed with the patient before implant placement.

The CBCT or three-dimensional (3D) imaging shows the alveolar bone in relation to the ideal tooth position with low radiation doses.[23] The radiation dose is reduced 98% when compared with the conventional fan-beamed computed tomography (CT) systems and a reported radiation dose equivalent to that needed for 4 to 15 panoramic radiographs.[24]

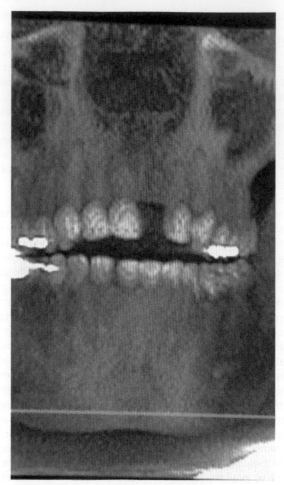

Fig. 2. Coronal view showing missing number 9 from CBCT.

Some surgeons prefer the use of computer-aided implant placement with or without the use of a surgical guide. The 3D implant planning software and CBCT with the "advances in CAD/CAM (Computer-Aided Design/Computer-Assisted Manufacturing) technique, digital data from the surgical plan can be transferred to the actual settings using computer-milled templates or stereolithographic surgical guides."[25] Feinerman[20] stated that "digital technology has provided the ability to more accurately assess the volume, height, and width of bone at proposed osteotomy sites as well as the location of key anatomical structures." Several systematic reviews have been published[25,26] regarding the accuracy of computer-aided implant placement to serve those who doubt their usefulness.

Hultin and colleagues[25] reported in their systematic review that "surgical guide fracture was the most common surgical complication and misfit of the prosthesis was the most common prosthetic complication." They went on to state that "Complications *after* guided implant placement were implant failures or referred to the prosthesis."[25]

Sanders[27] reported multiple risks associated with stereolithographic guided surgery, which include (1) the inability to determine high-level or low-level resistance

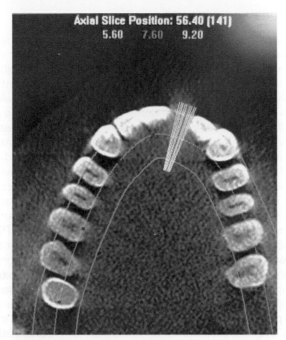

Fig. 3. Axial view of missing number 9 from CBCT.

during the osteotomy, (2) the use of mucosa-supported guides as the least accurate in terms of positioning, (3) a drill guide obscuring the view of the implant position, which can result in implants being placed deeper than planned, (4) the risk of overheating bone and the drill (not if the drill has internal irrigation), (5) lack of knowledge (an experienced clinician can adapt to conventional tactics when problems occur with the use of a guide).

Dental splints with radiopaque markers are intended to be used for the scanning procedure, to establish position, and inclination of the proposed implant.[28]

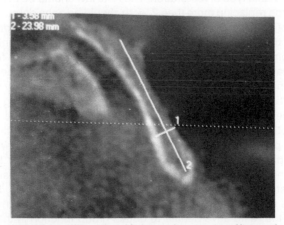

Fig. 4. Sagittal view of the maxillary alveolar bone showing insufficient facial-lingual width for implant placement at the site of missing number 9 from CBCT. This patient was treatment planned for a 3-unit all-ceramic bridge from numbers 8 to 10.

ORAL EXAMINATION AND OCCLUSION

A good clinician should have strong visual tactics. The restorative dentist should be able to visually see the outcome of a restoration or prosthesis. Barber and Seckinger[28] stated "The diagnosis and treatment planning of an implant patient should be a blueprint or a road map of where the patient is clinically, what the patient's expectations are, what the realistic treatment options are, and how those results will be achieved." They went on to say "these preimplant treatments should be under the guidance of the restorative doctor" and "the restorative dentist or the prosthodontist should be the leader of the team...." The restorative dentist should also be astute enough to be able to identify any problems that could arise surrounding a partially dentate or completely edentulous oral cavity. The clinician should be able to assess and diagnose (and document in the chart) periodontal disease (PD) in the dentate (and partially dentate) patient. The clinician should also be aware of the process of seeding, when bacteria from a periodontally diseased site incorporates the site of an implant, which can lead to inflammation and destruction of the surrounding bone. If PD is diagnosed, the patient should be asked if they are aware of it, or if they have ever been told. Time should be spent with the patient to explain the current status and progressive nature of this disease. The patient should have a good understanding in layman terms of their condition. It is important that patients are told the truth about their periodontal status and that radiographs and probing depths are documented in the chart to support the diagnosis. Some patients believe that if they do not have pain, then, there is no need to remove the tooth, even if it presents with a mobility of II or greater. Patients with moderate to severe chronic PD can be referred to a periodontist for a full diagnostic workup to obtain a nonbiased, medical-legal documentation of the prognosis of the remaining teeth, especially when there are gray areas or doubts that arise during the treatment plan phase. There are many patients who have never been told that they have PD and, therefore, have no knowledge or understanding of the slowly destructive process and believe that if they are not in pain, the tooth is "just fine as it is." This factor is especially important if a patient seeking a 6-unit fixed bridge, for example, presents with a Kennedy class IV (missing number 7 to number 10), trying to use tooth numbers 6 and 11 as abutments for a fixed partial denture (FPD). If teeth 6 and 11 have substantial gingival recession, plus pocket depth, it reduces the prognosis long-term for this type of restoration. The Ante law should be considered and the fact that any bridge replacing more than 2 teeth should be considered a high risk. Even in the absence of mobility, a patient has the right to know the periodontal status and the prognosis of the treatment planned. A patient should not be led into believing that periodontally compromised abutments support a long spanned fixed bridge for greater than 5 years. If a patient with chronic PD is not raised to a higher level of awareness, concern, and the ability to maintain their oral hygiene, then, they may opt to keep a removable partial denture or place implants in the areas of missing teeth, or transition into a complete denture with or without implants (considering the periodontal status is poor). Another concern not to be taken lightly by the restorative dentist is the partially dentate patient who wants to restore 1 quadrant at a time with implants. An example is the patient who presents with the Kennedy class I or II in the maxilla opposing a Kennedy class I in the mandible. This patient is interested in obtaining the ability to restore the function of chewing on 1 side at a time, but because of cost restraints is unable to put all 4 quadrants in function at the same time. It is the responsibility of the restorative dentist to obtain group function in the fixed prosthodontic cases, with the goal of achieving occlusion bilaterally in the removable prosthodontic cases. If the patient cannot afford fixed implants at various edentulous sites (quadrant therapy) at the time of the treatment plan phase, then, a removable partial denture should be suggested to the patient. If this option is not offered to the patient, then, simply allowing the patient to function on the side of the implants could lead to fractured porcelain or loosening of screws over time. Retreatment at any time or phase can be frustrating for the restorative dentist, and turn out to be costly for the patient, who in turn can become discouraged.

When a patient accepts the responsibility to manage their home care, then, they may be treatment planned for single or multiple implants. It is also important for patients to understand the carious process and the importance of daily flossing, especially when implants are placed next to natural teeth. The patient must know that they have a role and responsibility in maintaining their oral hygiene and recall visits. Implants can be used for single crown implants, FPDs, or removable partial dentures. An implant over-denture is the standard of care for patients who transition into a mandibular complete denture and for patients in the edentulous maxilla with substantial bone loss.

There are other notable findings that need to be discussed at the treatment plan phase, such as the supraeruption of opposing teeth. It is imperative for the restorative dentist to relay the proposed or foreseen treatment of extraction, enameloplasty, and also root canal treatment because of a foreseen encroachment of the nerve of a tooth or group of teeth to reduce the occlusal height of a tooth, by establishing a more ideal plane of occlusion. This effort benefits the esthetics of the restoration and prevents loosening/dislodgement of the crown, often as a result of lack of retention; otherwise, there is a need for a screw-retained crown when dealing with a short clinical crown.

All clinicians should evaluate patients in Kennedy class I, II, III, and IV to determine if teeth need to be altered or sacrificed (as mentioned earlier) or if an alveoplasty or augmentation with bone graft of the edentulous alveolus is needed as a result of loss of bone or excess of bone. The diagnosis of excessive or decreased interarch space is helpful to the surgeon. Another task of the restorative dentist is to identify teeth that are not in ideal occlusion. Teeth that are in cross-bite should be explained to patients, especially if they are in the esthetic zone. They should be made aware, before implant placement, so that patients can understand various malocclusions. The patient may not be aware of the malocclusion and problems that may present in the future. Those teeth In cross-bite along with the other remaining dentition should be assessed by allowing the patient to move in protrusive and lateral excursive movements. When doing so, the patient should be given a hand mirror, so that occlusal interferences and foreseen problems can be discussed and questions by the patient answered by the dentist. This dialogue with the patient builds trust; however, it should be documented in the chart to prevent any confusion in the future when modifications (ie, enameloplasty) need to be made. Barber and Seckinger[28] noted "The clinical examination should include oral hygiene, periodontal examination, evaluation of the remaining dentition, malocclusion or crowded or rotated teeth, incisal opening, vertical dimension, interarch space, temporomandibular joint examination, and width of available bone at edentulous sites." Klein[4] provided a list of things to observe while charting at the time of examination: (1) status of the remaining teeth, (2) mobility, (3) furcations, (4) probing depths, (5) keratinized tissue, (6) interarch space, (7) interteeth distance, (8) ridge width, (9) supraeruption, (10) tilting of adjacent teeth, (11) occlusal/incisal plane, (12) smile line, (13) does soft tissue appear in the smile?, (14) how many teeth appear in a wide smile?, (15) do the present teeth appear esthetic?, (16) is the current removable prosthesis stable and retentive?, (17) can the current denture be used as a provisional prosthesis?, and (18) are there any acute/chronic infections present?

Concerning esthetics and a beautiful smile, all uneven gingival margins should be assessed by the clinician and shared with the patient. A bilateral symmetric gingival framework needs to be the goal in esthetic cases, which enhances the smile. Rose and Mealy,[29] in describing the importance of an uneven smile to a treatment plan, give a list of causes such as "unfavorable tooth or implant position, previous crown margins or bridges with missing teeth, periodontal disease, recession, root exposure, or previous trauma resulting in gingival recession." Another problem that clinicians face with esthetics is the loss of interdental papilla, or open embrasure or black triangle. This condition occurs when the most apical extent of the contact point to crestal bone is greater than 5 mm, which creates a greater chance of recession of the papilla.[30] If the restorative dentist is not comfortable carrying out the osseous and gingival surgery needed for papillary reconstruction, then, the patient should be referred to a periodontist. Patients need to know in advance that it is a difficult task to recreate interdental papilla. Jivraj and colleagues[31] reported that "the predictability of the esthetic outcome of an implant restoration of an implant restoration is dependent on (1) patient selection and smile line, (2) tooth position, (3) root position of the adjacent teeth, (4) biotype of the periodontium and tooth shape, and (5) the bony anatomy of the implant site." As mentioned earlier, 1 problem for the restorative dentist is the prevention of black triangles in the esthetic zone. Tarnow and colleagues[30] studied implants placed adjacent to natural teeth and implants placed next to each other. They noted the difficulty of obtaining interdental papilla when implants are placed less than 3 mm apart; therefore, implants should be placed at least 3 mm apart to minimize the loss of vertical bone height. Obtaining or creating soft tissue interdental papilla in the esthetic zone is not a predictable outcome; therefore, the shape of clinical crown(s) with longer contact areas to improve the appearance may be an alternative treatment.

FIXED PROSTHODONTICS VERSUS REMOVABLE PROSTHODONTICS

There are a variety of prostheses to consider, based on the existing dentition or lack thereof, including (1) a single tooth replacement(s), (2) an FPD bridge or removable partial denture, (3) a full-arch fixed prosthesis roundhouse (in the completely edentulous dentition), or (4) an overdenture (implant retained overdenture or implant retained and supported overdenture).[4] The implant retained overdentures can have 2 to 6 implants. The placement of these implants is in the completely edentulous dentition. Babbush[32] showed how patient satisfaction in full-arch implant-supported fixed prosthesis improved comfort, speech, taste, function/chewing ability, denture stability, quality of life, and psychological well-being. The placement of the implants at times is determined by available bone. In these cases, the restorative dentist needs to understand the limitations of the surgeon and has an obligation to explain any additional costs to the patient. A good example is the patient who presents with substantial bone loss in the edentulous arch(es), which may involve superstructures (bars), which can be fabricated by a dental laboratory to give support where bone is lost and provide retention of the prosthesis, which greatly increases the cost of the treatment. This treatment can increase the cost from hundreds to thousands of dollars, which some patients may not be able to afford; therefore, a traditional denture may be the best option.

The restorative dentist should have determined the patient's skeletal jaw relationship at the initial consultation. This information should be shared with the surgeon. Diagnosis can be difficult in a completely edentulous patient without an existing denture. Sometimes, class III skeletal jaw relationships are not determined until the vertical dimension of occlusion (VDO) stage of making the prostheses. A mock setup to preview occlusion and lip support should be performed after the VDO stage; if there are any issues, they should be discussed and adjusted before delivery. If orthognathic surgery was not considered to correct a class II or III skeletal discrepancy, then, the positioning of implants or denture teeth to compensate for these relationships is needed.[33] The restorative dentist should be skilled enough to bring the patient close enough to an edge-to-edge bite; however, at the try-in stage, the patient should be allowed to judge the esthetic outcome (with the use of a hand mirror). This option is suggested because some patients who have been in class II or class III malocclusions all their life may want or choose to stay that way. If this is the patient's preference, then, necessary adjustments should be made at the try-in stage to avoid any changes in cost at delivery time.

The clinician should be wary of the patient who is anxious or eager to restore their implants. The restorative dentist should consult with the surgeon to find out the bone type in the patient, as analyzed at the time of implant placement. The second stage, placement of the healing cap, should be performed by the surgeon (this is not an issue if the surgeon is the restorative dentist) to evaluate the implant, bone, and peri-implant tissues. Papaspyridakos and colleagues[34] performed a systematic review of the 4 most frequently used parameters for measuring the success of dental implants: (1) the implant level, (2) peri-implant soft-tissue level, (3) prosthesis level, and (4) the patient's subjective assessment.

A recommended time to restore should come from the surgeon, based on the bone type determined (type I–IV), onlay bone grafting at the site, sinus lift, or distraction osteogenesis. Most cases can be restored at 3 months postoperatively; however, if there was a need for bone grafting, then, the surgeon may recommend 5 to 6 months or 6 to 9 months, depending if it was placed in the mandible or maxilla, respectively. The study and evaluation of preoperative CT is recommended to determine bone quality.[35] Some clinicians have embraced early loading of restorations, which satisfy the wants of the patient. Cochran and colleagues[36] recommended that the "Implant number and distribution are dependent on patient circumstances, including bone quality and quantity, number of missing teeth, condition of opposing dentition, type of occlusion, and bruxism. Implants must be characterized by a rough titanium surface, are allowed to heal for at least 6 weeks, and in type I, II, or III bone" as a protocol for early or immediate loading in the partially dentate maxilla awaiting a fixed prosthesis. Type IV bone has the highest failure rate and is not advised for immediate or early loading cases. Esposito and colleagues[37] in a Cochrane review expressed that as it pertains to immediate load (<1 week), early load (between 1 week and 2 months), and conventional (>2 months), clinicians should be cautious when interpreting the low failure rates that are being documented with publication bias. Many randomized clinical trials (RCTs) were excluded by the Cochrane Collaboration because "some of these trials were not actually randomized as described in the original articles." The documented success outcomes of immediate and early loaded implants relate to: (1) highly experienced clinicians, (2) the quality and quantity of bone, (3) the use of high insertion torques (ie, >80 N cm), (4) the diameter and length of implant, and (5) the use of nonocclusal loading (immediate provisionalization).[37] These topics are constantly up for debate; there is a need for more ethical RCTs to provide evidence that can be taken to the private practice. Otherwise, newly researched materials should be left out of what is already deemed successful in implantology. The recommendation is that immediate loaded implants should be restored by the clinicians who are both placing and restoring the implants. Every surgeon and clinician is free to decide their style of treatment. Most investigators recommend that patients wait for a more conventional healing period, which increases the chance of maximizing osteointegration and success of the implant.

The last topic to be considered in the treatment planning phase, which should not be overlooked, is dental implant maintenance. One aspect of implant maintenance that is occasionally encountered by the restorative dentist is when the crown becomes loose as a result of the screw. The causes of screw loosening are (1) lateral interference and (2) quality of the abutment implant interface. On removal of the crown and screw, it is recommended that the old screw be discarded and a new screw placed and torqued in (according to the manufacturer's recommendations). If the clinician decides to use the same old screw, they can run the risk of breaking the screw inside the implant, which results in the decision to (1) bury the implant, (2) the challenge of retrieving the screw, or (3) trephination (a trephine is used to cut the bone surrounding the implant), which can allow the opportunity to place a new implant in the future.

There are certain groups who because of their medical conditions cannot avoid a deterioration in their oral hygiene (eg, the elderly, patients with dementia, multiple sclerosis, or cerebral palsy); therefore, efforts by a caregiver or family member are needed. Then, there is the population of patients who neglect the maintenance of their dentition, whom dentists encounter on a daily basis. Furthermore, it should not be a surprise to see a patient with implants and a history of periodontitis or completely edentulous cases as a result of years of neglect to present at follow-up or recall appointments with poor oral hygiene. If they did not care for their natural teeth, this situation will probably continue, unless a disciplined oral hygiene regimen is introduced by the clinician/dentist, dental hygienist/dental therapist, and patient. The use of any metal instrument should be avoided while cleaning around the implant restoration, because it can scratch the implant surface and allow bacteria to manifest. There are several different implant instruments on the market (plastic, graphite, titanium-coated, and solid titanium); however, titanium is recommended because of its strength, which is needed to remove calculus.[38] This factor brings up the important aspect of implant scalers to clean around the implants and the use of plastic periodontal probes, but only when there is clinical or radiographic evidence of unhealthy tissue or abnormal bone loss, respectively. Precautions during recall visits should be taken to avoid disruption of the mucoperiosteal seal surrounding the implant. Wingrove[38] recommended that every clinician who is responsible for implant maintenance, "should have at least 1 go-to implant instrument set... needed to meet all implant maintenance challenges."

On recall visits (every 3 months within the first year, every 6 months in the partially dentate patient, annually in the completely edentulous patient), when it is determined by the dentist to take radiographs, then, measurements should be taken and the probing depths or any changes in bone height should be documented. Those patients with fixed implant bridges, roundhouse, or fixed hybrid dentures should be taught how to use and advised to use superfloss (Oral-B) or a floss threader. The use of a water flosser (Waterpik) can also be helpful in the cases described earlier; however, it should not be directed into the gingival sulcus. All advice for implant maintenance and good oral hygiene should be discussed at the beginning, throughout the delivery process, and during follow-up care.

From the beginning to the end of treatment and maintenance, there should be a satisfied patient, the dentist should have an interesting collection of histories and images, and most importantly, everyone should be... all smiles.

REFERENCES

1. Misch C, editor. Dental implant prosthetics. Rationale for dental implants. 2nd edition. St. Louis (MO): Elsevier(Mosby); 2015. p. 1–25.

2. Wood M, Vermilyea S. A review of selected dental literature on evidence-based treatment planning for dental implants: Report of the Committee on Research in Fixed Prosthodontics of the Academy of Fixed Prosthodontics. J Prosthet Dent 2004;92(5):447–62.

3. Lewis MB, Klineberg I. Prosthetic considerations designed to optimize outcomes for single-tooth implants. A review of the literature. Aust Dent J 2011; 56:181–92.

4. Klein M. Atlas of minor oral surgery. In: Dym H, Ogle O, editors. Evaluation and treatment planning for implants. Philadelphia: WB Saunders; 2001. p. 225–30.

5. American Dental Association principle of ethics and code of professional conduct. Available at: http:ada.org/. /code_of_ethics_2012.pdf. Accessed January 25, 2014.

6. Costello BJ, Barber HD, Betts NJ. Preprosthetic surgery: an overview and soft tissue procedures. In: Fonseca RJ, editor. Oral and maxillofacial surgery. St. Louis (MO): Saunders Elsevier; 2000. p. 37–58.

7. Henry PJ, Liddelow GJ. Immediate loading of dental implants. Aust Dent J 2008; 53(Suppl):S69–81.

8. Greenberg MS, Glick M, Ship JA. Burket's oral medicine. 11th edition. Hamilton (Ontario): BC Decker; 2008. p. 1–16.

9. Ganda K. Dentist's guide to medical conditions, medications, complications. 2nd edition. Ames (IA): Wiley Blackwell; 2013. p. 3–23.

10. Marder MZ. Medical conditions affecting the success of dental implants. Compendium 2004;25(10):735–56.

11. Wallace RH. The relationship between cigarette smoking and dental implant failure. Eur J Prosthodont Restor Dent 2000;8:103–6.

12. De Bruyn H, Colbert B. The effect of smoking on early implant failure. Clin Oral Implants Res 1994;5:260–4.

13. Lemons JE, Laskin DM, Roberts WE, et al. Changes in patient screening for a clinical study of dental implants after increased awareness of tobacco use as a risk factor. J Oral Maxillofac Surg 1997;55:72–5.

14. Gorman LM, Lambert PM, Morris HF, et al. The effect of smoking on implant survival at second-stage surgery: DICRG Interim Report #5. Dent Implant Clinical Research Group. Implant Dent 1994;3:165–8.

15. Ekfelt A, Christiansson U, Eriksson T, et al. A retrospective analysis of factors associated with multiple implant failures in the maxillae. Clin Oral Implants Res 2001;12:462–7.

16. Balshi TJ. An analysis and management of fractured implants: a clinical report. Int J Oral Maxillofac Implants 1996;11:660–6.

17. Abubaker AO, Benson KJ, Iuorno FP Jr. Oral and maxillofacial surgery secrets: dental implants. 2nd edition. St. Louis (MO): Saunders Elsevier; 2007. p. 410–7.

18. Soderstom JL, Mulligan JP, Ward J. Radiography for dental implantology. In: Fonseca, Marciani, Turvey, editors. Oral and maxillofacial surgery. (Section IV–implant surgery). 2nd edition. St. Louis (MO): Saunders Elsevier; 2009. p. 547–66.

19. Mupparapu M, Beideman R. Imaging for maxillofacial reconstruction and implantology: the relationship between the implant surgeon and the restorative doctor. In: Fonseca RJ, editor. Oral and maxillofacial surgery. St. Louis (MO): Saunders Elsevier; 2000. p. 17–34.

20. Feinerman D. Expanded dental implant treatment options through technology. Dental Learning: Knowledge for Clinical Practice 2013;2(4):3–12.

21. Tasoulis G, Yao SG, Fine JB. The maxillary sinus: challenges and treatments for implant placement. Compend Contin Educ Dent 2011;32(1):10–9.

22. Koo S, Dibart S, Weber HP. Ridge-splitting technique with simultaneous implant placement. Compend Contin Educ Dent 2008;29(2):106–10.

23. Loubele M, Bogarts R, Van Dijick E, et al. Comparison between effective radiation doses of cbCT and MSCT scanners for dentomaxillofacial applications. Eur J Radiol 2009;71:461–8.

24. Scarfe W, Farman A, Sukovic P. Clinical applications of cone-beamed computed tomography in the dental practice. J Can Dent Assoc 2006;72(1):75–80.

25. Hultin H, Svensson K, Trulsson M. Clinical advantages of computer-guided implant placement: a systematic review. Clin Oral Implants Res 2012;23(Suppl 6):124–38.

26. Van Assche N, Yercruyssen M, Coucke W, et al. Accuracy of computer-aided implant placement. Clin Oral Implants Res 2012;23(Suppl 6):112–23.

27. Sanders P. Guided surgery–understanding the risks. J Implant Pract 2013;6:18–20.

28. Barber HD, Seckinger RJ. Coordination in the comprehensive diagnosis and treatment of the implant patient: the relationship between the implant surgeon and the restorative doctor. In: Fonseca RJ, editor. Oral and maxillofacial surgery. St. Louis (MO): Saunders Elsevier; 2000. p. 14–6.

29. Genvo R, Rose L, Mealy B, et al. Periodontics, medicine, surgery, and implants. Elsevier Mosby; 2004.

30. Tarnow DP, Manger AW, Fletcher P. The effect of the distance from the contact point to the crest of bone on the presence or absence of the interproximal dental papilla. J Periodontol 1992;63:995–6.

31. Jivraj S, Reshad M, Chee W. Treatment planning of implants in the esthetic zone: part three. J Implant Pract 2013;6:32–5.

32. Babbush CA. Post-treatment quantification of patient experiences with full-arch implant treatment using a modification of the OHIP-14 questionnaire. J Oral Implantol 2012;38(3):251–60.

33. Block M. Surgery of the Anterior Mandible. Color atlas of dental implant surgery. 3rd edition. Maryland Heights (MO): Saunders Elsevier; 2011. p. 3–57.

34. Papaspyridakos P, Chen CJ, Singh M, et al. Success criteria in implant dentistry: a systemic review. J Dent Res 2012;91(3):242–8.

35. Ikumi N, Tsutsumi S. Assessment of correlation between computerized tomography values of bone and cutting torque values at implant placement: a clinical study. Int J Oral Maxillofac Implants 2005;20:253–60.

36. Cochran DL, Morton D, Weber HP. Consensus statements and recommended clinical procedures regarding loading protocols for endosseous dental implants. Int J Oral Maxillofac Implants 2004;19(Suppl):109–13.

37. Esposito M, Grusovin MG, Maghaireh H, et al. Interventions for replacing missing teeth: different times for loading dental implants [review]. Cochrane Database Syst Rev 2013;(3):CD003878.

38. Wingrove S. Dental implant maintenance: the role of the dental hygienist and therapist. Dent Health J of the Brit Soc of Dent Hygiene 2011;50(5):8–13.

Tissue Response:
Biomaterials, Dental Implants, and Compromised Osseous tissue

Arvind Babu RS, BDS, MDS, DFO*, Orrett Ogle, DDS

KEYWORDS

- Biomaterials • Dental implants • Tissue response • Osseous lesions

KEY POINTS

- Tissue (cellular and extracellular) responses following an implant surgery have greater influence over the better prognosis.
- Osseointegration is considered to be one of the important tissue responses that are expected following the dental implant surgery.
- Patient selection and critical evaluation of tissues need to be done in prior for the patients with compromised bone disorders.
- Following the proper guidelines in patients with compromised osseous tissue may help in better prognosis.

INTRODUCTION

Dental implants are one of the golden landmarks of modern dentistry. The treatment outcome of dental implants is determined by the degree and type of the tissue responses. The local and systemic responses of the tissue represent a feature of biocompatibility. The function and success of the dental implant rely on the tissue response. It is, therefore, essential to understand the fundamental characteristics of the tissue response to dental implants. This article reviews the tissue response to biomaterials and dental implants, specifically in compromised osseous tissues.

TISSUE RESPONSE TO BIOMATERIALS

Biomaterials are the biological or synthetic materials that are used to restore a part of a living system and/or to maintain contact with living tissue. The local and systemic responses of the tissue represent an important feature of biocompatibility.[1] Anderson[2] described the term, *biocompatibility*, as the ability of a biomaterial, prosthesis, or

The authors have nothing to disclose.
Dentistry Programme, Faculty of Medical Sciences, The University of the West Indies, Mona, Kingston 7, Jamaica, West Indies
* Corresponding author.
E-mail address: arvindbabu2001@gmail.com

medical device to perform with an appropriate host response in a specific application (i.e., the evaluation of biological responses is a measure of the magnitude and duration of the adverse alterations in homeostatic mechanisms that determine the host response). The fundamental characteristics of tissue response after implantation of the biomaterials are injury, blood material interactions, provisional matrix formation, acute and chronic inflammation, granulation tissue formation, foreign body reaction, and fibrous capsule development (**Fig. 1**).

An injury begins from the surgical intervention process of implantation and continues postoperatively.[3] Tissue injury predisposes blood vessel disruption with concomitant release of blood constituents. Immediately after the injury, the alterations in the vascular flow and permeability occur, thus initiating the inflammatory response by the escape of blood cells, fluids, and proteins from the vascular component. The injury and perturbation of homeostatic mechanism lead to the cellular cascades of the healing process. The initial acute inflammatory response is activated by injury to the vascular component of the tissue and the blood material interactions.[4]

Provisional matrix formation at the implant site is formed immediately after the injury of vascularized tissue. The provisional matrix is composed of inflammatory cells, fibrin, and endothelial cells. The mitogens, chemokines, cytokines, and growth factors are released in the provisional matrix and influence wound healing process.[5,6] The components of the provisional matrix initiate the resolution, reorganization, and repair processes.[6,7] During the process of acute inflammation, the major function of the neutrophils/microphages is to phagocytose microbes and foreign materials.[4,8] The engulfment and degradation of biomaterial may or may not occur and is greatly dependent on the property of the biomaterial. Generally, biomaterials are not engulfed by microphages/macrophages because of the size disparity. In certain biomaterials, phagocytosis may occur in which they are coated by natural

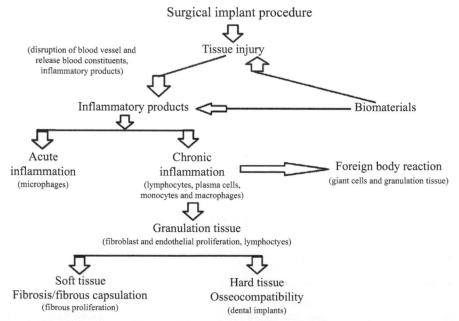

Fig. 1. Tissue response in biomaterial—implant surgical procedure.

substances, such as serum factors, known as opsonins. These opsonins are recognized by the host tissue and provoke degradation. Furthermore, this degradation process does not involve engulfment of the biomaterial but results in the extracellular release of leukocyte products in an attempt to degrade the biomaterial.[9–11] The neutrophils release enzymes, the amount of which depends on the size of the biomaterial particle, thus suggesting that activation of inflammatory response in the tissue depends on the size of the implant and the material of the implant, which is phagocytosable or nonphagocytosable. Persistent inflammation at the tissue injury of the implanted site results in chronic inflammation. The presence of lymphocytes, plasma cells, monocytes, and macrophages in the implant site designates the chronic inflammation. The physical and chemical properties of the biomaterial and movement of the implant material predispose the chronic inflammation process. The macrophages are important cells in chronic inflammation, because the macrophages process and present the antigen to the immunocompetent cells, thus initiating the immune reactions.[12,13]

The formation of the granulation tissue is considered a hallmark of the healing inflammation process. The initiation of granulation tissue formation depends on the site and size of the tissue injury, the formation of which can be anticipated in 3 to 5 days of the implantation. Foreign body reaction is characterized by foreign body giant cells and granulation tissue components. The physical and chemical properties of the biomaterial used, however, determine the composition of the foreign body reaction.[14] Anderson mentions that foreign body reaction in the implant site might be controlled by the surface properties of the biomaterial, form of the implant, and relationship between the surface area of the biomaterial and the volume of the implant.[3] Foreign body reaction with granulation tissue development is considered a normal wound healing response to the implanted biomaterials. Recent studies on oral implants report that osseointegration is a foreign body response to the implant and is a chronic inflammatory response characterized by bone embedding or separation of the implant from the host tissue.[15]

The end stage in the healing response to biomaterials is either fibrosis or fibrous encapsulation. The repair after the implant procedure usually involves 2 processes: regeneration and replacement of connective tissue that comprises the fibrous capsule. The Processes are controlled by the proliferative capacity of cells and persistence of tissue framework of the implant site.[3,16,17] The dental implants have a better compatibility with osseous tissue than with soft tissue. The bone bonding strength of the dental implants is high, but the bonding properties with soft tissue are poor and result in the fibrous encapsulation.[18]

TISSUE RESPONSE TO DENTAL IMPLANTS

The tissue involved in the implanted area shows a cascade of cellular and extracellular response at the bone–implant interface until the implant surface is covered with a newly formed bone.[19] The host response after the implantation procedure is modified by the physical and chemical properties of the implant material, stability of the fixation, heat injury, or death of osteocytes during implant procedure.[20,21] The blood is the first tissue component to come in contact with the implant surface. The blood cells and inflammatory cells from the severed vascular tissue migrate into the tissue around the implant.[22] The platelets are initiated and are responsible for forming a clot in the implant–tissue interface area. The fibrin matrix of the blood clot acts as a scaffold for osteoconduction, and migration of osteogenic cells takes place. Osteogenetic process, which is activated, is similar to bone healing process and is regulated by various growth factors that are released by the blood cells at the bone–implant interface.[23,24] The mesenchymal tissue formation begins and the osteogenetic process is character- ized by (1) woven formation through an intramembranous pathway and (2) lamellar bone formation on the spicules of woven bone.[22,25]

The blood cells at the implant–tissue interface are activated, resulting in the release of growth factors, cytokines. On initiation and activation of osteogenic cells, eventual differentiation results in osteoinduction at the tissue front, leading to the healing cascade. The newly formed osteoid tissues eventually come in direct contact with the implant surface and result in the osseointegration. The active osteogenic cells' and mesenchymal cells' migration to the implant surface starts after 24 hours of the implantation.[22,24,25] The cytokines liberated help in the signaling of the cell migration, cell adhesion, and cell proliferation. The signaling process leads to the bone proteins' deposition over the implant surface, thus creating a noncollagenous matrix scaffold over the implant surface and this regulates the cell adhesion and binds with the min- erals. The matrix formed is poorly mineralized bone tissue, and continuous apposition of calcium and phosphorus results in the integration of the implant with adjacent host tissue.[26]

TISSUE RESPONSE IN COMPROMISED OSSEOUS TISSUES

There is a new paradigm for dental implants in patients seeking oral rehabilitation needs. Dental implants in modern dentistry have gained a significant positive response from the partially or completely edentulous patients. The host response has a significant role in the successfulness of the implant treatment. The perturb- ance in physiologic conditions may have an impact on the treatment outcome and prognosis. Existing systemic diseases or systemic pharmacologic therapies can in- fluence dental implant treatment outcome. Thus, a preexisting systemic disease or systemic therapy may influence and complicate or contraindicate implant proce- dures in dental patients. Lesions (discussed later) are characterized according to the disease origin, such as developmental, metabolic, infection, and neoplastic. The recommendations for various osseous lesions for dental implant placement are represented in **Table 1**.

Osteogenesis Imperfecta

Osteogenesis imperfecta is characterized by impairment of collage maturation and enhanced bone fragility. Higher frequency of bone fractures are noted in type II osteo- genesis imperfecta. The wound healing is poor and fracture healing may be associ- ated with exuberant callus formation.[27] Cases have been reported of placement of osseointegrated dental implants in osteogenesis imperfecta that has been success- ful.[28–31] Prabhu and colleagues, reported a successful case of 9 years' follow-up; and Binger and colleagues, reported a successful case of follow-up of 4 years.[28,30] These data suggest that dental implants are not absolutely contraindicated in patients with osteogenesis imperfecta. Before placement of the dental implants, however, caution is needed regarding bone fragility and wound healing properties.

Hyperparathyroidism

Hyperparathyroidism is characterized by the excessive production of parathyroid hor- mone. Severe cases of hyperparathyroidism cause bone, renal, and gastric distur- bances. In skeletal depletion, it affects alveolar bone before rib, vertebrae, or long bones. The implant placement is contraindicated in the areas of active bony lesions. Implants may be placed after the successful treatment of hyperparathyroidism.[27,32]

| Table 1 Recommendations for dental implant placement in osseous lesions ||
Osseous Lesion	Recommendations for Dental Implant Placement
Osteogenesis imperfecta	Dental implant placement is not contraindicated; however, special attention needs to taken to evaluate bone fragility and wound healing properties.
Hyperparathyroidism	Dental implant placement is contraindicated in the areas of active bony lesions. In skeletal depletion, it more commonly affects the alveolar bone in comparison with rib, vertebrae, and long bones.
Osteoporosis	Dental implant placement is not contraindicated; however, special consideration is recommended in pre-, intra-, and postoperative periods.
Osteomyelitis	Dental implant placement is usually contraindicated due to the compromised vascular supply to the affected area of the bone. Dental implants may be placed, however, after the restoration of vascularity in the affected bone.
Fibrous dysplasia	Dental implant placement is contraindicated in the region of disorder. The dental implants may be placed after the completion of growth to avoid submerged implants and revision of prosthesis in young patients.
Cemento-osseous dysplasia	Dental implant placement is usually not contraindicated; however, a thorough radiographic evaluation is advised.
BP therapy	Dental implant may be placed, following the guidelines provided by the American Association of Oral and Maxillofacial Surgeons.
Paget disease	Dental implant placement is a relative contraindication due to the diminished bone quality and it interferes with osseointegration.
Multiple myeloma	Dental implant placement is a relative contraindication due to the severity of the disease and severe destruction of the bone.
Irradiated bone	Because of the higher incidence of dental implant failure, special caution needs to be taken with irradiated patients and a thorough evaluation is required with radiation exposure, type and total cumulative dose and timing, region of implant installation, quality of bone, implant length, and design prior to the implant procedure.

Cases have been reported of successful treatment of dental implants in patients with controlled and treated hyperparathyroidism.[33]

Osteoporosis

Osteoporosis is a metabolic bone disorder characterized by reduced mineral density of normally mineralized bone. The concern in this disorder for dental implants is due to the assumption that impaired bone metabolism may influence the osseointegration of implants.[34] Heersche and colleagues,[35] in 1998, discuss that bone remodeling is a nonuniform process; it varies between cortical and trabecular and from site to site. The studies on osteoporotic fractures suggested that, the healing are usually in better fashion which denotes a satisfactory healing and repair response. The study results denotes that the bone remodeling process in osteoporotic patients is not different from those of healthy individuals.[36,37] Holahan and colleagues,[38] in 2008, suggest that diagnosis of osteoporosis and osteopenia has not contributed to implant failure. Several case reports have indicated that successful placement of dental implants is possible in osteoporosis and steroid-induced osteoporosis, glucocorticoid dependent.[39–43] Reduced success rate was observed in patients who underwent maxillary sinus augmentation and in female patients without estrogen supplementation.[44,45] The bone density influences the treatment plan, surgical approach, length of healing, and progressive loading. Implant design needs to be considered with a greater width, and the surface conditions of the implant material need to be designed to increase bone contact and density.[32]

Beikler and Flemmings, discuss the pre-, intra-, and postoperative special considerations for dental implant therapy in patients with bone metabolic disease. The 2 considerations for pre- and intraoperative considerations are (1) thorough examination and evaluation of the causative factors for bone disease and treatment and (2) necessary bone augmentation procedures. The 3 postoperative considerations are (1) physiologic doses of vitamin D (400–800 IU/d) and calcium (1500 mg/d) in the postoperative period; (2) the healing period is increased by 2 to 8 months in maxillae and 6 months in mandible; and (3) careful occlusal adjustments and observation for the occlusal overload are required.[37]

Osteomyelitis

Osteomyelitis is inflammation in the medullary spaces or cortical surfaces of bone, histologically characterized by the sequestrum and involucrum.[27] Based on the duration, it can be an acute- or chronic-type osteomyelitis is usually contraindicated for placement of dental implants after the restoration of vascularity in the affected bone.[32]

Fibrous Dysplasia

Fibrous dysplasia is a developmental tumor-like condition affecting jaw bones, which is histologically characterized by replacement of normal osseous tissue by an excessive proliferation of fibrocellular connective tissue stroma intermixed with irregular-appearing bony trabeculae.[27] Lack of osseous tissue and increased amount fibrous tissue in these lesions predispose to decreased rigid fixation of the dental implant. The reduced fixation increases the chance of local infection and spread of the infection further complicates the dental implant treatment outcome.[32] On successful completion of treatment of fibrous dysplasias, patients may receive the implants. Case reports have shown successful dental implants in treated fibrous dysplasia and McCune-Albright syndrome.[46,47] Recommendations have been made for screening procedures and management of endocrinopathies associated with fibrous dysplasia.[48] The dental implants may be placed after a young patient has completed growth to avoid submerged implants and revision of prosthesis.[49]

Cemento-osseous Dysplasia

Cemento-osseous dysplasia is the most common fibro-osseous lesion in dental practice and the lesion is histologically characterized by the fibrocellular connective tissue stroma with avascular cementum–like areas. The 3 types of this disorder are focal, periapical, and florid cement osseous dysplasia.[27,33] Cases have been reported of dental implant placement and successful results in florid cemento-osseous dysplasia.[50] Recently, a case was reported of implant failure after 26 months in a patient, and the histopathologic evidence suggested concomitant florid cemento-osseous dysplasia with cemento-ossifying fibroma. The investigators of this report recommended a thorough radiographic evaluation of dental arch to locate suspected bony lesions that may lead to implant failure.[51] The dental implants are not contraindicated; however, radiographic evaluation for the presence of sclerotic bone is required, which indicates the hypovascularity. This bone has a chance of become infected and result in the failure of healing.[32]

Bisphosphonate-Treated Patients

Bisphosphonates (BPs) are drugs used in the management of osteoporosis, Paget disease, metastatic bone neoplasm, breast cancer, multiple myeloma, and malignant hypercalceima to increase survival and quality of life.[32,52] The oral and intravenous BPs bind with bone and inhibit the osteoclast activity and osteoclastic bone resorption and induce their apoptosis. The recent BPs include nitrogen in their molecules, which inhibits tumor proliferation and angiogenesis. Depending on the strength and half-life of BPs, the complication of osteonecrosis development may be observed.[53,54] The frequency of development of osteoradionecrosis are greater with intravenous therapy than oral delivery of BPs.[55] The fast development of osteoradionecrosis among intravenous BP users is due to higher and more rapid accumulation of these drugs in the bone.[56] The results of experimental studies on animals indicate a better osseointegration of dental implants with BPs.[57] Case reports of dental implant placement in patients receiving BPs have been reported, however, with development of osteoradionecrosis of jaw.[58] The inconsistent results obtained in animal experimental studies and human cases may be due to the short medication and follow-up period with BPs in animal studies.[54] Grant and colleagues,[55] in 2008, in their review of 115 cases, reveal that oral BPs do not seem to significantly affect implant success and suggest that all patients undergoing implant placement should be questioned about BP therapy, including drug taken, drug dosage, and length of treatment prior to surgery.

The American Association of Oral and Maxillofacial Surgeons has provided guidelines for patients treated with BPs. (1) If BP is administered intravenously in cancer patients, dental implant placement is contraindicated. (2) If BP is taken orally, 3 possibilities exist: (a) In patients treated with BPs for less than 3 years who have no clinical risks, dental implants can be placed without altering the conventional surgical treatment; (b) If patients have been treated for fewer than 3 years and are treated jointly with corticoids, BPs must be removed 3 months before and not administered again, until the bone has completely healed; and (c) If patients have taken BPs for more than 3 years, it is possible to place dental implants if BPs are removed for 3 months before surgery and not administered again until the bone has completely healed.[59]

Paget Disease

Paget disease of bone is characterized by abnormal and anarchic resorption and deposition of bone, resulting in distortion and weakening of the affected bones.[27] Paget disease is a relative contraindication for dental implant placement due to the diminished bone quality and it interferes with osseointegration.[32] Cases have been reported of placement and survival of dental implants in remission cases of Paget disease and patients under BP therapy.[60,61] Rasmussen and Hopfensperger,[60] in 2008, report that on surgical placement of dental implants, poor quality of bone was observed.

Multiple Myeloma

Multiple myeloma is a malignant neoplasm of plasma cell origin that often seems to have a multicentric origin within the bone, with osteolytic destruction of the bone. Pathologic fractures are often noted in some cases due to the osteolytic destruction.[27] The dental implant placements in this neoplastic condition are a relative contraindication due to the severity of the disease and severe destruction of the bone. A case was reported of dental implant placement in a patient with multiple myeloma who wished to maximize his quality of life. The reported case was reported as successful.[62]

Irradiated Bone

Radiotherapy results in the hypovascular, hypoxic, and hypocellular state of hard and soft tissue.[27] Caution needs to be taken prior to the placement of dental implants. The radiation exposure, type of and total cumulative dose and timing, region of implant installation, quality of bone, implant length, and design need to be evaluated prior to implant therapy. Implant prostheses are recommended rather than soft tissue prosthesis in irradiated patients, which reduce the possible soft tissue irritation in these patients.[32,63,64] The failure rate of dental implants in irradiated patients may be reduced by adjunctive hyperbaric oxygen therapy.[63]

SUMMARY

Dental implant placement requires thorough patient examination and selection. The success of the treatment relies on the tissue response. Although lesions (discussed previously) are relative contraindications, the published literatures are available for successful placement and treatment of dental implants. Thorough examination and evaluation of patients with a specific disorder/disease process may alter patient selection. Following the proper guidelines in patients with specific types of disorder or disease is, therefore, recommended.

ACKNOWLEDGMENTS

The authors are thankful for the support from Professor Archibald McDonald, Principal, University of the West Indies at Mona (UWI-Mona); Professor Horace Fletcher, Dean, Faculty of Medical Sciences (FMS), UWI-Mona; Professor Russell Pierre, Programme Director, Undergraduate Medical Programme, FMS, UWI-Mona; and Dr Thaon Jon Jones, Programme Director, Undergraduate Dental Programme, FMS, UWI-Mona.

REFERENCES

1. Park J, Lakes RS. Biomaterials an introduction. Tissue response to implants. 3rd edition. New York: Springer; 2007. p. 265–90.
2. Anderson JM. Biological responses to materials. Annu Rev Mater Res 2001;31: 81–110.
3. Clark RA, Henson PM. The molecular and cellular biology of wound repair. 2nd edition. New York: Springer; 1996. p. 3–10.
4. Kumar V, Abbas AK, Aster J. Robbins basic pathology. 8th edition. Philadelphia: Elsevier; 2013. p. 29–74.
5. Tang L. Mechanisms of fibrinogen domains: biomaterial interactions. J Biomater Sci Polym Ed 1998;9:1257–66.
6. Villar CC, Huynh-Ba G, Mills MP, et al. Wound healing around dental implants. Endod Topics 2011;25:44–62.
7. Shaw TJ, Martin P. Wound repair at a glance. J Cell Sci 2009;122:3209–13.
8. Broadley KN, Aquino AM, Woodward SC, et al. Monospecific antibodies implicate basic fibroblast growth factor in normal wound repair. Lab Invest 1989;61: 571–5.
9. Ratner BD, Hoffman AS, Schoen FJ, et al. Biomaterials science: an introduction to materials in medicine. 3rd edition. Oxford (UK): Elsevier; 2013. p. 503–11.

10. Henson PM. The immunologic release of constituents from neutrophil leukocytes. II. Mechanisms of release during phagocytosis, and adherence to nonphagocytosable surfaces. J Immunol 1971;107:1547–57.
11. Katzenmeyer KN, Bryers JD. Multivalent artificial opsonin for the recognition and phagocytosis of gram-positive bacteria by human phagocytes. Biomaterials 2011;32:4042–51.
12. Bridges AW, Whitmire RE, Singh N, et al. Chronic inflammatory responses to microgel based implant coatings. J Biomed Mater Res 2010;94:252–8.
13. Tang L, Eaton JW. Inflammatory responses to biomaterials. Am J Clin Pathol 1995; 103:466–71.
14. Anderson JM, Rodriguez A, Chang DT. Foreign body reaction to biomaterials. Semin Immunol 2008;20:88–100.
15. Albrektsson T, Dahlin C, Jemt T, et al. Is marginal bone loss around oral implants the result of a provoked foreign body reaction? Clin Implant Dent Relat Res 2013. http://dx.doi.org/10.1111/cid.12142.
16. Grainger DW. All charged up about implanted biomaterials. Nat Biotechnol 2013; 31:507–9.
17. Higgins DM, Basaraba RJ, Hohnbaum AC, et al. Localized immunosuppressive environment in the foreign body response to implanted biomaterials. Am J Pathol 2009;175:161–70.
18. Johnson R, Harrison D, Tucci M, et al. Fibrous capsule formation in response to ultrahigh molecular weight polyethylene treated with peptides that influence adhesion. Biomed Sci Instrum 1997;34:47–52.
19. Fini M, Giavaresi G, Torricelli P, et al. Osteoporosis and biomaterial osteointegration. Biomed Pharmacother 2004;58:487–93.
20. Rigo EC, Boschi AO, Yoshimoto M, et al. Evaluation in vitro and in vivo of biomimetic hydroxyapatite coated on titanium dental implants. Mater Sci Eng C Mater Biol Appl 2004;24:647–51.
21. Soballe K. Hydroxyapatite ceramic coating for bone implant fixation. Mechanical and histological studies in dogs. Acta Orthop Scand Suppl 1993;255:1–58.
22. Davies JE. Mechanisms of endosseous integration. Int J Prosthodont 1998;11: 391–401.
23. Berglundh T, Abrahamsson I, Lang NP, et al. De novo alveolar bone formation adjacent to endosseous implants. Clin Oral Implants Res 2003;14:251–62.
24. Meyer U, Joos U, Mythili J, et al. Ultrastructural characterization of the implant/bone interface of immediately loaded dental implants. Biomaterials 2004;25: 1959–67.
25. Mavrogenis AF, Dimitriou R, Parvizi J, et al. Biology of implant osseointegration. J Musculoskelet Neuronal Interact 2009;9:61–71.
26. Murai K, Takeshita F, Ayukawa Y, et al. Light and electron microscopic studies of bone-titanium interface in the tibiae of young and mature rats. J Biomed Mater Res 1996;30:523–33.
27. Neville D, Allen B. Fibro osseous lesions. Oral and maxillofacial pathology. 2nd edition. Philadelphia: Elsevier; 2002. p. 553–6.
28. Prabhu N, Duckmanton N, Stevenson AR, et al. The placement of osseointegrated dental implants in a patient with type IV B osteogenesis imperfecta: a 9-year follow-up. Oral Surg Oral Med Oral Pathol Oral Radiol Endod 2007; 103:349–54.
29. Payne MA, Postlethwaite KR, Smith DG, et al. Implant-supported rehabilitation of an edentate patient with osteogenesis imperfecta: a case report. Int J Oral Maxillofac Implants 2008;23:947–52.

30. Binger T, Rücker M, Spitzer WJ. Dentofacial rehabilitation by osteodistraction, augmentation and implantation despite osteogenesis imperfecta. Int J Oral Maxillofac Surg 2006;35:559–62.

31. Lee CY, Ertel SK. Bone graft augmentation and dental implant treatment in a patient with osteogenesis imperfecta: review of the literature with a case report. Implant Dent 2003;12:291–5.

32. Misch CE. Medical evaluation of the dental implant patient. Contemporary implant dentistry. 3rd edition. Canada: Elsevier; 2008. p. 421–66.

33. Flannagan D, Mancini M. Bimaxillary full arch fixed dental implant supported treatment for a patient with renal failure and secondary hyperparathyroidism and osteodystrophy. J Oral Implantol 2013. http://dx.doi.org/10.1563/AAID-JOI-D-13-00188.

34. Mori H, Manabe M, Kurachi Y, et al. Osseointegration of dental implants in rabbit bone with low mineral density. J Oral Maxillofac Surg 1997;55:351–61.

35. Heersche JN, Bellows CG, Ishida Y. The decrease in bone mass associated with aging and menopause. J Prosthet Dent 1998;79:14–6.

36. Dao TT, Anderson JD, Zarb GA. Is osteoporosis a risk factor for osseointegration of dental implants? Int J Oral Maxillofac Implants 1993;8:137–44.

37. Beikler T, Flemming TF. Implants in the medically compromised patient. Crit Rev Oral Biol Med 2003;14:305–16.

38. Holahan CM, Koka S, Kennel KA, et al. Effect of osteoporotic status on the survival of titanium dental implants. Int J Oral Maxillofac Implants 2008;23:905–10.

39. Shibli JA, Aquiar KC, Melo L, et al. Histologic analysis of human perii-implant bone in type 1 osteoporosis. J Oral Implantol 2008;34:12–6.

40. Fujimoto T, Niimi A, Nakai H, et al. Osseointegrated implants in a patient with steoporosis: a case report. Int J Oral Maxillofac Implants 1996;11:539–42.

41. Fujimoto T, Niimi A, Sawai T, et al. Effects of steroidinduced osteoporosis on osseointegration of titanium implants. Int J Oral Maxillofac Implants 1998;13:183–9.

42. Eder A, Watzek G. Treatment of a patient with severe osteoporosis and chronic polyarthritis with fixed implant-supported prosthesis: a case report. Int J Oral Maxillofac Implants 1999;14:587–90.

43. Friberg B. Treatment with dental implants in patients with severe osteoporosis: a case report. Int J Periodontics Restorative Dent 1994;14:348–53.

44. Blomqvist JE, Alberius P, Isaksson S, et al. Factors in implant integration failure after bone grafting: an osteometric and endocrinologic matched analysis. Int J Oral Maxillofac Surg 1999;25:63–8.

45. August M, Chung K, Chang Y, et al. Influence of estrogen status on endosseous implant osseointegration. J Oral Maxillofac Surg 2001;59:1285–9.

46. Monje A, Monje F, Suarez F, et al. Oral rehabilitation with dental implants for teeth involved in a maxillary firbous dsyplasia. Clin Adv Periodontics 2013;3:208–13.

47. Bajwa MS, Ethunandan M, Flood TR. Oral rehabilitation with endosseous implants in a patient with fibrous dysplasia (McCune-Albright syndrome): a case report. J Oral Maxillofac Surg 2008;66:2605–8.

48. Dobbs RN, S A, Lee JS. Indications for and management of implants in children. Selected Readings in Oral & Maxillofacial Surgery 2010;18:1–20.

49. Lee JS, FitzGibbon EJ, Chen YR, et al. Clinical guidelines for the management of craniofacial fibrous dysplasia. Orphanet J Rare Dis 2012;7:S2.

50. Bencharit S, Schardt-Sacco D, Zuniga JR, et al. Surgical and prosthodontic rehabilitation for a patient with aggressive florid cemento-osseous dysplasia: a clinical report. J Prosthet Dent 2003;90:220–4.

51. Gerlach RC, Dixon DR, Goksel T, et al. Case presentation of florid cemento-osseous dysplasia with concomitant cemento-ossifying fibroma discovered

during implant explantation. Oral Surg Oral Med Oral Pathol Oral Radiol 2013; 115:e44–52.

52. Heymann D, Ory B, Gouin F, et al. Bisphosphonates: new therapeutic agents for the treatment of bone tumors. Trends Mol Med 2004;10:337–43.

53. Wood J, Bonjean K, Ruetz S, et al. Novel antiangiogenic effects of the bisphosphonate compound zoledronic acid. J Pharmacol Exp Ther 2002;302:1055–61.

54. Flichy Fernandez AJ, Balaguer Martinez J, Penarrocha Diago M, et al. Bisphosphonates and dental implants: current problems. Med Oral Pathol Oral Cir Bucal 2009;14:E355–60.

55. Grant BT, Amenedo C, Freeman K, et al. Outcomes of placing dental implants in patients taking oral bisphosphonates: a review of 115 cases. J Oral Maxillofac Surg 2008;66:223–320.

56. Palaska PK, Cartsos V, Zavras AI. Bisphosphonates and time to osteonecrosis development. Oncologist 2009;14:1154–66.

57. Meraw SJ, Reeve CM, Wollan PC. Use of alendronate in periimplant defect regeneration. J Periodontol 1999;70:151–8.

58. Wang HL, Weber D, McCauley LK. Effect of long-term oral bisphosphonates on implant wound healing: literature review and a case report. J Periodontol 2007; 78:584–94.

59. Advisory Task Force on Bisphosphonate-Related Ostenonecrosis of the Jaws. American Association of Oral and Maxillofacial Surgeons. American Association of Oral and Maxillofacial Surgeons position paper on bisphosphonate-related osteonecrosis of the jaws. J Oral Maxillofac Surg 2007;65:369–76.

60. Rasmussen JM, Hopfensperger ML. Placement and restoration of dental implants in a patient with Paget's disease in remission: literature review and clinical report. J Prosthodont 2008;17:35–40.

61. Torres J, Tamimi F, Garcia I, et al. Dental implants in a patient with Paget disease under bisphosphonate treatment: a case report. Oral Surg Oral Med Oral Pathol Oral Radiol Endod 2009;107:387–92.

62. Sager RD, Theis RM. Dental implants placed in a patient with multiple myeloma: report of case. J Am Dent Assoc 1990;121:699–701.

63. Granstrom G. Placement of dental implants in irradiated bone: the use for using hyperbaric oxygen. J Oral Maxillofac Surg 2006;64:812–8.

64. Buddula A, Assad DA, Salinas TJ, et al. Survival of dental implants in native and grafted bone in irradiated head and neck cancer patients: a retrospective analysis. Indian J Dent Res 2011;22:644–8.

Short Implants
Are They a Viable Option in Implant Dentistry?

Steven Richard Schwartz, DDS[a,b,c],*

KEYWORDS

- Short implant • Maxilla • Mandible • Grafting

KEY POINTS

- Short-length implants (<10 mm) can be used effectively in atrophic maxillae or mandibles even with crown/implant ratios that previously would have been considered excessive.
- Short implants can support either single or multiple units and can be used for fixed prostheses or overdentures.
- The use of short-length implants may obviate complicated bone augmentation procedures, thus allowing patients who are either unwilling or unable for financial or medical reasons to undergo these advanced grafting techniques to be adequately treated.

BRIEF HISTORY OF IMPLANTS

People's desire to replace missing teeth predates all recorded treatises on dentistry. Human osseous remains carbon dated as far back as 600 AD show the Mayan practice of using seashells carved into tooth-shaped pieces placed into empty sockets.[1]

The modern era of root form endosseous implants begins with Dr P.I. Brånemark's discovery of osseointegration in 1952[2] and subsequent placement of the first Brånemark implants in human patients in 1965.[2] Dr Brånemark's presentation in 1982 at the Toronto Osseointegration Conference in Clinical Dentistry included incomparable scientific documentation going back to 1952 and data on human research from 1965. Such data in implantology had never before been collected.

The author has nothing to disclose.
[a] Woodhull Medical and Mental Health Center, Department of Dentistry, Division of Oral and Maxillofacial Surgery, 760 Broadway, Brooklyn, New York 11206, USA; [b] The Brooklyn Hospital Center, Department of Dentistry, Division of Oral and Maxillofacial Surgery, 121 Dekalb Avenue, Brooklyn, New York 11026, USA; [c] Private Practice, New York Oral and Maxillofacial Surgeon, P.C. 2844 Ocean Parkway B2, Brooklyn, New York 11235, USA
* New York Oral & Maxillofacial Surgeon, P.C. 2844 Ocean Parkway B2, Brooklyn, New York 11235, USA
E-mail address: office@nyomsurgeons.com

EARLY HISTORY OF IMPLANT LENGTHS

Early implants ranged in length from 7 mm to 20 mm. The most widely available implant diameter at the time was 3.75 mm with a machined or turned surface. At first, the implant length was considered paramount and the diameter not as important, even though a linear relationship between length and success had not been proved.[3]

WHAT ARE SHORT IMPLANTS?

There is no general consensus in dentistry as to what constitutes a short versus a long implant. Various investigators have considered various lengths of less than or equal to 7 mm up to 10 mm as short.[4–9] For the purposes of this article, lengths less than 10 mm are considered short. Implants 10 mm or greater in length are considered long or standard length.

WHY LONG IMPLANTS WERE PREFERRED

As stated earlier, long implants were considered most desirable.[4] Reasons for this opinion was probably 2-fold.

First there was early evidence that short Brånemark implants (6–10 mm) with traditional turned/machine surfaces had inferior success rates compared with longer fixtures.[5,10–14]

Friberg and colleagues[10] reported on 4641 consecutively placed Brånemark machined implants that were followed from implant surgery to prosthesis insertion. They concluded that, "A preponderance of failures could also be seen among the shortest fixtures (7 mm)" compared with the longer 10-mm to 20-mm fixtures.

Wyatt and colleagues[11] reported in 1998 on 230 machined Brånemark implants followed for up to 12 years (mean 5.4 years). Of the 7-mm implants placed, 25% failed, whereas the 10-mm fixtures had an 8% failure rate and the 13-mm and 15-mm implants had failures rates of only 5% and 2% respectively.

Bahat[12] followed a total of 660 implants placed in the posterior maxilla from 5 to 12 years. Of the 3.75-mm diameter short implant fixtures, including 7 and 8.5 mm, 17% failed.

In 2003, Attard and Zarb[13] showed a 15% failure rate for 7-mm implants, whereas 10-mm and 13-mm implants had failure rates of 6% to 7%.

Weng and colleagues[14] reported in 2003 on a multicenter prospective clinical study evaluating the success of 1179 3i machined surface implants for up to 6 years. Of the 1179 implants, 48.5% were considered short (≤10 mm). These short implants (7–10 mm) accounted for 60% of all failed implants, with a cumulative success rate of only 88.7%. The 10-mm long implants accounted for 10% of the failures, whereas the 8.5-mm and 7-mm implants accounted for 19% and 26% of failures respectively. The cumulative success rate for the long implants (>10 mm) was 93.1%. The overall cumulative success rate was only 89%.

Herrmann and colleagues[5] described in 2005 a multicenter analysis of 487 Brånemark System; Nobel Biocare implants followed for 5 years in the hope of predicting implant failures based on patient and implant characteristics. They found a 10.1% failure rate for 10-mm implants and a 21.8% failure rate for the 7-mm implants.

Second, dental training in conventional fixed prosthodontics, specifically Ante's law, possibly skewed clinicians' thought processes. Ante's law states that the total periodontal membrane area of the abutment teeth must equal or exceed that of the teeth to be replaced.[15] From that law, the radiographic calculation of the crown/root ratio (CRR) was used to decide a tooth's suitability as an abutment. A variety of ratios are reported in the literature. A CRR of 1:2 was considered ideal, but is seldom found in clinical practice.[16] Shillingburg and colleagues[17] suggested that a CRR of 1:1.5 was optimal and a ratio of at least 1:1 necessary for a satisfactory result. Even though Ante's law has subsequently been disproved,[18] the concept of longer roots being better abutments than short roots still prevails. With these ideas already established, short implants just looked wrong and, whenever possible, long implant fixtures were placed.

So why, after so many of the early studies showed generally decreased success with short implants, did researchers and clinicians continue to pursue the idea of short implant fixtures? The answer is because there are numerous clinical situations in which the placement of long implants is problematic because of anatomic boundaries. Some of the more commonly encountered problems are the position of the inferior alveolar nerve and canal, low-lying maxillary sinuses with insufficient residual alveolar bone height, and alveolar ridge deficiencies.[4,19] In an effort to overcome these anatomic problems, advanced surgical techniques were developed. To increase the alveolar bone height, guided bone regeneration, block grafting, maxillary sinus floor grafting, and distraction osteogenesis procedures were performed. To bypass vital structures such as the inferior alveolar nerve, nerve transpositioning techniques were used. All of these advanced surgical procedures can be challenging, technique sensitive, time consuming, and costly, and can increase surgical morbidity and prolong overall treatment time.[4,19–22]

With early disappointing results such as these, why would anyone want to continue to use short implants? The answer lies in improvements in surface technology, implant to abutment connections, a better understanding of implant to bone biomechanics using finite elemental analysis (FEA), and weighing the risks versus benefits of advanced bone augmentation procedures as opposed to using short implants.

COST/BENEFIT AND RISK/BENEFIT OF ADVANCED BONE GRAFTING SURGERY VERSUS SHORT IMPLANTS

A systematic review by Milinkovic and Cordaro[21] of different alveolar bone augmentation procedures for partially edentulous and fully edentulous jaws documented the mean implant survival rate (MISR) and the mean complication rate (MCR) for vertical augmentation procedures, including guided bone regeneration (GBR), bone blocks (BBs), and distraction osteogenesis (DO). In partially edentulous patients with GBR, the MISR ranged from 98.9% to 100%, with an MCR 13.1% to 6.95%. BBs had an MISR of 96.3% and MCR of 8.1%. The greatest vertical gain was noted with DO, but it also had the highest MCR (22.4%) and MISR (98.2%). In fully edentulous patients, the BB MISR was only 87.75%. The complication rate was highly variable, contingent on whether the different donor sites or recipient sites were being analyzed. The overall MCR was calculated as 21.9%. For Le Fort? I grafts, the MISR was 87.9%, with complications ranging from 24% to 30%. With sinus graft there are multiple different complications possible, including intraoperative and postoperative complications. Vasquez and colleagues[23] documented the complication rate in 200 consecutive sinus lift procedures. They reported that the most common intraoperative complication, at 25.7%, was schneiderian membrane perforation. Previous reports note a range of 7% to 56% in the rate of perforation. After surgery, 19.7% had some type of complication. The most frequent were wound infection (7.1%), sinusitis (3.9%), and graft loss (1.6%).

For atrophic mandibles, it is the posterior segment, distal to the mental foramen, that poses the greatest challenge. When the remaining posterior vertical alveolar bone is deemed inadequate for 10-mm or longer implants, the only option is either vertical grafting as outlined previously or inferior alveolar nerve transpositioning surgery. Hassani and colleagues[22] documented initial postoperative sensory impairment after inferior alveolar nerve transposition of almost 100%. Normal sensory function returned in 84% of cases, with 16% of patients left with a permanent and irreversible condition. Neurosensory disturbances are so prevalent with this procedure that many surgeons consider sensory disorders such as these to represent a normal and predictable postsurgical state and that they should not be considered untoward sequelae of treatment.

The concept of placing short implants was introduced as a way to avoid the need for advanced surgical procedures and their associated risks.[6,7]

Nisand and Renouard[29] in 2014 reviewed multiple studies comparing short implants with standard-length implants with various vertical augmentation procedures and found similar survival rates. However, the use of short implants resulted in faster and lower-cost treatment with reduced morbidity (**Table 1**).[29]

ROUGH/TEXTURED SURFACE VERSUS MACHINE/TURNED SURFACE

Over the years research progressed on the surface technology of implant fixtures, leading to textured or rough-surface implants.

Table 1
Short implants versus standard-length implants with various vertical augmentation procedures

Author/Year	Patients/ Implants	Follow-up (mo)	Test Implant	Control Implant/Sx	Cumulative Success Rate
Penarrocha-Oltra et al,[8] 2014	37/80	12	5.5 mm (intrabony length)	≥10 mm + block vertical graft (≥8.5 mm intrabony length)	T: 1 short failed C: 2 long failed (preload); 7 grafts deficient needed to use short implants; 21 needed additional grafting
Gulje et al,[24] 2013	95/208	12	6 mm	11 mm	T: 3 short failed; 2 preloading; 1 postloading C: 1 long failed
Pieri et al,[25] 2012	68/144	36	6 mm	≥11 mm + sinus graft	T: 98.6% success C: 96% success
Esposito et al,[26] 2011	60/121	36	6.3 mm	≥9.3 mm + vertical bone graft	T: 2 short failed C: 3 long failed; 2 grafts failed
Felice et al,[27] 2011	28/178	5	5.0–8.5 mm	≥11.5 mm + vertical bone graft	T: 2 short failed C: 1 long failed; 2 grafts failed
Felice et al,[28] 2010	60/121	12	7 mm	≥10 mm+ vertical bone graft	T: 1 short failed C: 3 long failed; 2 grafts failed

Abbreviations: C, control; Sx, surgery; T, test.
Adapted from Nisand D, Renouard F. Short implant in limited bone volume. Periodontology 2000, 2014;66:77; with permission.

If clinicians were to still accept 1.5 mm of crestal bone loss in the first year and no more than 0.2 mm of bone loss per year in succeeding years,[30] then short implants would effectively become even shorter, potentially increasing the negative effects. These criteria for success were written in 1989, at a time when most implants had only a machined/turned surface. With the advent of rough/textured surfaces, these old criteria are no longer valid.

Renouard and Nisand[7] reviewed 53 human studies of the impact of implant length and diameter on survival rates. They found that 12 of the studies indicated an increased failure rate with short implants, which was associated with operator experience, routine surgical preparation (irrespective of bone density), machined surface implants, and placement in areas of poor bone density. Twenty-two later publications showed comparable survival rates between short and long implants when rough-surface implants and adapted surgical protocols based on bone density were used.

Pommer and colleagues[4] indicated that rough-surfaced implants showed significantly lower failure rates than machined implants. Balshe and colleagues[31] found in their retrospective study of 2182 smooth (machined) surface implants versus 2425 rough-surfaced implants that there was no statistical difference in the 5-year survival rates (94% vs 94.5% respectively). However, when implants of less than or equal to 10 mm were evaluated separately, the estimate of survival for rough-surface implants was 93.7%, whereas for smooth-surface implants it was only 88.5%. A prospective study by Nedir and colleagues[36] on a 7-year life table analysis on International Team for Implantology of Institute Straumann (ITI) rough-surface (titanium plasma-sprayed [TPS] and sandblasted, large grit, acid-etched [SLA]) implants loaded for at least 1 year showed that the cumulative success rate for short implants (8–9 mm) was as high as for the longer implant groups (10–11 mm and 12–13 mm).

ABUTMENT CONNECTION: EXTERNAL HEX TO INTERNAL

The evolution of the abutment to implant interface from the flat-top external hex to an internal connection of varying designs, including the Morse taper or cone connection, also had a bearing on the survivability of short implants. The Morse taper connection has been shown to incur less marginal bone loss than external hex abutment connections and may even promote bone growth over the implant shoulder in close approximation with the abutment.[32] Weng and colleagues[37] compared implants with an internal Morse taper connection placed 1.5 mm subcrestally and additional fixtures placed at the bony crest with external hex implant fixtures placed subcrestally and at the crest. The greatest crestal bone loss occurred when external hex implants were placed subcrestally. The reduced bone loss noted with the internal connection implants was statistically significant.

Crestal bone loss is therefore not a significant factor in the success of short implant fixtures.

FINITE ELEMENT ANALYSIS AND ITS IMPORTANCE FOR SHORT IMPLANTS

FEA is a type of computer program that uses the finite element method to analyze an object (in this case a dental implant) and predict how applied stresses will affect the object (implant) or its relationship to adjacent structures (bone). The analysis is done by creating a mesh of points in the shape of the implant that contains information about the material and the object at each point for analysis. FEA is a computer model to allow clinicians to observe the bone-implant interface. By changing variables such as implant length, diameter, and bone density, clinicians can try to determine what will happen to the bone interface under varying conditions.

Himmlova and colleagues[33] studied the stress occurring at the bony interface with FEA using three-dimensional computer models. Their simulated implants varied in length from 8 mm to 18 mm and diameters ranged from 2.9 mm to 6.5 mm. The maximum stress concentration was at the top 5 to 6 mm of the implant and there was little difference in area affected by maximum stress with the 8-mm versus the 17-mm implant. The difference in stress was only 7.3%. In contrast, stress reduction continued to decrease as implant diameter increased. Maximum stress values in the 6.5-mm diameter implant were almost 60% less than those of the narrow 2.9-mm implant. This simulation showed that implant diameter was more important for stress distribution than length.

Baggi and colleagues[34] analyzed the effect of implant diameter and length on stress distribution, including crestal bone loss, using 5 commercially available implant designs. The implants tested included diameters of 3.3 mm to 4.5 mm and lengths of 7.5 mm to 12 mm. The investigators concluded that "to control the risk of bone overload and to improve implant biomechanical stress-based performance, numerical results from the current study suggest that implant diameter can be considered to be a more effective design parameter than implant length."

CROWN/IMPLANT RATIOS: ARE THEY IMPORTANT?

Multiple studies and case series are available that deal with the question of increased crown/implant ratios (CIRs) by virtue of using short implants. In a systematic review that included machined surface, solid implants, and rough-surface hollow cylinder and solid implants, Blanes[35] addressed the issue of CIR affecting implant survival and crestal bone loss. He found a 94.1% survival rate of implants with CIRs greater than or equal to 2 after a mean follow-up of 6 years. In addition, this review concluded that the CIR did not affect peri-implant crestal bone loss.

Tawil and Younan[38] followed 269 Brånemark system implants (machined surface) placed in 111 patients for 12 to 992 months. The lengths were 6 mm, 7 mm, 8 mm, 8.5 mm, and 10 mm. The diameters were 3.3 mm, 3.75 mm, 4 mm, and 5 mm. The 6-mm to 8.5-mm lengths were designated as short implants, compared with the standard 10-mm long implant. There was an overall survival rate of 95.5%. In comparing the short with the standard length implants there was no statistical difference in survival (93.1% vs 97.4%). Furthermore, there was no statistical difference between the diameters 3.75 mm (96.3%), 4.0 mm (96.0%), and 5 mm (94.5%). There was no analysis for the lone 3.3-mm implant. In addition, the mean crestal bone loss was 0.71 ± 0.65 mm, with only 8.9% of the sites losing more than 1.5 mm of bone height. In their 7-year life table analysis of 528 rough-surface implants (including titanium plasma sprayed and sandblasted and etched), Nedir and colleagues[36] included a breakdown of the CIR by implant length. The short implants (6, 8, 9 mm) had CIRs ranging from 1.45 to 1.97. The long implants (10–13 mm) had CIRs ranging from 1.05 to 1.3. There was a cumulative success rate of 99.4% and short implants did not fail more than longer ones despite the greater CIRs with the short implants. Atieh and colleagues[39] conducted a systematic review for the treatment of partial posterior edentulism. They included 33 studies totaling 3573 short (≤8.5 mm) implants. Thirty-eight percent were in the maxilla, 51% were mandibular, and the remaining 11% were unknown. The follow-up ranged from 1 to 7 years with an average of 3.9 years. There were 67 failures in total, with 71% occurring before loading. This finding of early failure before loading is consistent with other studies,[6,10,37,38] and implies that the forces associated with implant loading and reduced bone-to-implant contact are not the primary determinants in the ultimate success or failure of short implants.[39]

CURRENT LITERATURE VALIDATES THE USE OF SHORT IMPLANTS, BUT THERE ARE RISK FACTORS: SMOKING, LOW DENSITY BONE (TYPE IV), OPERATOR EXPERIENCE

Telleman and colleagues[45] conducted a systematic review of the posterior zone of partially edentulous patients. Their report included 29 studies totaling 2611 short (5–9.5 mm) implants. They analyzed multiple variables including implant length, rough versus machined surface, maxilla versus mandible, and smokers versus nonsmokers. They concluded that increasing length from 5 mm to 9.5 mm improved overall survival. The survival rates were 5 mm (93.1%), 6 mm (97.4%), 7 mm (97.6%), 8 mm (98.4%), 8.5 mm (98.8%), 9 mm (98.0%), and 9.5 mm (98.6%). There was a 29% improvement of rough surfaces compared with machined surfaces. The difference in the failure rate of maxillary implants (generally lower density/lower quality bone) than mandibular implants was substantial at 100%. When studies including heavy smokers ($\geq$15 cigarettes/d) versus strictly excluding smokers were examined, the estimated failure rate was 57% lower.

Atieh and colleagues[39] showed a noteworthy increase in the 3-year to 4-year cumulative survival rate as implant length increased from 5-mm implants (89.9%) to 6 mm (96.6%), 7 mm (95.6%), 8 mm (99.2%), and 8.5 mm (98.2%) lengths. There was an overall acceptable 5-year cumulative survival rate of 98.3% for short implants compared with 97.7% for long implants.

Nisand and Renouard[29] recently reported a structured review of short (European Association of Osseointegration definition $\leq$8 mm) versus longer length implants. For the short implants they included 29 case series for a total of 9780 implants. They found an overall cumulative survival rate of 96.67%. They also studied long implants, analyzing 5 reviews comprising 58,953 implants with cumulative survival rates ranging from 93.1% to 99.1%. These results are consistent with previous evaluations corroborating the efficacy of short implants when used in the appropriate clinical circumstances.

Table 2 lists several recent studies with mean follow-ups ranging from 24 months to more than 10 years with favorable success rates. These 4 studies totaled 493 short implants ranging in length from 5.5 mm to 10 mm and including both machined and rough-surface implants, posterior maxilla and mandible, smokers and nonsmokers, and bone types I to IV. The overall success rate for the short (5.5–10 mm) implants was still 95.5%.

Table 2
Recent studies with favorable success rates

Author/Year	Mean Follow-up (mo)	No. of Patients/Implants	CSR (%)	No. of Failed Implants	Prosthesis Failures
Anitua et al,[40] 2014	24	34/45 $\leq$6.5 mm	100	0	0
Anitua et al,[41] 2014	123.3	75/111 (94 were splinted to longer implants)	98.90	1	NR
Lai et al,[42] 2013	86 (range 60–120)	168/231	98.7 at 5 y 98.3 at 10 y	4	11
Sanchez-Garces et al,[43] 2012	81	136/273 (total) 167 10 mm 106 short	92.67 92.82 92.5	20 (total) 12 8	NR — —

Abbreviations: CSR, cumulative success rate; NR, not recorded.

Adapted from Nisand D, Renouard F. Short implant in limited bone volume. Periodontology 2000, 2014;66:76; with permission.

The last 2 factors to consider when evaluating the success of short implants are the surgical protocol and operator experience. Adapted surgical protocols to increase the primary mechanical stability have been suggested by several investigators, including Tawil and Younan[38] (2003), Fugazzotto and colleagues[44] (2004), Renouard and Nisand[7] (2006), and Nisand and Renouard[29] (2014). Although slightly different in the specifics, the overall theme is similar: to enhance initial stability. This outcome might be accomplished by eliminating a step in the standard protocol, such as eliminating the countersink drill or eliminating the final drill in the standard drilling sequence. Many implant companies have manufactured narrower final drills than their standard final drill for drilling in soft bone (the so-called soft bone drilling protocol).

Operator experience is probably the most difficult variable to account for. It has been suggested that operator experience, or lack thereof, with short implants may be a reason for the different reported outcomes with short implants between studies.[7]

Although it may seem to require a simpler procedure than a long implant, there is a learning curve and short implants are best not attempted by novice surgeons. Surgeons must be totally comfortable with the basics of implant surgery so that attention can be directed toward modification of the drilling protocol as needed to compensate for changes in bone density while still being acutely aware of implant three-dimensional positioning.[7,29]

When deciding whether or not to use short implants some guidelines have been suggested by Nisand and Renouard[29] (2014) based on available bone height, bone quality, and risk factors such as smoking, history of periodontal disease, and advanced patient age, which can all affect marginal bone loss over the long term.

At this time, if 6 mm is accepted as the minimum implant length, because of its acceptable success rates (Telleman,[45] 97.4%; and Atieh and colleagues,[39] 96.6%), then the minimum height of remaining bone that would be acceptable can be calculated backwards. In the maxilla the minimum height below the maxillary sinus is 6 to 7 mm to use a short implant without additional grafting. Once the height decreases to 5 to 6 mm, the other risk factors, including bone quality, smoking, history of periodontal disease, and advanced patient age, must be taken into consideration. With less than 5-mm bone height, some sort of sinus graft surgery is suggested. Whether it is a lateral window graft or vertical crestal uplift graft is up to the individual operator.

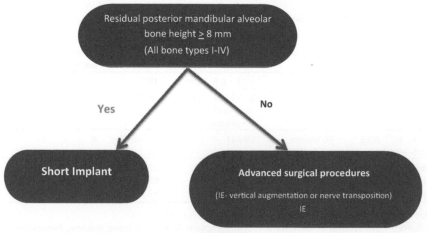

Fig. 1. Treatment guidelines for atrophic mandibles.

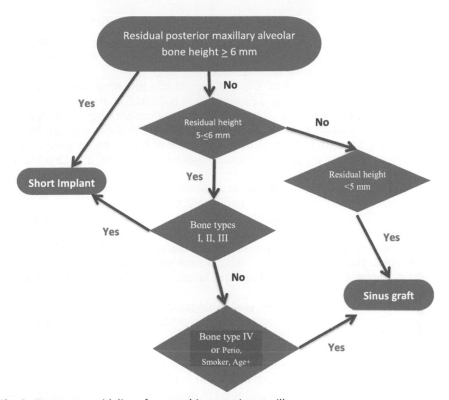

Fig. 2. Treatment guidelines for atrophic posterior maxillae.

In the mandible, the residual bone height superior to the inferior alveolar nerve canal needs to be greater than or equal to 8 mm. This height includes 6 mm for the implant length and 2 mm as a safety zone above the inferior alveolar nerve canal. With less than 8 mm of bone height, an advanced surgical procedure such as onlay or interpositional grafting, distraction osteogenesis, or nerve transposition would be necessary. Other factors to consider are using the appropriate drilling protocol to maximize primary stability and using an implant with a moderate rough surface to speed up the secondary biological healing (osseointegration) as primary stability wanes. It is this author's opinion that using an implant design that already incorporates platform switching with a tapered internal connection may also prove to be beneficial in the long term. These height recommendations are for residual alveolar ridges that are wide enough to accommodate a 4-mm diameter implant. **Figs. 1** and **2** summarize the recommendations enumerated earlier.[29]

SUMMARY

Short-length implants (<10 mm) can be used effectively in atrophic maxillae or mandibles even with crown/implant ratios that previously would have been considered excessive. Short implants can support either single or multiple units and can be used for fixed prostheses or overdentures. The use of short-length implants may avoid the need for complicated bone augmentation procedures, thus allowing patients who were either unwilling or unable for financial or medical reasons to undergo these advanced grafting techniques to be adequately treated.

REFERENCES

1. Ring ME. Dentistry: an illustrated history. New York: Harry N Abrams; 1985.
2. Brånemark PI, Zarb GA, Albrektsson T. Tissue-integrated prostheses: osseointegration in clinical dentistry. Quintessence (IL): 1985.
3. Lee JH, Frias V, Lee KW, et al. Effect of implant size and shape on implant success rates: a literature review. J Prosthet Dent 2005;94:377–81.
4. Pommer B, Frantal S, Willer J, et al. Impact of dental implant length on early failure rates: a meta-analysis of observational studies. J Clin Periodontol 2011;38:856–63.
5. Herrmann I, Lekholm U, Holm S, et al. Evaluation of patient and implant characteristics as potential prognostic factors for oral implant failures. Int J Oral Maxillofac Implants 2005;20:220–30.
6. Neves FD, Fones D, Bernardes SR, et al. Short implants—an analysis of longitudinal studies. Int J Oral Maxillofac Implants 2006;21:86–93.
7. Renouard F, Nisand D. Impact of implant length and diameter on survival rates. Clin Oral Implants Res 2006;17(Suppl 2):35–51.
8. Penarrocha-Oltra D, Aloy-Prosper A, Cervera-Ballester J, et al. Implant treatment in atrophic posterior mandibles: vertical regeneration with block bone grafts versus implants with 5.5-mm intrabony length. Int J Oral Maxillofac Implants 2014;29:659–66.
9. Hagi D, Deporter DA, Pilliar RM, et al. A targeted review of study outcomes with short (<7 mm) endosseous dental implants placed in partially edentulous patients. J Periodontol 2004;75:798–804.
10. Friberg B, Jemt T, Lekholm U. Early failures in 4,641 consecutively placed Brånemark dental implants: a study from stage 1 surgery to the connection of completed prostheses. Int J Oral Maxillofac Implants 1991;6:142–6.
11. Wyatt CC, Zarb GA. Treatment outcomes of patients with implant-supported fixed partial prostheses. Int J Oral Maxillofac Implants 1998;13:204–11.
12. Bahat O. Brånemark system implants in the posterior maxilla: clinical study of 660 implants followed for 5 to 12 years. Int J Oral Maxillofac Implants 2000;15:646–53.
13. Attard NJ, Zarb GA. Implant prosthodontic management of partially edentulous patients missing posterior teeth: the Toronto experience. J Prosthet Dent 2003;89:352–9.
14. Weng D, Jacobson Z, Tarnow D, et al. A prospective multicenter clinical trial of 3i machined-surface implants: results after 6 years of follow-up. Int J Oral Maxillofac Implants 2003;18:417–23.
15. Ante IH. The fundamental principles of abutments. Mich State Dent Society Bulletin 1926;8:14–23.
16. Dykema RW, Goodacre CJ, Phillips RW. Johnston's modern practice in fixed prosthodontics. 4th edition. Philadelphia: WB Saunders; 1986. p. 8–21.
17. Shillingburg HT Jr, Hobo S, Whitsett LD. Fundamentals of fixed prosthodontics. 3rd edition. Chicago: Quintessence Publishing; 1997. p. 89–90.
18. Lulic M, Bragger U, Lang NP, et al. Ante's (1926) law revisited: a systematic review on survival rates and complications of fixed dental prostheses (FDPs) on severely reduced periodontal tissue support. Clin Oral Implants Res 2007; 18(Suppl 3):63–72.
19. Kotsovilis S, Fourmousis I, Karoussis I, et al. A systematic review and meta-analysis on the effect of implant length on the survival of rough-surface dental implants. J Periodontol 2009;80:1700–18.
20. Esposito M, Grusovin M, Felice P, et al. The efficacy of horizontal and vertical bone augmentation procedures for dental implants–a Cochrane systematic review. Eur J Oral Implantol 2009;2(3):167–84.

21. Milinkovic I, Cordaro L. Are there specific indications for the different alveolar bone augmentation procedures for implant placement? A systematic review. Int J Oral Maxillofac Surg 2014;43:606–25.
22. Hassani A, Motamedi M, Saadat S. Inferior alveolar nerve transpositioning for implant placement, a textbook of advanced oral and maxillofacial surgery. Rijeka, Croatia: InTech Publishing; 2013. p. 659–93.
23. Vasquez JC, Rivera AS, Gil HS, et al. Complication rate in 200 consecutive sinus lift procedures: guidelines for prevention and treatment. J Oral Maxillofac Surg 2014;72:892–901.
24. Gulje F, Abrahamsson I, Chen S, et al. Implants of 6 mm vs. 11 mm lengths in the posterior maxilla and mandible: a 1-year multicenter randomized controlled trial. Clin Oral Implants Res 2013;24:1325–31.
25. Pieri F, Aldini N, Fini M, et al. Preliminary 2-year report on treatment outcomes for 6-mm-long implants in posterior atrophic mandibles. Int J Prosthodont 2012;25:279–89.
26. Esposito M, Cannizzaro G, Soardi E, et al. 3-year post-loading report of a randomized controlled trial on the rehabilitation of posterior atrophic mandibles: short implants or longer implants in vertically augmented bone? Eur J Oral Implantol 2011;4(4):301–11.
27. Felice P, Soardi E, Pellegrino G, et al. Treatment of the atrophic edentulous maxilla: short implants versus bone augmentation for placing longer implants. Five-month post-loading results of a pilot randomized controlled trial. Eur J Oral Implantol 2011;4(3):191–202.
28. Felice P, Pellegrino G, Checchi L, et al. Vertical augmentation with interpositional blocks of anorganic bovine bone vs. 7-mm-long implants in posterior mandibles: 1-year results of a randomized clinical trial. Clin Oral Implants Res 2010;21:1394–403.
29. Nisand D, Renouard F. Short implant in limited bone volume. Periodontol 2000, 2014;66:72–96.
30. Smith DE, Zarb GA. Criteria for success of osseointegrated endosseous implants. J Prosthet Dent 1989;62:567–72.
31. Balshe AA, Assad DA, Eckert SE, et al. A retrospective study of the survival of smooth-and rough-surface dental implants. Int J Oral Maxillofac Implants 2009;24:113–8.
32. de Castro D, de Araujo M, Benfatti C, et al. Comparative histological and histomorphometrical evaluation of marginal bone resorption around external hexagon and Morse cone implants: an experimental study in dogs. Implant Dent 2014;23:270–6.
33. Himmlova L, Dostalova T, Kacovsky A, et al. Influence of implant length and diameter on stress distribution: a finite element analysis. J Prosthet Dent 2004;91:20–5.
34. Baggi L, Cappelloni I, Di Girolamo M, et al. The influence of implant diameter and length on stress distribution of osseointegrated implants related to crestal bone geometry: a three-dimensional finite element analysis. J Prosthet Dent 2008;100:422–31.
35. Blanes RJ. To what extent does the crown-implant ratio affect survival and complications of implant-supported reconstructions? A systematic review. Clin Oral Implants Res 2009;20(Suppl 4):67–72.
36. Nedir R, Bischof M, Briaux JM, et al. A 7-year life table analysis from a prospective study on m implants with special emphasis on the use of short implants. Results from a private practice. Clin Oral Implants Res 2004;15:150–7.

37. Weng D, Nagata M, Bosco A, et al. Influence of microgap location and configuration on radiographic bone loss around submerged implants: an experimental study in dogs. Int J Oral Maxillofac Implants 2011;26:941–6.
38. Tawil G, Younan R. Clinical evaluation of short, machined-surface implants followed for 12 to 92 months. Int J Oral Maxillofac Implants 2003;18:894–901.
39. Atieh M, Zadeh H, Stanford C, et al. Survival of short dental implants for treatment of posterior partial edentulism: a systematic review. Int J Oral Maxillofac Implants 2012;27:1323–31.
40. Anitua E, Alkhraist M, Pinas L, et al. Implant survival and crestal bone loss around extra-short implants supporting a fixed denture: the effect of crown height space, crown-to-implant ratio, and offset placement of the prosthesis. Int J Oral Maxillofac Implants 2014;29:682–9.
41. Anitua E, Pinas L, Begona L, et al. Long-term retrospective evaluation of short implants in the posterior areas: clinical results after 10–12 years. J Clin Periodontol 2014;41:404–11.
42. Lai HC, Si MS, Zhuang LF, et al. Long-term outcomes of short dental implants supporting single crowns in posterior region: a clinical retrospective study of 5–10 years. Clin Oral Implants Res 2013;24:230–7.
43. Sanchez-Garces MA, Costa-Berenguer X, Gay-Escoda C. Short implants: a descriptive study of 273 implants. Clin Implant Dent Relat Res 2012;14:508–16.
44. Fugazzotto P, Beagle J, Ganeles J, et al. Success and failure rates of 9 mm or shorter implants in the replacement of missing maxillary molars when restored with individual crowns: preliminary results 0 to 84 months in function. A retrospective study. J Periodontol 2004;75:327–32.
45. Telleman G, Raghoebar GM, Vissink A, et al. A systematic review of the prognosis of short (<10 mm) dental implants placed in the partially edentulous patient. J Clin Periodontol 2011;38:667–76.

Treatment of Peri-Implantitis and the Failing Implant

 CrossMark

Kevin Robertson, DDS, Timothy Shahbazian, DDS*,
Stephen MacLeod, BDS, MD

KEYWORDS

- Peri-implantitis • Peri-implant mucositis • Implant failure • CIST

KEY POINTS

- Appropriate supportive treatment of implants is becoming increasingly important for the general dentist as the number of implants placed per year continues to increase.
- Early diagnosis of peri-implantitis is imperative, and initiating the correct treatment protocol depends on a proper diagnosis.
- Several risk factors exist for the development of peri-implantitis, which can guide patient selection and treatment planning.
- Treatment of peri-implantitis should be tailored to the severity of the lesion (as outlined by the cumulative interceptive supportive treatment protocol), which ranges from mechanical debridement to explantation.
- Several surgical and nonsurgical treatment alternatives exist, and there is little consensus on superior treatment methods.

INTRODUCTION

Dental implants have revolutionized the treatment of tooth loss to the extent that they are now considered the standard of care in many circumstances. Although implants are now a very predictable treatment option, occasionally they fail for a variety of reasons. Peri-implantitis is a late complication of dental implants and is the primary process that leads to late failure. This article reviews definitions, risk factors, diagnosis, and therapy for peri-implantitis.

Since the first dental implants were placed by Brånemark in 1965, they have experienced enormous success and growth. The number of implants placed in the United States increased more than 10-fold from 1983 to 2002 and increased another 10-fold

The authors have nothing to disclose.
Division of Oral and Maxillofacial Surgery and Dental Medicine, Department of Surgery, Loyola University Medical center, 2160 S. First Ave., Maywood, Illinois 60153, USA
* Corresponding author.
E-mail address: timothy.shahbazian@va.gov

from 2000 to 2010. The number of dental implants placed in the United States per year is roughly 5 million, and this number is projected to sustain yearly growth at 12% to 15% for the next several years.[1] With the ever-increasing number of implants, management of attendant complications (such as peri-implantitis) will become increasingly important for all clinicians involved in the patient's care.

DEFINITION OF TERMS

To discuss peri-implantitis, it is important to briefly differentiate it from other forms of bone loss around implants. These other forms of bone loss include those that could be primarily biomechanical in nature (eg, implant fracture, occlusal overload, and marginal bone loss) as well as those that are primarily inflammatory in nature (eg, peri-implant mucositis and retrograde peri-implantitis). Although bone loss is a shared end result, there are distinctions of probable cause, probable course, and current treatments. The ongoing process of reaching consensus is important,[2–5] because it will affect reporting of prevalence, as well as the inclusion of studies in systematic reviews and the use of data in meta-analyses.

Marginal Bone Loss

As originally described in 1986 by Albrektsson and colleagues,[6] marginal bone loss allowed for 1.2 mm of bone loss the first year following abutment connection and 0.2 mm per year thereafter, later to be modified as 1.5 mm of bone loss in the first year followed by 0.2 mm per year thereafter.[2] This bone loss occurs in the absence of clinical symptoms, and, as is the case with peri-implant mucositis and peri-implantitis, has multiple potential contributing factors.[7]

Retrograde Peri-Implantitis

First described by McAllister and colleagues,[8] retrograde peri-implantitis is a radiographically diagnosed, periapical, lucent lesion that is symptomatic and that develops shortly after implant placement. The coronal portion of the implant appears to have a normal relationship to bone.[9,10] In some cases, a fistula may develop. It is likely related to microbiological conditions at the implant site and has been shown to be related to distance from site and time since endodontic therapy.[11]

Peri-Implant Mucositis

Peri-implant mucositis is an inflammatory process around a functioning implant characterized by bleeding on probing (BOP), with depths of 4 mm or more. There is no indication of bone loss other than that which would normally be expected with marginal bone loss and it may or may not be accompanied by suppuration. It is considered to be reversible without procedural intervention, other than perhaps scaling and root planing. Although it is generally considered to be the precursor to peri-implantitis, it is not necessarily true that it will progress to peri-implantitis.[3]

Peri-Implantitis

Similar to peri-implant mucositis, peri-implantitis is inflammatory in nature, but is considered distinct in that it is not considered to be reversible without surgical intervention and has bone loss around a functioning implant beyond that which would be expected by normal bone remodeling.[3,12] The bone loss threshold used to make that distinction lacks consensus, as reflected by the fact that prevalence can vary as much as 47% to 11%, depending on where the threshold is set (Table 1).[13]

Table 1
Diagnostic comparison of peri-implantitis versus peri-implant mucositis

	BOP ± Suppuration	Probing Depth ≥4 mm	Radiographic Bone Loss
Peri-implant mucositis	+	+	–
Peri-implantitis	+	+	+

The earlier in its progression that peri-implant disease can be identified, the better the prognosis for the implant in question, thus underscoring the importance of periodontal probing.

RISK FACTORS

A risk factor is any attribute, characteristic, or exposure of an individual that increases the likelihood of developing a disease or injury. Elucidating risk factors and the conditions predisposing to peri-implantitis gives insight into the pathophysiology of the disease and will allow for the eventual development of concepts of disease prevention and logical treatment strategies.

Numerous contributing factors for peri-implantitis have been considered.[14–19] A limited number have been selected for discussion. Nevertheless, arriving at a clear and evident cause, or causes, remains elusive.

Diabetes

Although periodontal disease is considered to be a complication of diabetes,[20,21] the relationship between diabetes and peri-implantitis remains unclear.[3]

In rodent studies, sustained hyperglycemia as a result of type 1 or type 2 diabetes mellitus will lead to deleterious changes in the periodontium, including impairment of host defense against pathogens, prolonged inflammatory response, microvascular alterations, impairment of new bone formation and repair, and impaired wound healing.[22–25] As similarly explained for the human model,[20] these changes have the potential to result in increased susceptibility of diabetics to periodontitis, which can be explained by multiple mechanisms in both models. Hyperglycemia is also known to delay wound healing, supporting the recommendation for allowing extended osseointegration periods for diabetics.[26]

Given the similarities between periodontitis and peri-implantitis[3,27–29] and the deleterious effect that diabetes has been noted to have on soft tissue, periodontal membranes, and alveolar bone, it would be reasonable that studies would demonstrate a relationship between diabetes and peri-implantitis.[30] Nevertheless, despite these similarities, systematic reviews[31–33] of studies attempting to demonstrate a possible relationship do not show a clear linkage between them; this could be due to an inadequate number of studies actually assessing glycemic control as part of the study, because chronic hyperglycemia is the underlying issue, as opposed to a diagnosis of diabetes, which can be well-controlled. Although the intricacies of a possible relationship may eventually become apparent, (ie, quality of normoglycemic control, other comorbidities), it remains to be seen if future studies and systematic reviews will reconcile this apparent lack of correlation.

Occlusal Overload

Occlusal overload is another risk factor influenced by prosthetic design; however, it is very difficult to define and quantify clinically over the lifetime of an implant. Thus, it is a very difficult risk factor to study (especially across different studies that all may have different definitions and methods of quantifying occlusal overload). However, a systematic review by Fu and colleagues[34] concluded that occlusal overloading was associated with peri-implant marginal bone loss because this type of bone loss is likely caused directly by microtrauma and because occlusal load is concentrated at the marginal bone, this bone loss is likely to occur via a different pathophysiologic process than other forms of peri-implantitis. Again, more studies with more uniform criteria for occlusal loading are necessary.

Genetic Factors

The host response to bacterial insult is extremely complex and influenced by many host genes. Pathogenic species stimulate proinflammatory cytokines, such as interleukin (IL)-1β, IL-6, and tumor necrosis factor (TNF)-α, which coordinate many aspects of the local inflammatory response.[35] TNF-α subsequently induces more adhesion molecules, proinflammatory cytokines, and chemokines as well as induces osteoclast function resulting in bone loss. Peri-implant crevicular fluid TNF-α may be an indicator for peri-implant inflammation and may precede indicators such as BOP increased probing depth (PD), providing for an earlier diagnosis.[35]

There is potential for genetic alterations of any of the above factors to influence peri-implantitis. IL-1 is a group of 11 cytokines that are involved in the regulation of immune and inflammatory responses. There is conflicting evidence regarding IL-1 gene polymorphism and its link to peri-implantitis. Several studies suggest a link between the two, for example, as shown with polymorphism of the Interleukin-1 receptor antagonist gene (IL-1RN).[14] However, a 2010 systematic review[36] found no consensus among the studies reviewed. Further studies are necessary to determine which genetic markers, if any, can be used to predict patient susceptibility to peri-implantitis.

Residual Cement

Restoration design influences several of the known peri-implantitis risk factors, including plaque control, occlusal overload, and also the likelihood of residual cement. Unfortunately, the vast majority of cements used for implant restorations are radiolucent; thus, clinicians cannot reply on radiographic confirmation of clean margins. Stock abutments that do not follow the gingival contours make interproximal cement removal difficult or impossible, and accessible margins can become esthetic issues. It is unclear whether the progression to peri-implantitis results from the roughness of the cement (which alone can cause inflammation) or from providing a suitable environment for bacterial attachment. A study by Wilson[37] evaluated 42 implants with signs of peri-implantitis and compared them to 20 other asymptomatic implants in the same patients. Using endoscopic visualization of the margins, he found that 0% of the asymptomatic implants had extruded cement, whereas 81% of the symptomatic implants had extruded cement. Of these with extruded cement, 76% had resolution of symptoms with removal of cement (either as a closed procedure with endoscopy, or rarely, requiring flap reflection to achieve complete removal); this underscores the importance of techniques to avoid cement extrusion at the time of cementation and suggests screw-retained restorations as the ideal restoration if possible.

Smoking

The numerous deleterious effects of cigarette smoking on health are well-documented[38–41] and appear in most cases of smoking-related pathoses to share a common pathway of alterations in the immune-inflammatory system.[42]

The literature is replete with reports from various disciplines documenting the negative effects of smoking on multiple organs and body systems. For example, it has been shown that osteotomies in smokers require a 42% increase in time over nonsmokers to achieve radiographic bone consolidation.[43] There is a strong association between smoking and dermatologic conditions, including skin wound healing, wrinkling, and the effects of premature aging as well as other conditions.[44] Smokers showing impaired wound healing after breast reduction surgery also have higher levels of urine cotinine both preoperatively and postoperatively than do nonsmokers.[45]

In order for any wound to heal properly, the 4 stages of healing (hemostasis, inflammation, proliferation, and remodeling) need to occur in the proper sequence and be of proper duration.[46] Although smoking has been shown to attenuate the normal inflammatory healing response by a reduction in inflammatory chemotactic responsiveness, migratory function, and oxidative bactericidal mechanisms,[47] there is also evidence that in both diabetes and periodontal disease,[48] a condition of hyperinflammation is established. These immunomodulatory effects of smoking, either pro-inflammatory or suppressive, can lead to an altered inflammatory response, including chronic inflammation, at mucosal surfaces.[49]

In recognizing the documented effects that smoking has on healing tissues, it would be reasonable to assume that cigarette smoking would have similar negative effects in the oral cavity[48] as it has with periodontal disease.[48,50–52]

Combining this information with the findings that smoking cessation mitigates against the progression and incidence of periodontitis,[53] a compelling argument can be made for the negative effects of smoking on periodontal disease. However, recent studies have suggested that smoking has been shown to be a weak predictor of periodontitis and that it may take up to 30 years or more of smoking before its impact becomes clinically significant.[54]

The attempt to delineate the relationship of smoking to peri-implantitis shows that it runs a similar course as that with periodontitis. There are ample studies to show that there is a negative effect of smoking on implants,[31,55–58] including contributing to peri-implantitis.

Nevertheless, although these studies arrive at the logical conclusion linking smoking to peri-implantitis, there are other reports that confound this assumption. A recent systematic review and meta-analysis by Sgolastra and colleagues[59] brings that association into question. This study states that while an implant-based meta-analysis reveals a higher risk of peri-implantitis in smokers compared with nonsmokers, the patient-based meta-analysis did not reveal any significant differences in risk of peri-implantitis. This finding could be due to a small number of studies fulfilling the inclusion criteria, and further studies are suggested to prove or disprove the link. Prior studies help support this conclusion.[54,60,61]

Just as with diabetes, a clear linkage of cigarette smoking to peri-implantitis is problematic both at the level of individual studies and at the level of systematic reviews and meta-analyses.

Periodontal Disease

Intuitively, the patient population with dental implants would have a higher than average history of periodontal disease, because periodontal disease is the most common reason for teeth to be extracted and subsequently replaced with implants. Systematic reviews have shown that a history of periodontitis increases the likelihood that an implant will have peri-implantitis.[3] Interestingly, these systematic reviews suggest that this does not appear to negatively influence the implant survival rate; however, several recent long-term prospective cohort studies indicate decreased implant survival when implants are placed to replace teeth lost due to periodontal lesions compared with other reasons.[19,62]

Another important consideration is how the existing periodontal disease affects the "quality" of the patient's biofilm. Healthy peri-implant biofilms consist of low total bacterial loads that are primarily gram-positive cocci (similar to natural teeth). The progression to peri-implantitis follows the same general course as the progression to periodontitis, resulting in increased total bacterial load and, specifically, increased proportions of *Aggregatibacter actinomycetemcomitans*, *Fusobacterium* species, *Prevotella intermedia*, *Porphyromonas gingivalis*, mobile organisms, and spirochetes (ie, *Treponema denticola*). Specifically, *A actinomycetemcomitans* and *P gingivalis*, which can be found in healthy peri-implant biofilms in small numbers, have been suggested to be the predominant pathogens implicated in peri-implant destruction.[63]

A major difference between implants and teeth (in a partially edentulous case) is that with implants, one is introducing a sterile object into an environment of widely variable existing microbiota, so the most important question to answer is whether the existing microbiota influences the progression to peri-implantitis. Quirynen and colleagues[64] showed that colonization of an implant occurs within 2 weeks of healing abutment placement, and that this flora was nearly identical to the adjacent teeth (same quadrant). Another indirect finding that would suggest the existing microbiota influences the likelihood of peri-implantitis is that implants in partially edentulous environments harbor more pathogenic peri-implant microflora than do their counterparts in fully edentulous environments. Also, higher plaque levels in fully edentulous sulci do not lead to impaired peri-implant conditions when compared with partially edentulous sulci.[65] Further studies are necessary to determine if the presence of specific microbiological characteristics before implant placement can predict future peri-implantitis, or whether it is a concomitant finding that peri-implant microflora closely resembles that of periodontal lesions through its own separate pathway.

Poor Plaque Control

There are many factors that can lead to poor plaque control, although the one most unique to implant restorations (compared with natural teeth) is prosthetic design. The design of the prosthesis (whether single unit or full arch) has the potential to create uncleansable situations, and this must be considered when treatment planning (often there is a compromise between esthetics and cleansability). The surgical implant position must also be in harmony with the planned prosthesis to attain planned cleansability. Prosthesis design also has the potential to preclude clinical evaluation with periodontal probing, which may delay diagnosis of peri-implant mucositis or early peri-implantitis. Depending on the "quality" of the patient's biofilm (discussed above), plaque control can potentially be more or less crucial for success in different patients.

THERAPEUTIC RATIONALE AND TREATMENT APPROACHES

In the broadest sense, the goal of treatment of peri-implant diseases should be at a minimum to restore the implant and patient to a state of acceptable health and function. Although all the variables of success have yet to be agreed on, there are logical and generally accepted quantifiable clinical parameters that can be used as monitors. These clinical parameters include reduction of periodontal PD, improvement in clinical attachment level, reduction of BOP, and radiographic bone fill.[12,66] It may or may not be possible, or even necessary, to re-establish osseointegration[67]; it may only be possible to fill the osseous defect or to simply arrest the disease. As more cases of peri-implant disease are treated by the various modalities and protocols, relapse and the need for re-treatment may become considerations as well. Also, given the large constellation of possible contributing factors, successful treatment may take on different meanings for various factors unique to the patient, the lesion, and the design of the implant. As further progress is made, the use of biomarkers[68] may go hand in hand with clinical parameters, allowing for better predictability and selection of appropriate treatment rationale.

The cumulative interceptive supportive treatment (CIST) protocol was designed to tailor treatment of peri-implant lesions as related to easily measured clinical parameters and has been generally accepted since its introduction in 2000.[69] It provides a progressive algorithm of treatment recommendations depending on the severity of the lesion. This protocol is briefly reviewed as well as alternatives to each aspect.[70] It is important to remember that these protocols are additive (ie, the success of protocol C depends on the successful implementation of protocols A + B, and so on) (**Fig 1**).

Protocol A

Protocol A (mechanical cleansing) is designed for implant restorations with PD less than 3 mm with the presence of plaque and/or calculus, with or without BOP. It calls for nonsurgical mechanical debridement of the implant surface, focusing on both plaque use of a Prophy cup and calculus by scaling. The difficulty with mechanical debridement lies in the roughened surfaces of most implants, which promote colonization and bacterial adhesion.[71] Steel curettes or ultrasonic instruments are contraindicated against the implant surface because they can alter the implant surface to promote bacterial colonization.[71] Several alternative instruments have been suggested (plastic curettes, carbon fiber–reinforced plastic curette, Prophy brush/cup,

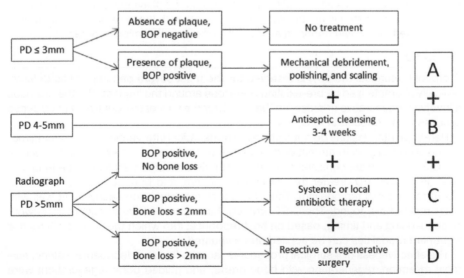

Fig. 1. CIST protocol. (*Adapted from* Algraffee H, Borumandi F, Cascarini L. Review: peri-implantitis. Br J Oral Maxillofac Surg 2012;50(8):689–94; with permission.)

sonic or ultrasonic-driven polyetheretherketone plastic tip [PEEK], air polishing with glycine powder), and a recent study found oscillating PEEK plastic tips and air polishing methods to be most effective for both acid-etched and polished implant surfaces, while the standard plastic curette was comparatively ineffective.[72]

Protocol B

Protocol B (antiseptic therapy) is used for lesions with PD from 3 to 5 mm, or greater than 5 mm without radiographically identifiable bone cratering around the implant. Although chlorhexidine is described in the CIST protocol,[69] the most effective treatment to detoxify the implant surface has not been identified.[73] Many other surface treatments aimed at eradication of the biofilm have been described[73–78]; these include EDTA, citric acid, hydrogen peroxide, local anesthetic, cetylpyridinium chloride, and tetracycline, among others. Mechanical debridement alone, as described in protocol A, is considered to be inadequate for this group of lesions as a result of the increased pocket depth, thus necessitating the effort at antisepsis. Antiseptic treatment with chlorhexidine is recommended twice per day for 3 to 4 weeks to achieve positive results, at which time the lesion is reclassified and treated according to the outlined diagnostic parameters.

Protocol C

Protocol C (antibiotic therapy) involves the addition of systemic or local antibiotics and is recommended for lesions with PD greater than 5, BOP, and an identifiable bone defect up to 2 mm loss on radiograph. As larger periodontal pockets around implant restorations are conducive to colonization with primarily anaerobic gram-negative bacteria, antibiotic therapy is focused on these microorganisms. Antibiotic treatment is typically instituted during the last week of antiseptic treatment per protocol B. Systemic antibiotic options include amoxicillin, metronidazole, clindamycin, augmentin, tetracycline, bactrim, and ciprofloxacin (or a combination of the above) with no clear preferred therapy.[79] Local antibiotic delivery methods appear to have similar effectiveness as systemically administered antibiotics as long as they remain at the site of action for at least 7 to 10 days and can have the advantage of avoiding adverse reactions associated with systemic antibiotics. Such products with these desirable characteristics include tetracycline periodontal fibers and minocycline microspheres.[70]

Protocol D

Protocol D (surgical therapy) is reserved for the most severe peri-implantitis defects, typically characterized by pre-existing bone loss around the implant. Per the protocol, it involves regenerative or resective therapy after the successful control of the disease process with protocols A to C.

Peri-implantitis lesions do not respond to nonsurgical intervention[3,80] (including mechanical nonsurgical treatment or debridement). The lesions marked for protocol D of the CIST protocol are consistent with the generally accepted definition of peri-implantitis[3] (ie, +BOP, PD greater than or equal to 4 mm, and bone loss beyond that expected for normal remodeling). Thus, the escalatory approach seems to fit well with what others have found. The CIST protocol furthermore offers a rational framework of sequencing and timing, based on host response, into which the various alternative treatment modalities can be applied and evaluated.

The effectiveness of 4 surgical procedures (access flap and debridement alone, surgical resection, regeneration with bone grafts, and guided bone regeneration) were studied in a systematic review and meta-analysis of peri-implantitis treatment option outcomes. Although the first 2 of these would not be classified into the CIST protocol

D, each of the 4 procedures yielded roughly 2 to 3 mm PD reduction based on short-term outcomes, and 2-mm increase in bone height was associated with the regenerative procedures in a systematic review.[66]

Notwithstanding the numerous case studies, clinical series, and systematic reviews showing favorable results and effectiveness with surgical approaches,[66,76,77,81–86] it should be mentioned that there are reports in which the rigors of systematic review do not allow for the identification of the most effective option.[87–89]

At the time of treatment decision, the choice of the procedure should be guided by clinical judgment, esthetic considerations, patient input, clinician experience, and treatment goals. In those instances whereby an increase in bone height has been observed, it is difficult to determine whether this is reosseointegrated bone or merely bone filling a space. However, in an animal model, reosseointegration has been shown to be possible after peri-implantitis treatment on sand-blasted, large-grit, acid-etched implant surfaces, but not smooth collars.[89] Regardless, even nonosseointegrated bone in a treated lesion could be an achievable treatment goal that would provide for more favorable maintenance, esthetics, and implant stability compared with a lack of new bone.

Lasers

Lasers exert their effects on the offending bacteria thermally, which denatures proteins and causes cellular necrosis.[71] There are many different types of lasers with unique properties and subsequently differing effects on both bacterial contamination and the implant surface itself. The CO_2 laser and the Er:YAG laser have been shown to be acceptable choices because they do not damage the implant surface, or significantly increase the body temperature of the implant. However only the Er:YAG laser appears capable of removing bacterial deposits from both smooth and rough titanium implants without damaging their surfaces.[90] Although a diode laser alone causes an unacceptable increase in implant body temperature, it can be used in conjunction with a photosensitizing substance (phenothiazine chloride dye), which fixes itself to bacteria and is then activated by a diode laser (increasing its efficacy at lower power), making it a viable option.[91]

In vitro studies indicate that several lasers have the ability to achieve 100% bacterial elimination without damaging the implant surface.[92] However, nonsurgical laser therapy has been shown to be minimally successful (decreases in clinical attachment level and pocket depths generally less than 1 mm) in a systematic review.[93,94] When used appropriately, nonsurgical laser therapy is beneficial in reducing mucosal inflammation, and to some extent, PD around implants diagnosed with peri-implantitis. However, this appears to be a transient benefit that wanes after 12 months,[93] indicating it should be used as an adjunctive therapy rather than as definitive therapy. As an adjunctive therapy, lasers may be useful in conjunction with guided bone regeneration, as they may improve clinical and radiographic findings up to 5 years after therapy.[95]

Based on current evidence, the following conclusions can be made for lasers at this point in time:

- Lasers are *not* a *substitute* for surgical therapy for advanced lesions.
- Lasers have *not* been shown to be any more effective than other methods of surface decontamination (mechanical, antiseptic, antibacterial).[96]
- Lasers may be useful as an adjunctive treatment (especially in initial reduction of peri-implant inflammation, and in conjunction with guided bone regeneration (GBR)).

Implant Removal

The notion of "repair" should encompass any efforts with an acceptable chance of restoring the patient to a state of well-being, with or without implant retention. Regardless of the degree to which it may be technically possible or predictable, treatment of peri-implantitis aimed at retaining the implant may not be the best option. Explantation should be a consideration and may be arrived at for different reasons by either the patient or the clinician.

Implant fracture is an example of a biomechanical cause of bone loss that is irreparable and that will clearly lead to worsening conditions for the patient,[97,98] including loss of integration sufficient to result in implant mobility. Without the possibility of repair, the lesion will not heal and conditions will almost definitely worsen with time. Explantation becomes the evident and clear choice in this situation.

Although the surgical technique of implant removal in most cases is not difficult,[99] the process by which the surgeon and patient arrive at a mutually acceptable approach to peri-implantitis may prove to be more challenging than in the case of implant fracture with mobility. Unless obviously mobile, attempts at implant retention are a technical option. Continued efforts in the research community will be needed to arrive at a consensus as to the best approach given the probable contributing factors and ability of the patient to respond positively. For example, the committed smoker with a history of aggressive periodontitis, diabetes, and poor oral hygiene may not be the best candidate for surgical repair of peri-implantitis. Just as important, each clinician must weigh his or her ability to meet the technical demands of the procedure. Finally, the patient will also need to make an informed and personal decision based on possible risks and benefits, financial resources, time, and intensity of effort involved in attempting to repair peri-implantitis in contrast to the option of explantation.[87]

SUMMARY

- Appropriate supportive treatment of implants is becoming increasingly important for the general dentist as the number of implants placed per year continues to increase.
- Early diagnosis of peri-implantitis is imperative, and initiating the correct treatment protocol depends on a proper diagnosis.
- Several risk factors exist for the development of peri-implantitis, which can guide patient selection and treatment planning.
- Treatment of peri-implantitis should be tailored to the severity of the lesion (as outlined by the CIST protocol), which ranges from mechanical debridement to explantation.
- Several surgical and nonsurgical treatment alternatives exist, and there is little consensus on superior treatment methods.

REFERENCES

1. Misch CE. Dental implant prosthetics. St. Louis, Missouri: Elsevier; 2015.
2. Albrektsson T, Isidor F. Consensus report: implant therapy. In: Lang NP, Karring T, editors. Proceedings of the 1st European workshop on periodontology. London: Quintessence Publishing; 1994. p. 365–9.
3. Academy report: peri-implant mucositis and peri-implantitis: a current understanding of their diagnoses and clinical implications. J Periodontol 2013;84(4): 436–43.

4. Sanz M, Chapple IL. Clinical research on peri-implant diseases: consensus report of working group 4. J Clin Periodontol 2012;39(Suppl 12):202–6.
5. Zitzmann NU, Berglundh T. Definition and prevalence of peri-implant diseases. J Clin Periodontol 2008;35(Suppl 8):286–91.
6. Albrektsson T, Zarb G, Worthington P, et al. The long-term efficacy of currently used dental implants: a review and proposed criteria of success. Int J Oral Maxillofac Implants 1986;1:11–25.
7. Valderrama P, Bornstein MM, Jones AA, et al. Effects of implant design on marginal bone changes around early loaded, chemically modified, sandblasted acid-etched-surfaced implants: a histologic analysis in dogs. J Periodontol 2011;82:1025–34.
8. McAllister BS, Masters D, Meffert RM. Treatment of implants demonstrating periapical radiolucencies. Pract Periodontics Aesthet Dent 1992;4:37–41.
9. Quirynen M, Gijbels F, Jacobs R. An infected jawbone site compromising successful osseointegration. Periodontol 2000, 2003;33:129–44.
10. Chan HL, Wang HL, Bashutski JD, et al. Retrograde peri-implantitis: a case report introducing an approach to its management. J Periodontol 2011;82:1080–8.
11. Zhou W, Han C, Li D, et al. Endodontic treatment of teeth induces retrograde peri-implantitis. Clin Oral Implants Res 2009;20:1326–32.
12. Lagervall M, Jansson LE. Treatment outcome in patients with peri-implantitis in a periodontal clinic: a retrospective study. J Periodontol 2013;84(10):1365–73.
13. Koldsland OC, Scheie AA, Aass AM. Prevalence of peri-implantitis related to severity of the disease with different degrees of bone loss. J Periodontol 2010; 81(2):231–8.
14. Laine ML, Leonhardt A, Roos-Jansåker AM, et al. IL-1RN gene polymorphism is associated with peri-implantitis. Clin Oral Implants Res 2006;17:380–5.
15. Lin GH, Chan HL, Bashutski JD, et al. The effect of flapless surgery on implant survival and marginal bone level: a systematic review and meta-analysis. J Periodontol 2014;85(5):e91–103.
16. Chaves ES, Lovell JS, Tahmasebi S. Implant-supported crown design and the risk for peri-implantitis. Clin Adv Periodontics 2014;4(2):118–26.
17. Silva ES, Feres M, Figueiredo LC, et al. Microbiological diversity of peri implantitis biofilm by Sanger sequencing. Clin Oral Implants Res 2013;25:1–8.
18. Fransson C, Wennström J, Tomasi C, et al. Extent of peri-implantitis-associated bone loss. J Clin Periodontol 2009;36:357–63.
19. Swierkot K, Lottholz P, Flores-de-Jacoby L, et al. Mucositis, peri-implantitis, implant success, and survival of implants in patients with treated generalized aggressive periodontitis: 3- to 16-year results of a prospective long-term cohort study. J Periodontol 2012;83:1213–25.
20. Iacopino AM. Periodontitis and diabetes interrelationships: role of inflammation. Ann Periodontol 2001;6:125–37.
21. Taylor GW, Borgnakke WS. Periodontal disease: associations with diabetes, glycemic control and complications. Oral Dis 2008;14(3):191–203.
22. Pontes Andersen CC, Flyvbjerg A, Buschard K, et al. Relationship between periodontitis and diabetes: lessons from rodent studies. J Periodontol 2007;78(7):1264–75.
23. Allen EM, Matthews JB, O'Halloran DJ, et al. Oxidative and inflammatory status in Type 2 diabetes patients with periodontitis. J Clin Periodontol 2011;38:894–901.
24. Katz J, Bhattacharyya I, Farkhondeh-Kish F, et al. Expression of the receptor of advanced glycation end products in gingival tissues of type 2 diabetes patients with chronic periodontal disease: a study utilizing immunohistochemistry and RT-PCR. J Clin Periodontol 2005;32:40–4.

25. Venza I, Visalli M, Cucinotta M, et al. Proinflammatory gene expression at chronic periodontitis and peri-implantitis sites in patients with or without type 2 diabetes (hyperinflammatory). J Periodontol 2010;81(1):99–108.
26. Oates TW, Huynh-Ba G, Vargas A. A critical review of diabetes, glycemic control, and dental implant therapy. Clin Oral Implants Res 2013;24(2):117–27.
27. Meffert RM. Periodontitis vs. peri-implantitis: the same disease? The same treatment? Crit Rev Oral Biol Med 1996;7(3):278–91.
28. Heitz-Mayfield LJ, Lang NP. Comparative biology of chronic and aggressive periodontitis vs. peri-implantitis. Periodontol 2000, 2010;53:167–81.
29. Mombelli A, Lang NP. The diagnosis and treatment of peri-implantitis. Periodontol 2000, 1998;17:63–76.
30. Ferreira SD, Silva GL, Cortelli JR, et al. Prevalence and risk variables for peri-implant disease in Brazilian subjects. J Clin Periodontol 2006;33:929–35.
31. Heitz-Mayfield LJ, Huynh-Ba G. History of treated periodontitis and smoking as risks for implant therapy. Int J Oral Maxillofac Implants 2009;24(Suppl):39–68.
32. Bornstein MM, Cionca N, Mombelli A. Systemic conditions and treatments as risks for implant therapy. Int J Oral Maxillofac Implants 2009;24(Suppl):12–27.
33. Mombelli A, Cionca N. Systemic diseases affecting osseointegration therapy. Clin Oral Implants Res 2006;17(Suppl 2):97–103.
34. Fu JH, Hsy YT, Wang HL. Identifying occlusal overload and how to deal with it to avoid marginal bone loss around implants. Eur J Oral Implantol 2012;5(Suppl): S91–103.
35. De Mendonca A, Santos V, Cesar-Neto J. Tumor necrosis factor-alpha levels after surgical anti-infective mechanical therapy for peri-implantitis: a 12-month follow-up. J Periodontol 2009;80(4):693–9.
36. Bormann KH, Stuhmer C, Z'Graggen M, et al. IL-1 polymorphism and peri-implantitis. A literature review. Schweiz Monatsschr Zahnmed 2010;120:510–20.
37. Wilson T. The positive relationship between excess cement and peri-implant disease: a prospective clinical endoscopic study. J Periodontol 2009;80(9):1388–92.
38. Yanbaeva DG, Dentener MA, Creutzberg EC, et al. Systemic effects of smoking. Chest 2007;131:1557–66.
39. The health consequences of smoking—50 years of progress: a report of the surgeon general. Atlanta (GA): U.S. Department of Health and Human Services, Centers for Disease Control and Prevention, National Center for Chronic Disease Prevention and Health Promotion, Office on Smoking and Health; 2014.
40. Mallampalli A, Guntupalli KK. Smoking and systemic disease. Med Clin North Am 2004;88:1431–51.
41. Sørensen LT. Wound healing and infection in surgery (the clinical impact of smoking and smoking cessation: a systematic review and meta-analysis). Arch Surg 2012;147:373.
42. Rom O, Avezov K, Aizenbud D, et al. Cigarette smoking and inflammation revisited. Respir Physiol Neurobiol 2013;187(1):5–10.
43. Krannitz KW, Fong HW, Fallat LM, et al. The effect of cigarette smoking on radiographic bone healing after elective foot surgery. J Foot Ankle Surg 2009;48: 525–7.
44. Freiman A, Bird G, Metelitsa AI, et al. Cutaneous effects of smoking. J Cutan Med Surg 2004;8:415–23.
45. Bartsch RH, Weiss G, Kästenbauer T, et al. Crucial aspects of smoking in wound healing after breast reduction surgery. J Plast Reconstr Aesthet Surg 2007;60: 1045–9.
46. Guo S, Dipietro LA. Factors affecting wound healing. J Dent Res 2010;89:219–29.

47. Sørensen LT. Wound healing and infection in surgery: the pathophysiological impact of smoking, smoking cessation, and nicotine replacement therapy: a systematic review. Ann Surg 2012;255(6):1069–79. http://dx.doi.org/10.1097/SLA.0b013e31824f632d.

48. Johannsen A, Susin C, Gustafsson A. Smoking and inflammation: evidence for a synergistic role in chronic disease. Periodontol 2000, 2014;64:111–26.

49. Kou YR, Kwong K, Lee LY. Airway inflammation and hypersensitivity induced by chronic smoking. Respir Physiol Neurobiol 2011;178:395–405.

50. Albandar JM, Streckfus CF, Adesanya MR, et al. Cigar, pipe, and cigarette smoking as risk factors for periodontal disease and tooth loss. J Periodontol 2000;71(12):1874–81.

51. Tomar SL, Asma S. Smoking-attributable periodontitis in the United States: findings from NHANES III. National Health and Nutrition Examination Survey. J Periodontol 2000;71(5):743–51.

52. Han DH, Lim S, Kim JB. The association of smoking and diabetes with periodontitis in a Korean population. J Periodontol 2012;83(11):1397–406.

53. Fiorini T, Musskopf ML, Oppermann RV, et al. Is there a positive effect of smoking cessation on periodontal health? A systematic review. J Periodontol 2014;85(1):83–91.

54. Persson RE, Kiyak AH, Wyatt CC, et al. Smoking, a weak predictor of periodontitis in older adults. J Clin Periodontol 2005;32:512–7.

55. Haas R, Haimböck W, Mailath G, et al. The relationship of smoking on peri-implant tissue: a retrospective study. J Prosthet Dent 1996;76:592–6.

56. Strietzel FP, Reichart PA, Kale A, et al. Smoking interferes with the prognosis of dental implant treatment: a systematic review and meta-analysis. J Clin Periodontol 2007;34:523–44.

57. Mombelli A, Müller N, Cionca N. The epidemiology of peri-implantitis. Clin Oral Implants Res 2012;23(Suppl 6):67–76.

58. Heitz-Mayfield LJ. Peri-implant diseases: diagnosis and risk indicators. J Clin Periodontol 2008;35:292–304.

59. Sgolastra F, Petrucci A, Severino M, et al. Smoking and the risk of peri-implantitis. A systematic review and meta-analysis. Clin Oral Implants Res 2014;1–6.

60. Renvert S, Aghazadeh A, Hallström H, et al. Factors related to peri-implantitis - a retrospective study. Clin Oral Implants Res 2014;25:522–9.

61. Koldsland OC, Scheie AA, Aass AM. The association between selected risk indicators and severity of peri-implantitis using mixed model analyses. J Clin Periodontol 2011;38:285–92.

62. Karoussis IK, Salvi GE, Heitz-Mayfield LJ, et al. Long-term implant prognosis in patients with and without a history of chronic periodontitis: a 10 year prospective cohort study of the ITI Dental Implant System. Clin Oral Implants Res 2003;14:329–39.

63. Ata-Ali J, Candel-Marti M, Flichy-Fernandez A, et al. Peri-implantitis: associated microbiota and treatment. Med Oral Patol Oral Cir Bucal 2011;16(7):e937–43.

64. Quirynen M, Vogels R, Peeters W, et al. Dynamics of subgingival colonization of 'pristine' peri-implant pockets. Clin Oral Implants Res 2006;17(1):25–37.

65. De Waal Y, Winkel E, Meijer H, et al. Differences in peri-implant microflora between fully and partially edentulous patients: a systematic review. J Periodontol 2014;85(1):68–82.

66. Chan HL, Lin GH, Suarez F, et al. Surgical management of peri-implantitis: a systematic review and meta-analysis of treatment outcomes. J Periodontol 2014;85:1027–41.

67. Renvert S, Polyzois I, Maguire R. Re-osseointegration on previously contaminated surfaces: a systematic review. Clin Oral Implants Res 2009;20(Suppl 4): 216–27.

68. Rakic M, Struillou X, Petkovic-Curcin A, et al. Estimation of bone loss biomarkers as a diagnostic tool for peri-implantitis. J Periodontol 2014;85:1566–74.

69. Lang NP, Wilson TG, Corbet EF. Biological complications with dental implants: their prevention, diagnosis and treatment. Clin Oral Implants Res 2000;11:146–55.

70. Froum S. Dental implant complications: etiology, prevention, and treatment. Chichester United Kingdom: Blackwell Publishing; 2010.

71. Mellado A, Buitrago P, Sola MF, et al. Decontamination of dental implant surface in peri-implantitis treatment: a literature review. Med Oral Patol Oral Cir Bucal 2013;18(6):e869–76.

72. Schmage P, Kahili F, Nergiz I, et al. Cleaning effectiveness of implant prophylaxis instruments. Int J Oral Maxillofac Implants 2014;29(2):331–7.

73. Suarez F, Monje A, Galindo-Moreno P, et al. Implant surface detoxification: a comprehensive review. Implant Dent 2013;22:465–73.

74. De Waal YC, Raghoebar GM, Huddleston Slater JJ, et al. Implant decontamination during surgical peri-implantitis treatment: a randomized, double-blind, placebo-controlled trial. J Clin Periodontol 2013;40:186–95.

75. Khoury F, Buchmann R. Surgical therapy of peri-implant disease: a 3-year follow-up study of cases treated with 3 different techniques of bone regeneration. J Periodontol 2001;72:1498–508.

76. Froum SJ, Froum SH, Rosen PS. Successful management of peri-implantitis with a regenerative approach: a consecutive series of 51 treated implants with 3- to 7.5-year follow-up. Int J Periodontics Restorative Dent 2012;32:11–20.

77. Schmidt EC, Papadimitriou DE, Caton JG. Surgical management of peri-implantitis: a clinical case report. Clin Adv Periodontics 2014;4(1):31–7.

78. Roccuzzo M, Bonino F, Bonino L, et al. Surgical therapy of peri-implantitis lesions by means of a bovine-derived xenograft: comparative results of a prospective study on two different implant surfaces. J Clin Periodontol 2011;38:738–45.

79. Heitz-Mayfield L, Mombelli A. The therapy of peri-implantitis: a systematic review. Int J Oral Maxillofac Implants 2014;29(Suppl):325–45.

80. Renvert S, Roos-Jansåker AM, Claffey N. Non-surgical treatment of peri-implant mucositis and peri-implantitis: a literature review. J Clin Periodontol 2008; 35(Suppl 8):305–15.

81. Roos-Jansåker AM, Lindahl C, Persson GR, et al. Long-term stability of surgical bone regenerative procedures of peri-implantitis lesions in a prospective case-control study over 3 years. J Clin Periodontol 2011;38:590–7.

82. Nguyen-Hieu T, Borghetti A, Aboudharam G. Peri-implantitis: from diagnosis to therapeutics. J Investig Clin Dent 2012;3(2):79–94.

83. Froum SJ. Regenerative treatment for a peri-implantitis-affected implant: a case report. Clin Adv Periodontics 2013;3(3):140–6.

84. Faggion CM Jr, Chambrone L, Listl S, et al. Network meta-analysis for evaluating interventions in implant dentistry: the case of peri-implantitis treatment. Clin Implant Dent Relat Res 2011;15:576–88.

85. Serino G, Turri A. Outcome of surgical treatment of peri-implantitis: results from a 2-year prospective clinical study in humans. Clin Oral Implants Res 2011;22: 1214–20.

86. Lorenzoni M, Pertl C, Keil C, et al. Treatment of peri-implant defects with guided bone regeneration: a comparative clinical study with various membranes and bone grafts. Int J Oral Maxillofac Implants 1998;13:639–46.

87. Esposito M, Grusovin MG, Worthington HV. Treatment of peri-implantitis: what interventions are effective? A Cochrane systematic review. Eur J Oral Implantol 2012;5(Suppl 1):21–41.

88. Byrne G. Effectiveness of different treatment regimens for peri-implantitis. J Am Dent Assoc 2012;143:391–2.

89. Persson LG, Berglundh T, Lindhe J. Re-osseointegration after treatment of peri-implantitis at different implant surfaces. An experimental study in the dog. Clin Oral Implants Res 2001;12:595–603.

90. Schwarz F, Nuesry E, Bieling K. Influence of an erbium, chromium-doped yttrium, scandium, gallium, and garnet (Er,Cr:YSGG) laser on the reestablishment of the biocompatibility of contaminated titanium implant surfaces. J Periodontol 2006; 77(11):1820–7.

91. Bassetti M, Schar D, Wicki B, et al. Anti-infective therapy of peri-implantitis with adjunctive local drug delivery or photodynamic therapy: 12-month outcomes of a randomized controlled clinical trial. Clin Oral Implants Res 2014;25:279–87.

92. Tosun E, Tasar F, Strauss R, et al. Comparative evaluation of antimicrobial effects of Er:YAG, diode, and CO2 lasers on titanium discs: an experimental study. J Oral Maxillofac Surg 2012;70:1064–9.

93. Kotsakis G, Konstantinidis I, Karoussis IK, et al. A systematic review and meta-analysis of the effect of various laser wavelengths in the treatment of peri-implantitis. J Periodontol 2014;85:1203 13.

94. Algraffee H, Borumandi F, Cascarini L. Review: peri-implantitis. Br J Oral Maxillofac Surg 2012;50:689–94.

95. Geisinger M, Holmes C, Vassilopoulos P. Is laser disinfection an effective adjunctive treatment to bone augmentation for peri-implantitis? A review of current evidence. Clin Adv Periodontics 2013;4:274–9.

96. Mailoa J, Lin G, Chan G, et al. Clinical outcomes of using lasers for peri-implantitis surface detoxification: a systematic review and meta-analysis. J Periodontol 2014; 85:1194–202.

97. Al Quran FA, Rashan BA, Al-Dwairi ZN. Management of dental implant fractures. A case history. J Oral Implantol 2009;35:210 4.

98. Gealh WC, Mazzo V, Barbi F, et al. Osseointegrated implant fracture: causes and treatment. J Oral Implantol 2011;37:499–503.

99. Muroff FI. Removal and replacement of a fractured dental implant: case report. Implant Dent 2003;12:206–10.

Immediate Placement and Immediate Loading
Surgical Technique and Clinical Pearls

James Parelli, DMD, MD, MS.Ed[a], Shelly Abramowicz, DMD, MPH[b],*

KEYWORDS

• Immediate implants • Provisionalization • Abutment

KEY POINTS

• Immediate placement and immediate loading of dental implants is a safe and successful option for replacement of teeth in newly edentulous areas.
• There are specific conditions in which immediate placement and immediate loading are not recommended, including bony wall defects, poor bone quality, and acute infection.
• There are multiple techniques that practitioners can choose from when deciding to place immediate implants with immediate loading, all of which can provide more convenience for the patient and practitioner.
• Immediate implants can be performed for single-unit restorations in partial edentulism, or for fixed prostheses in complete edentulism.

Dental implants are the preferable method of rehabilitation of partially or completely edentulous patients.[1,2] Traditionally, implant placement follows a nonloading period of 3 to 6 months for osseointegration.[3,4] However, in recent years, the viability of immediate implant loading has been researched in an attempt to shorten the waiting period for osseointegration.

Immediate loading is defined as a restoration placed on the endosseous implant structure within 72 hours of placement.[5] Multiple prospective studies and systematic reviews have shown that immediately loaded implants successfully integrate at least 95% of the time.[6–8] This integration depends on several factors: surgical technique, primary stability of the implant, quality and quantity of available bone, minimal postoperative occlusal loading, and patient selection. Patients with comorbidities, such as uncontrolled diabetes, osteoporosis, heavy smoking, immunocompromise, and malnutrition, may experience delayed healing or poorer outcomes.[9,10]

The author has nothing to disclose.
[a] Department of Surgery, Division of Oral and Maxillofacial Surgery, Emory University, 1365 Clifton Road, Building B, Suite 2300, Atlanta, GA 30322, USA; [b] Department of Surgery, Division of Oral and Maxillofacial Surgery, Emory University, 1365 Clifton Road, Building B, Suite 2300, Atlanta, GA 30322, USA
* Corresponding author.
E-mail address: sabram5@emory.edu

Dent Clin N Am 59 (2015) 345–355
http://dx.doi.org/10.1016/j.cden.2014.10.002
0011-8532/15/$ – see front matter © 2015 Elsevier Inc. All rights reserved.

Immediate-loading implants are generally versatile and can be used in various locations and conditions, such as a healed edentulous area, a fresh extraction socket, posterior maxilla in the area of the maxillary sinus, and a narrow-ridge anterior mandible. To maximize the potential for success, multiple factors must be must be considered when treatment planning. In an ideal situation, an implant would be placed into a well-healed ridge with sufficient bone quantity and quality, in a healthy, nonsmoking patient. This, unfortunately, is not always the case, and preoperative planning is paramount for optimizing the outcome. There are specific indications (**Box 1**) and contraindications (**Box 2**) for immediate implant placement.

IMMEDIATE PLACEMENT OF IMPLANTS INTO EXTRACTION SITES

The optimal treatment consists of tooth extraction, immediate implant placement, and immediate loading. This is ideal because it eliminates the need for a period of edentulism and reduces the steps required to reach the final result. In addition, placement of an immediate implant allows for preservation of associated hard and soft tissues and minimizes ridge resorption.[11,12] Typically, resorption is more pronounced on the buccal aspect than the lingual/palatal aspects, resulting in a bony crest that is no longer on the same level of adjacent teeth. This complicates subsequent implant placement and restoration and may lead to future bone grafts.[13]

There are bone preservation and augmentation techniques associated with immediate implant placement: bone grafts using autogenous bone,[14] bone substitutes,[15–18] or platelet concentrates,[19] and guided bone regeneration with membrane placement.[20–23] There are several factors that influence postsurgical hard and soft tissue remodeling, such as initial reason for extraction (eg, periodontal disease, endoperio lesion, root fracture), position of implant within the socket,[24] and thickness of alveolar bone on the facial aspect of the socket.[25–28]

The timing of placement of implants in extraction sockets is the basis for the current classification system (**Table 1**).[13] From a patient convenience perspective, type I immediate implant placement and loading is most desirable. However, studies show that single implants placed into extraction sockets and loaded immediately have higher failure rates than those placed into healed extraction sites, particularly in the maxilla.[29,30] Nevertheless, success rates often still exceed 95%.[13]

SURGICAL TECHNIQUE

Implant placement cannot take place in a sterile environment, but is considered a clean contaminated procedure. When extracting teeth with the intention of immediately placing an implant, it is important to extract the tooth as atraumatically as feasible. The goals of this method are to retain as much bone and adjacent soft tissue as possible. If the tooth is extracted because of an infection, thorough curettage and

---

Box 1
Indications for immediate implant placement

1. Traumatic avulsion, reimplantation not possible

2. Nonrestorability of tooth because of caries

3. Tooth malposition

4. Failed endodontic therapy

5. External or internal root resorption

Box 2
Contraindications for immediate implant placement
1. Bony wall defects (that preclude primary stability)
2. Poor quality of bone
3. Acute infection or periodontitis
4. Aesthetic areas that require hard/soft tissue grafting before implantation
5. Inadequate root trajectory

irrigation of the socket with normal saline should be performed before implant placement. Perioperative and postoperative antibiotics are recommended, although more quality studies are needed for definitive guidelines.[11,31]

Following an extraction, implant positioning does not depend on the orientation of the root socket, but rather on the axial position that allows maximum primary stability and restorability.[11] The remaining periodontal ligament should be removed with a curette, periotome, or round bur. A round bur should be used to score the appropriate wall of the socket where the osteotomy will commence. It is important to ensure copious irrigation while performing the osteotomy to prevent bony tissue damage. Careful attention should be given to angulation of each drill as they are advanced; perforation of the thin buccal wall could compromise the success of the implant. Once the series of drills create the appropriate osteotomies for the implant, the implant should be seated with a torque of approximately 30 Ncm. However, the torque value depends on the specific implant's design, surface treatment, and screw thread geometry.[12] Most implants placed in extraction sites have gaps between the implant and the bone because of the difference in size and shape between the implant body and the extraction socket. In those situations, a concurrent bone graft can be used (eg, autogenous, bovine, porous cancellous particulate allograft).

Whatever restorative option is chosen for the single immediate implant, the "immediate-loading" aspect should be nonfunctional. The restored implant should be out of occlusion so as to not sustain the force of the opposing dentition for 2 to 3 months. This allows for maximum potential for successful osseointegration.[32,33]

PROVISIONALIZATION
Partial Edentulism

There are multiple options for provisionalization of immediate-loading single implants. Typically, a laboratory fabricates the abutment and provisional restoration preoperatively. This reduces the chairside time of the restorative dentist. Preoperative impressions are taken and models fabricated. If the site is already edentulous, an implant

Table 1	
Classification of immediate implant placement	
Type	**Description**
I	Implants placed into sockets immediately after extraction
II	Implants placed after soft tissue coverage of the socket (4–8 wk after extraction)
III	Implants placed in a socket with clinical or radiographic bone fill (12–16 after extraction)
IV	Implants placed in a completely healed edentulous site (>16 wk after extraction)

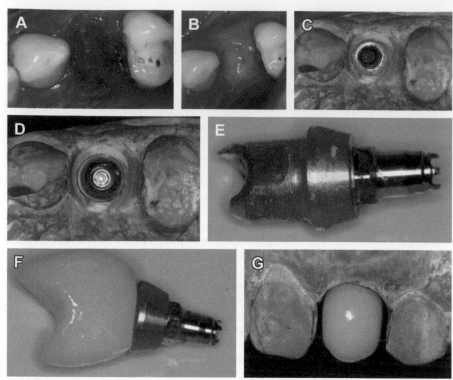

Fig. 1. (*A*) Tooth has been extracted and the site grafted with human mineralized bone. A membrane can be used to hold the graft in position. (*B*) Four months after the tooth extraction, the ridge has excellent width. (*C*) Models are made, and an implant analog is position with the labial surface of the implant approximately 2 mm palatal to a line drawn from the labial surface of the adjacent teeth. The internal flat surface of the hex is placed directly labial. (*D*) Abutment chosen has a gingival collar height of approximately 2 to 3 mm. The abutment is prepared vertically with minimal change in the wall parallelism to ensure retention of the provisional crown. (*E*) Modified fixed abutment. Note that the flat surface has not been removed so as to improve provisional crown retention. The parallel walls also provide retention of the provisional crown. (*F*) Provisional crown on the abutment. (*G*) Provisional crown on the model. Note the 0.5-mm gap between adjacent contact points to allow surgical flexibility and passive seating of the crown. The gingival margin has been prepared to match the gingival margin of the tooth before extraction. (*H*) After administration of a local anesthetic, a tissue punch is used in the exact location where the crown will emerge. (*I*) After the tissue punch has been used, a small incision is made across the crest and around the adjacent teeth within the gingival sulcus. Elevation of the periosteum is limited to the superior aspect of the crest. Vertical incisions are not recommended. (*J*) Circle of tissue created with the tissue punch is removed. (*K*) A round bur is used to create the entry hole for the first drill. The round bur sets the position of the implant between the teeth, in the middle of the crest, and in the appropriate buccal-palatal direction. (*L*) Implant is properly positioned according to the prescription from the model. Note that the internal flat surface of the hex is directly labial. Also note the excellent bone contour over the area. (*M*) Abutment previously prepared in the laboratory is passively seated and secured with a screw. After cotton has been placed, the provisional crown is tried. (*N*) Provisional crown is placed in position, and after occlusal clearance has been confirmed, it is cemented in position with temporary cement. Vertical mattress sutures are used to place the gingival margin back in the correct position. (*From* Block MS. Color atlas of dental implant surgery. 3rd edition. Maryland Heights (MO): Saunders, an imprint of Elsevier; 2011. Figure 7.1, p. 310–2; with permission.)

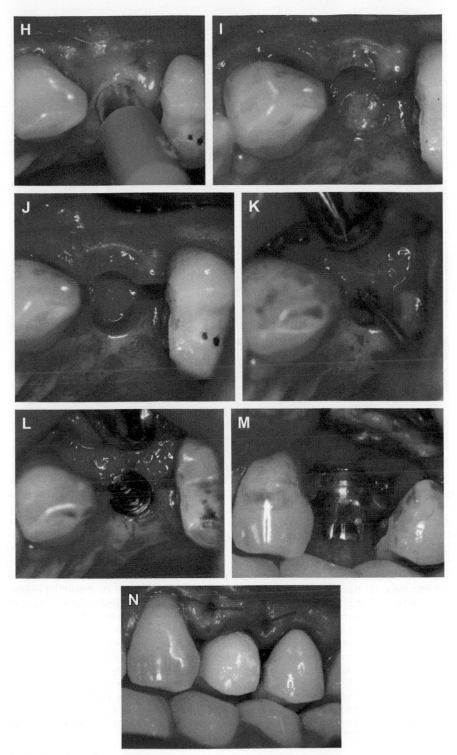

Fig. 1. (*continued*).

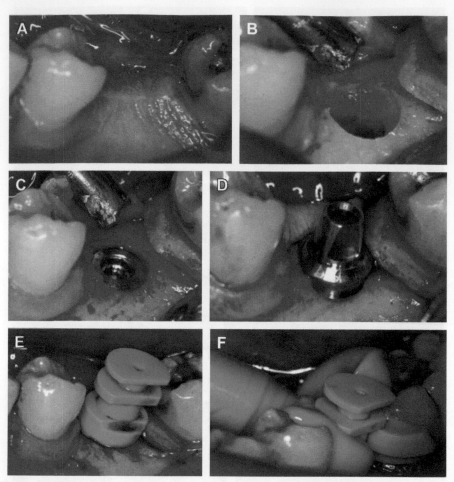

Fig. 2. (*A*) Treatment plan for this patient calls for the placement of one implant in the first molar location with immediate placement of a final, "nonprepable" abutment. Before surgery, the gingival collar height is chosen to match the 2-mm gingival thickness; the interocclusal space allowed an abutment 5 mm tall. (*B*) Implant site is prepared for an expanded platform type of implant. (*C*) Implant is placed level with the crestal bone. A radiofrequency index of 75 indicates excellent implant stability. (*D*) Abutment is placed and secured with a gold screw. The margins of the abutment are predetermined, which allows the transfer to snap into place. (*E*) Transfer coping is snapped over the margins of the abutment. (*F*) Impression is taken by first placing the less viscous material around the transfer coping (Aquasil; Dentsply/Caulk, Milford, Delaware). (*G*) Rim of impression material is placed over the putty, which has been mixed and placed in an impression tray. (*H*) After removal of the impression from the mouth, a protection cap is placed over the abutment to prevent trauma to the patient's tongue. (*I*) Impression with the transfer copings in place. This patient had bilateral implants placed. (*J*) Abutment analog snapped into the transfer coping in the impression. (*K*) Impression with the analog in place is poured in the laboratory. (*L*) Provisional crown can be made using a hollowed denture tooth or a hollow-shell crown. (*M*) Provisional restoration out of occlusion is positioned within days of implant placement. (*From* Block MS. Color atlas of dental implant surgery. 3rd edition. Maryland Heights (MO): Saunders, an imprint of Elsevier; 2011. Figure 7.4, p. 321–3; with permission.)

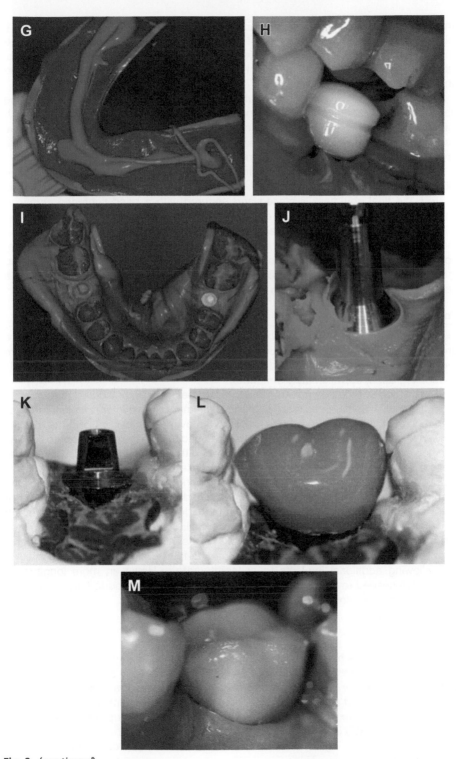

Fig. 2. (*continued*).

analog is placed into the model. The abutment is then prepared, and the laboratory fabricates the provisional restoration. If a tooth is present at the area to receive the implant, the tooth on the model is removed, the implant analog placed, and provisional fabricated. Following implant placement, the abutment and provisional can be placed and adjusted chairside, respecting the concept of nonfunctional loading (**Fig. 1**).

Another option is to prepare the abutment and provisional chairside on the same day as implant placement. After the implant is seated, the abutment is placed with minimal adjustments by the surgeon or restorative dentist. A hollow shell can be used for fabrication of the provisional restoration chairside. This reduces preoperative preparation and laboratory costs, but increases time at chairside.

A third option involves implant and final abutment placement by the surgeon. The laboratory or restorative dentist then fabricates the provisional. After the implant is seated, the final abutment is placed and secured with a hand-tightened screw. A snap-on transfer coping is placed over the abutment, and a closed-tray impression is taken using less viscous impression material around the transfer coping, and more viscous impression material in the tray. The impression then has the transfer coping imbedded in the implant location. An abutment analog is then placed into the transfer coping, and sent to the laboratory or restorative dentist. In the mouth, a cap is placed over the abutment to prevent trauma to the tongue (**Fig. 2**).[33]

Complete Edentulism

In the completely edentulous patient, nonfunctional loading is difficult because there are no natural teeth to bear the occlusal load. Instead, it is recommended to splint the implants to distribute the load. The patient should adhere to a soft diet until osseointegration, approximately 3 months.[11]

Rehabilitation of the edentulous mandible has been well-studied and renders predictable results. Some authors recommend placement of two interforaminal mandibular implants followed by immediate loading with overdentures.[12,34–36] In the maxilla, however, immediate rehabilitation is challenging because of the specific anatomy. The location of the maxillary sinus and nasal cavity and the fact that the maxilla has thinner cortical bone and less dense trabecular bone make achieving primary stability more arduous. To increase success, the surgeon may choose to place additional implants than may be needed; the surgeon and restorative dentist can then plan to load some while allowing the other implants to remain unloaded and thereby osseointegrate. If any of the immediately loaded implants were to fail, the remaining unloaded implants will be viable because they were given a less stressful environment for osseointegration. Good results have been reported by loading four to six implants in the maxilla, and allowing additional implants to osseointegrate.[11] However, more longitudinal studies are needed to assess immediately loaded, implant-supported maxillary prostheses in the edentulous patient.[35,36]

SUMMARY

Dental implants have had tremendous improvement since their initial introduction into clinical practice. With ongoing advances in implant technology and materials, better data emerge to allow shorter time between placement and restoration. This allows the restorative dentist and surgeon to provide improved treatment options to patients. Most evidence that exists supports the practice of immediately placed (after extraction) and immediately loaded implants. Additional high-quality studies are still needed to develop specific guidelines for a standardized approach to immediate rehabilitation.

REFERENCES

1. Adell R, Lekholm U, Rockler B, et al. A 15-year study of osseointegrated implants in the treatment of the edentulous jaw. J Int Oral Surg 1981;10:387–416.
2. Kammeyer G, Proussaefs P, Lozada J. Conversion of a complete denture to a provisional implant-supported, screw-retained fixed prosthesis for immediate loading of a completely edentulous arch. J Prosthet Dent 2002;87:473–6.
3. Branemark PI, Hansson BO, Adell R, et al. Osseointegrated implants in the treatment of the edentulous jaw. Experience from a 10-year period. Scand J Plast Reconstr Surg 1977;16:1–132.
4. Branemark PI. Osseointegration and its experimental background. J Prosthet Dent 1983;50:399–410.
5. Nkenke E, Fenner M. Indications for immediate loading of implants and implant success. Clin Oral Implants Res 2006;17(Suppl 2):19–34.
6. Strub JR, Jurdzik BA, Tuna T. Prognosis of immediately loaded implants and their restorations: a systematic literature review. J Oral Rehabil 2012;39:704–17.
7. Banemark PI, Engstrand P, Ohrnell LO, et al. Branemark Novum: a new treatment concept for rehabilitation of the edentulous mandible. Preliminary results from a prospective clinical follow-up study. Clin Implant Dent Relat Res 1999;1:2–16.
8. Testori T, Meltzer A, Del Fabbro M, et al. Immediate occlusal loading of Osseotite implants in the lower edentulous jaw. A multicenter prospective study. Clin Oral Implants Res 2004;15:278 84.
9. Clarizio LF. Immediate implant loading. In: Fonseca RJ, Barber HD, Matheson JD, editors. Oral and maxillofacial surgery. St. Louis (MO): Saunders Elsevier; 2009. p. 511–24 Chapter 31.
10. Goiato MC, Bannwart LC, Pesqueira AA, et al. Immediate loading of overdentures: systematic review. Oral Maxillofac Surg 2013;18(3):259–64.
11. Botticelli D, Berglundh T, Lindhe J. Hard-tissue alterations following immediate implant placement in extraction sites. J Clin Periodontol 2004;31:820–8.
12. Caneva M, Salata LA, De Souza SS, et al. Influence of implant positioning in extraction sockets on osseointegration: hisomorphometric analyses in dogs. Clin Oral Implants Res 2010;21:43–9.
13. Del Fabbro M, Ceresoli V, Taschieri S, et al. Immediate loading of postextraction Implants in the esthetic area: systematic review of the literature. Clin Implant Dent Relat Res 2013. [Epub ahead of print].
14. Becker W, Becker BE, Polizzi G, et al. Autogenous bone grafting of defects adjacent to implants placed into immediate extraction sockets in patients: a prospective study. Int J Oral Maxillofac Implants 1994;9:389–96.
15. Artzi Z, Tal H, Dayan D. Porous bovine bone mineral in healing of human extraction sockets. Part 1: histomorphometric evaluations at 9 months. J Periodontal 2000;71:1015–23.
16. Artzi Z, Tal H, Dayan D. Porous bovine bone mineral in healing of human extraction sockets: Part 2. Histochemical observations at 9 months. J Periodontol 2001; 72:152–9.
17. Lasella JM, Greenwell H, Miller RL, et al. Ridge preservation with freeze-dried bone allograft and a collagen membrane compared to extraction alone for implant site development: a clinical and histologic study in humans. J Periodontol 2003;74:990–9.
18. Barone A, Aldini NN, Fini M, et al. Xenograft versus extraction alone for ridge preservation after tooth removal: a clinical and histomorphometric study. J Periodontol 2008;79:1370–7.

19. Rutkowski JL, Johnson DA, Radio NM, et al. Platelet rich plasma to facilitate wound healing following tooth extraction. J Oral Implantol 2010;36:11–23.

20. Lekovic V, Kenney EB, Weinlaender M, et al. A bone regenerative approach to alveolar ridge maintenance following tooth extraction. Report of 10 cases. J Periodontol 1997;68:563–70.

21. Lekovic V, Camargo PM, Klokkevold PR, et al. Preservation of alveolar bone in extraction sockets using bioabsorbable membranes. J Periodontol 1998;69: 1044–9.

22. Lang NP, Lui P, Lau KY, et al. A systematic review on survival and success rates of implants placed immediately into fresh extraction sockets after at least 1 year. Clin Oral Implants Res 2012;23(Suppl 5):39–66.

23. Nowzari H, Molayem S, Chiu CH, et al. Cone beam computed tomographic measurement of maxillary central incisors to determine prevalence of facial alveolar bone width ≥ 2mm. Clin Implant Dent Relat Res 2010. http://dx.doi.org/10.1111/j.1708–8208.2010.00287.x.

24. Braut V, Bornstein MM, Belser U, et al. Thickness of the anterior maxillary facial bone wall: a retrospective radiographic study using cone beam computed tomography. Int J Periodontics Restorative Dent 2011;31:125–31.

25. Hammerle CH, Chen ST, Wilson TG Jr. Consensus statements and recommended clinical procedures regarding the placement of implants in extraction sockets. Int J Oral Maxillofac Implants 2004;19(Suppl):26–8.

26. Chen ST, Beagle J, Jensen SS, et al. Consensus statements and recommended clinical procedures regarding surgical techniques. Int J Oral Maxillofac Implants 2009;24(Suppl):272–8.

27. Atieh MA, Payne AGT, Duncan WJ, et al. Immediate restoration/loading of immediately placed single implants: is it an effective bimodal approach? Clin Oral Implants Res 2009;20:645–59.

28. Testori T, Zuffetti F, Caelli M, et al. Immediate vs conventional loading of post-extraction implants in the edentulous jaws. Clin Implant Dent Relat Res 2013. http://dx.doi.org/10.111/cid.12055.

29. Chrcanovic BR, Martins MD, Wennerberg A. Immediate placement of implants into infected sites: a systematic review. Clin Implant Dent Relat Res 2013. http://dx.doi.org/10.1111/cid.12098.

30. Kim SJ, Ribeiro ALV, Atlas AM, et al. Resonance frequency analysis as a predictor of early implant failure in the partially edentulous posterior maxilla following immediate nonfunctional loading or delayed loading with single unit restorations. Clin Oral Implants Res 2013. http://dx.doi.org/10.1111/clr.12310.

31. Block MS. Immediate provisionalization of implant restorations. Color atlas of dental implant surgery. 3rd edition. St. Louis (MO): Saunders Elsevier; 2011. p. 308–55 Chapter 7.

32. Tawse-Smith A, Payne AG, Kumara R, et al. Early loading of unsplinted implants supporting mandibular overdentures using a one-stage operative procedure with two different implant systems: a 2-year report. Clin Implant Dent Relat Res 2002; 4:33–42.

33. Turkyilmax I, Tozum TF, Tumer C, et al. A 2-year clinical report of patients treated with two loading protocols for mandibular overdentures: early versus conventional loading. J Periodontol 2006;77(12):1998–2004.

34. Buttel AE, Gratwohl DA, Sendi P, et al. Immediate loading of two unsplinted mandibular implants in edentulous patients with an implant-retained overdenture: an observational study over two years. Schweiz Montasschr Zahnmed 2012; 122(5):392–7.

35. Glauser R, Ree A, Lundgren A, et al. Immediate occlusal loading of Branemark implants applied in various jawbone regions: a prospective, 1-year clinical study. Clin Implant Dent Relat Res 2001;3:204–13.
36. Gallucci GO, Morton D, Weber HP. Loading protocols for dental implants in edentulous patients. Int J Oral Maxillofac Implants 2009;24(Suppl):132–46.

Implant-related Nerve Injuries

Mark J. Steinberg, DDS, MD[a,b], Patrick D. Kelly, DDS[c],*

KEYWORDS

- Dental implants • Nerve injuries • Neurosensory disturbance • Management
- Atrophic mandible • Seddon • Sunderland

KEY POINTS

- Implant-related nerve injuries are typically permanent compared with other dentoalveolar procedural causes, which are more likely to be transient.
- Many implant-related nerve injuries are caused by inadequate planning and can be avoided with appropriate imaging and preprocedural assessment.
- Techniques to avoid nerve injuries include using local anesthetic infiltration rather than regional blocks, implementing short implants to maintain appropriate safety zones from neurovascular structures, applying bone augmentation techniques to increase available bone, cantilevering hybrid restorations to avoid placing implants in atrophic posterior mandibles, and conducting a nerve lateralization procedure as a final option.
- A suspected nerve injury or a patient presenting with numbness following an implant procedure should be managed in a systematic manner to allow timely referral when appropriate.

INTRODUCTION

Nerve injuries in the maxillofacial region may happen as a result of trauma, neoplasms, infections, or secondary to a surgical procedure. Studies investigating the incidence of nerve injury have many inconsistencies in classifying nerve impairment, rely on varying sample sizes, use differing methods for evaluation, or are retrospective in nature. Because of the limitations of such investigations there is a large range in the rates of injury reported from study to study.[1] To complicate the issue further, the data are usually stratified, separating transient impairment from permanent loss of function, and only occasionally is the presence or absence of painful neuralgias or dysesthesia included.

Disclosure: The authors have nothing to disclose.
[a] Division of Oral and Maxillofacial Surgery, Loyola University Stritch School of Medicine, 2160 South First Avenue, Maywood, IL 60153, USA; [b] Private Practice, Northbrook, 1240 Meadow Rd, IL 60062, USA; [c] Division of Oral and Maxillofacial Surgery, Loyola University Stritch School of Medicine, Loyola University Medical Center, 2160 South First Avenue, Maguire Building #105, Room 1814, Maywood, IL 60153, USA
* Corresponding author.
E-mail address: patrkelly@lumc.edu

Dent Clin N Am 59 (2015) 357–373
http://dx.doi.org/10.1016/j.cden.2014.10.003
0011-8532/15/$ – see front matter © 2015 Elsevier Inc. All rights reserved.

dental.theclinics.com

The studies of the incidence of trigeminal nerve injuries related to dentoalveolar surgery go back decades.[2] Nonsurgical procedures such as endodontic treatment or local anesthesia administration have also been implicated.[3,4] From the literature, the incidence of inferior alveolar nerve (IAN) injury following removal of third molars has been reported to be 0.26% to 8.4%,[1] of which 0.81% to 5.7%[5] are transient and 0.7%[6] permanent. Lingual nerve (LN) sensory disturbance is typically reported between 0.1% and 8%[1] with transient injury as high as 23%.[7] A recent study showed permanent damage in more than one-third of injured trigeminal nerve injuries.[1]

The convention of placing osseointegrated implants for tooth replacement in the United States started in the early 1980s and became increasingly routine in the 1990s.[8] The first prospective studies of the rate of nerve injury related to implant placement were conducted in the early 1990s. As the frequency of placing osseointegrated implants increased, more investigations of nerve injury were undertaken.[9] Similar to the literature concerning nerve injuries secondary to third molar surgery, these studies show great variability in the stated incidence. Published studies of the rate of nerve injury related to implant placement show a range of incidence from 0% to 13%.[10] One outlier article places an incidence rate at 44%.[11]

Unlike nerve injuries as a result of most oral surgical procedures, which tend to be mostly transient, implant-related nerve injuries are typically permanent. Libersa and colleagues[12] investigated transient versus permanent injuries sustained during various procedures, with a notable 75% incidence of implant-related nerve injuries being permanent (**Fig. 1**). The reason for the higher percentage of permanent injury is explained later in the article.

CLASSIFICATION OF NERVE INJURIES

It is important to be familiar with the various classifications for nerve injuries, and therefore to understand the severity and expected clinical course. The 2 most widely used descriptions of nerve injuries are by Seddon and Sunderland (**Fig. 2**). They classify based on the level of disruption of anatomic structures. Seddon broadly classifies by severity using descriptors that include neuropraxia, axonotmesis, and neurotmesis.[13] Sunderland focuses on the fascicular construct of nerves and the

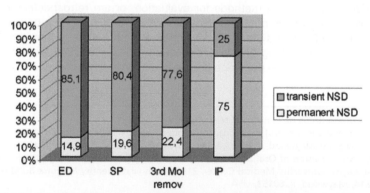

Fig. 1. Distribution (%) of the transient and permanent neurosensory disturbances (NSD) related to the various procedures. ED, endodontic procedures; IP, implant placement; SP, surgical procedures other than third molar removal (3rd Mol remov). (*From* Libersa P, Savignat M, Tonnel A. Neurosensory disturbances of the inferior alveolar nerve: a retrospective study of complaints in a 10-year period. J Oral Maxillofac Surg 2007;65(8):1487; with permission.)

Nerve Injury in Compression Neuropathy

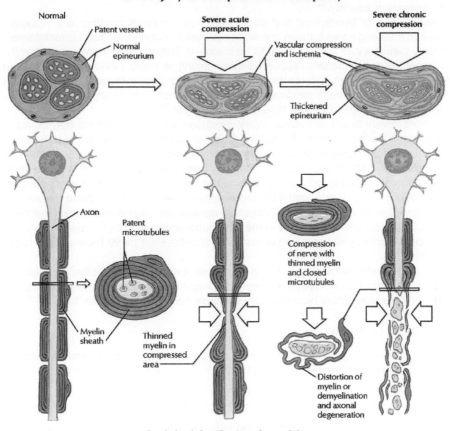

Normal

Patent vessels

Normal epineurium

Severe acute compression

Vascular compression and ischemia

Severe chronic compression

Thickened epineurium

Axon

Patent microtubules

Compression of nerve with thinned myelin and closed microtubules

Myelin sheath

Thinned myelin in compressed area

Distortion of myelin or demyelination and axonal degeneration

Sunderland classification of nerve injury

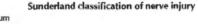

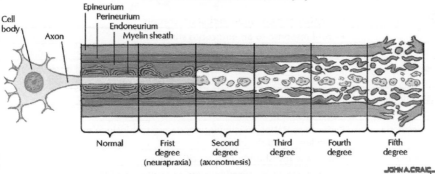

Cell body

Axon

Epineurium
Perineurium
Endoneurium
Myelin sheath

| Normal | First degree (neurapraxia) | Second degree (axonotmesis) | Third degree | Fourth degree | Fifth degree |

Classification of nerve injury by degree of involvement of various neural layers

JOHN A.CRAIG—AD

Fig. 2. The destruction of the neural layers as severity progresses through the Seddon and Sunderland classifications. (Netter illustration from www.netterimages.com. © Elsevier Inc. All rights reserved.)

remaining integrity following the injury. He expands on Seddon through 5 categories with increasing severity.[14]

Neuropraxia, or Sunderland first-degree injury, is an insult resulting in conduction blockade following nerve traction or mild compression. Axonal continuity is maintained. Sensory disturbances are expected to be transient, lasting a few months or more.[14]

Axonotmesis (Sunderland second-degree injury) is more severe, with wallerian degeneration occurring distal to the site of a crush injury. Axon regeneration can occur because the endoneurium remains undisrupted. Complete recovery occurs normally within several months, but may take 1 year or longer.[14]

A more severe crush or traction injury produces a Sunderland third-degree injury that disrupts the fascicular endoneurium. Complete axonal regeneration is hampered, and a form of permanent sensory disturbance is expected.[14]

Sunderland fourth-degree injury additionally disrupts the perineurium with the likelihood of fibrosis, scarring, or neuroma formation further impeding regeneration efforts.[14]

Neurotmesis and Sunderland fifth-degree injuries result from complete transection of the peripheral nerve structure, including epineurium, perineurium, and endoneurium. Complete anesthesia occurs in the distribution innervated by the specified nerve. Neuropathic pain syndromes can occur, with spontaneous nerve regeneration being unlikely.[13,14]

The patient returns following a nerve injury with a myriad of subjective descriptions for hypoesthesia, paresthesia, anesthesia, and dysesthesia. A list of these descriptive terms and the associated neurosensory disturbance is given in **Table 1**.[15]

MECHANISM OF INJURY

The mechanism of injury occurring secondary to most other dentoalveolar procedures is usually nerve compression or stretching; a neuropraxia-type injury (**Fig. 3**). These

Table 1
Definition of neurosensory disturbances and verbal descriptions commonly associated with pain typology

Pain Term	Definition and Common Verbal Descriptors
Allodynia	Painful response to an innocuous stimulus
Analgesia	Absence of pain to a noxious stimulus
Dysesthesia	Unpleasant abnormal sensation (spontaneous or evoked); descriptors include tender, pricking, stinging, burning, electric, cold
Hyperalgesia	Increased painful response to a noxious stimulus
Hyperpathia	Explosive abnormal pain that outlasts a noxious stimulus
Hypoesthesia	Reduced sensation to stimulation; descriptors include numb, rubbery, swollen, wooden
Neuralgia	Pain in the distribution of a specific nerve
Neuropathic pain	Spontaneous pain caused by a lesion or disease of the somatosensory nervous system. Involves sharp paroxysmal pain not associated with painful stimuli; descriptors include throbbing, electric shock, burning, excruciating, wrenching
Paresthesia	Abnormal sensation (spontaneous or evoked) that is not unpleasant; descriptors include tingling, tickling, itching, crawling

From Marchiori EC, Barber JS, Williams WB, et al. Neuropathic pain after mandibular sagittal split ramus osteotomy of the mandible: prevalence, risk factors, and clinical course. J Oral Maxillofac Surg 2013;71:2115–22; with permission.

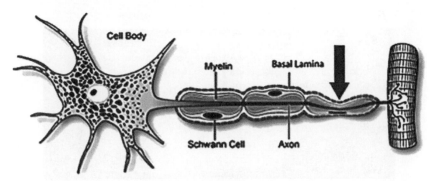

Fig. 3. The arrow indicates the site of compression from a neuropraxia-type injury. The epineurium, perineurium, endoneurium, myelin sheath, and axon remain intact. This type of injury has the potential to undergo spontaneous nerve regeneration and recovery of function. (*Adapted from* Steed M. Peripheral nerve response to injury. Atlas Oral Maxillofac Surg Clin North Am 2011;19(1):1–13; with permission.)

types of injuries have the potential to undergo nerve regeneration and recover function. The chances are higher that an implant-related injury will be permanent because the mechanism of injury usually involves the nerve being cut or severely damaged by the drill during preparation; partial or complete transections (axonotmesis or neurotmesis). Severe compression of the neurovascular bundle caused by implants compressing the bony housing of the nerve canal may cause an injury consistent with axonostenosis. In addition to the direct pressure on the nerve, the resulting stenosis of the canal may cause further ischemic injury. This injury results in demyelination of the nerve, causing impairment of nerve conduction and possibly painful neuropathic symptoms.

Implant-related nerve injuries can be from drilling the osteotomy, placement of the implant, or both. If the site is not overprepared vertically, then it is unlikely that the implant will enter the nerve canal and directly injure the neurovascular bundle[16]; this is true for normal to dense bone. In situations in which the bone quality is poor, implants may be placed apical to the prepared osteotomy and directly compress or injure the nerve.

In patients with neurosensory impairment, postoperative radiographs do not always show the implant to be near or in contact with the nerve canal. The osteotomy site may have been unknowingly overprepared; however, if the clinician places the appropriate-length implant based on preoperative imaging, a false impression results. A case demonstration of this scenario is shown in **Fig. 4**.

In such situations in which the nerve has been transected by the drill, the injury has occurred before the placement of the implant. Backing out or removing the implant based on the presence of postoperative numbness does not serve any purpose. The nerve could be surgically repaired while keeping the implant in place (**Fig. 5**).

Plain radiographs or computed tomography (CT) scans are useful in situations in which postoperative neurosensory disturbances are present following implant placement. If the imaging shows that the canal is intact or the superior border of the canal has been minimally violated, backing out or removing the implant is advised to decompress the neurovascular bundle. In addition, surgical decompression and adjunctive medical management may also be beneficial. Treatment with steroids or nonsteroidal antiinflammatory agents is recommended to reduce the intraneuronal edema that can lead to further ischemic axonal damage.[17]

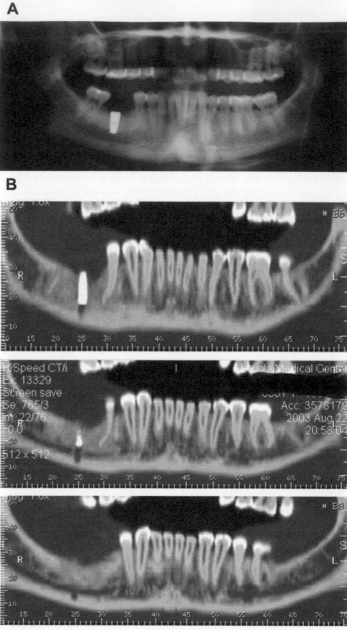

Fig. 4. A patient who had complete anesthesia after implant placement in the tooth number 30 edentulous site. The postoperative radiograph (*A*) shows the implant superior to the inferior alveolar canal; however, there is a vague radiolucency inferior to the implant that was an indication to image further with a computed tomography (CT) scan. (*B*) The subsequent CT scan, which shows the drill channel traversing through the inferior alveolar canal and approaching the inferior border.

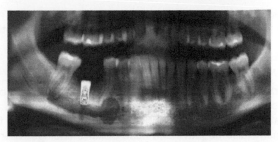

Fig. 5. The patient from **Fig. 4** after surgical repair of the IAN. An osteotomy of the lateral cortex, including the mental foramen, is made and a primary neurorrhaphy is performed with the implant in place.

REASONS FOR NERVE INJURY

Many implant-related nerve injuries are the result of inadequate planning. These injuries are principally caused by not having an awareness of the amount of bone available for implant placement or knowledge of the location of the neurovascular canal. Coincident with this is also a lack of understanding of bone quality at the implant site.

Careful preoperative planning and the availability of appropriate radiographs are important not only for the proper placement of implants for restorative reasons but also to avoid injuries to the important structures in the surgical region. For many cases, plain radiographs, clinical measurements, and direct surgical visualization are sufficient for judicious implant placement.[16] In situations involving complex cases or when the measures discussed earlier do not generate clear enough results, a CT scan and three-dimensional planning may be prudent. Although not necessary for all cases, the use of three-dimensional planning with the construction of a computer-generated surgical guide adds another level of safety in cases in which the planned implant will be close to the neurovascular bundle. Many of these systems incorporate depth control in the computer-generated guide, which further aids in avoidance of injuries to adjacent structures.

The bone quality at the site of the implant is also a factor contributing to nerve injuries. If a surgeon puts pressure on the implant drill while preparing the osteotomy and encounters an unexpected change in bone density, the drill will be inserted deeper than intended.[8] Awareness of the density may be gained when drilling the initial pilot osteotomy with the 2-mm twist drill. Experienced operators can ascertain valuable information from this initial pilot channel. This information is then used to gauge the pressure needed to prepare the remaining osteotomy, avoiding excessive pressure as penetration into less dense spongiosa is encountered. As an alternative, many third-party CT implant planning programs allow users to measure the Hounsfield units of the bone at the implant site, which also helps gauge the density of the bone in that area.[18]

Another cause of nerve injuries is the overzealous use of immediate implants in areas that are too close to the neurovascular structures. Many immediate implants require drill preparation and implant placement apical to the extraction socket in order to gain primary stability. If the neurovascular bundle is close to the apex of the tooth that was removed, overdrilling apically may violate the canal and injure the nerve.[19] This possibility is important in the second premolar region where the apex of the tooth socket may be close to the mental foramen.[20] If there is concern for the proximity of the neurovascular structures in an area of a proposed immediate implant, the possibility of delaying the implantation should be considered. This delay would remove the need for drilling deeper than the natural apex of the tooth socket.

AREAS OF CONCERN

First Bicuspid Region, Anterior Loop of Mental Branch

Radiographic and cadaveric evidence indicates that an anterior loop of the mental branch exists. Its size and how often it is present are not clear. Greenstein and Tarnow[20] associated both radiographic and cadaver dissections and found that radiographs provide many false-negative and false-positive findings. There was poor correlation between radiographic and cadaver studies. They determined that the size of the loop from cadaver dissections ranged from 0.5 to 3.31 mm. The investigators recommended 2-mm clearance coronal from an area of suspected anterior loop, as shown in **Fig. 6**.[20]

The anterior loop region is of concern when placing implants in the first premolar or between the first and second premolars. It also is a consideration when planning angled implants for fixed-hybrid cases (**Fig. 7**). In these cases the distal implants are strategically angled around the mental foramen to increase the anterior-posterior spread. The presence and size of the anterior loop becomes a factor in treatment planning these cases. Intraoperative direct visualization of the mental foramen is helpful in placing the distal implants. However, if a loop of significant size is present, the apex of the implant may cause injury even though the coronal aspect of the implant is at a safe distance from the mental foramen. Appropriate radiographic imaging is useful in planning these cases.

Second Premolar, Mental Foramen Region

The second premolar region is of concern because of the proximity of the mental foramen. The mental foramen is located inferior to the second premolar 73.8% of

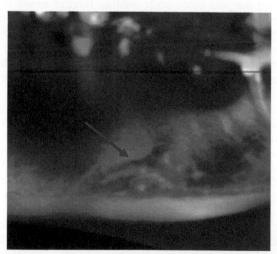

Fig. 6. Periapical radiograph showing an atrophic mandible with the mental foramen indicated by an arrow. Location of the foramen must be considered when placing implants in the mandibular premolar region because 2 mm of coronal clearance from the anterior loop is suggested. (*Data from* Alhassani A, AlGhamdi A. Inferior alveolar nerve injury in implant dentistry: diagnosis, causes, prevention, and management. J Oral Implantol 2010;36(5):401–7.)

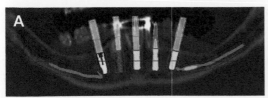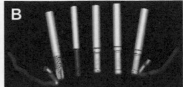

Fig. 7. (*A, B*) CT-guided planning software provides visualization of the anterior loop of the mental branch and allows the greatest anterior-posterior spread when planning cantilevered fixed-hybrid prosthesis while avoiding nerve injury.

the time according to cadaver studies. The second most common location is between the first and second premolars.[21]

This finding is of importance when planning implants in this region, especially immediate implants in a second premolar extraction socket. When placing an implant in this region, overdrilling the preparation intentionally, for primary stability of an immediate implant, or unintentionally in a healed site may cause direct trauma to the contents of the mental foramen (**Fig. 8**). Accurate measurement preoperatively, or by intraoperative radiographs, and/or by direct visualization of the mental foramen is advised when placing implants in this region of the mandible.[10]

The mental foramen can be imaged on both plain radiographs and CT scans. It also can be directly visualized during the surgical procedure by reflecting the subperiosteal flap enough to see the superior aspect of the foramen. Direct measurement of the foramen to the crest of the alveolar ridge can then be made. Localization of the mental foramen by any of these methods is helpful when placing implants in this region, particularly immediate implants.

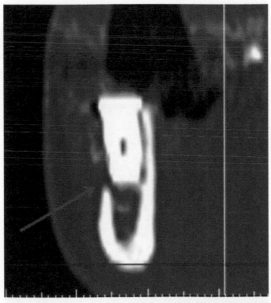

Fig. 8. CT cross section showing an implant placed in the second premolar area that has penetrated into the mental foramen. The arrow points to the location of the mental foramen.

Posterior Mandible Associated with Atrophy

Many patients have missing posterior mandibular teeth with a dentate anterior segment. Conventional prosthodontic treatment of this situation usually involves fabricating a bilateral distal extension partial denture. Patients subsequently present for implant evaluation after significant atrophy of the posterior ridges occurs causing loss of denture stability (**Fig. 9**).

Atrophy, which makes it difficult to wear partial dentures, also affects the ability to place implants. In order to avoid injury to the inferior alveolar bundle, patients with posterior ridge atrophy typically require other procedures to facilitate implant placement. These options are discussed later in this article.

Anterior Maxilla, Nasopalatine Nerve

Although not common, implant-related nerve injuries can also occur in the anterior maxilla, involving the nasopalatine nerve. The injury could occur where the neurovascular bundle traverses the nasopalatine canal or where it exits the incisive foramen in the anterior maxilla. Using two-dimensional and three-dimensional radiology techniques, Mraiwa and colleagues[22] found the anatomy of the nasopalatine canal to be variable in its dimensions and morphology (**Fig. 10**). The clinical significance of this study's finding affects treatment planning of implants in the central incisor region of the maxilla. A common variant is the presence of a wide canal, which reduces the volume of bone present in the premaxillary region, limiting the placement of implants in this situation. Scher[23] and Misch[24] suggested using the incisive foramen as a site for implant placement in atrophic maxillae. Reports of failure caused by ingrowths of soft tissue or complications including development of neurosensory disturbances must be considered before implementing this option.

STRATEGIES TO AVOID INJURY
Local Anesthesia Administration

When placing mandibular implants, it is not necessary to administer an inferior alveolar block injection for adequate local anesthesia. The primary advantage of not giving a block injection is that the patient has some awareness and perception around the IAN. If the site preparation is drilled too close to the neurovascular bundle, the patient

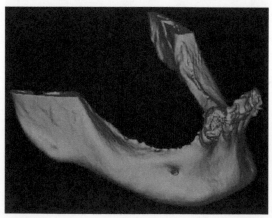

Fig. 9. Bilateral edentulous posterior mandible regions with atrophy. The loss of bone in both vertical and horizontal planes limits the ability to place implants in this situation.

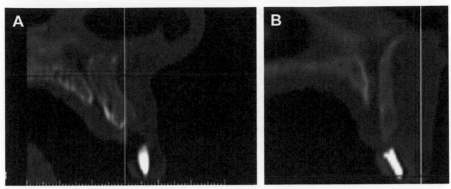

Fig. 10. (*A*) Cross-sectional view of a narrow nasopalatine canal. (*B*) A significantly wider, more cylindrical nasopalatine canal. The wider dimension of the canal decreases bony volume of the premaxilla, limiting available bone for implant placement.

may be able to provide feedback to the surgeon. In addition, not giving a regional block injection eliminates the risk of a needle-stick injury to the IAN trunk. If the patient has numbness following implant placement with an IAN block administered, there is confusion about the mechanism of injury because of the possibility of a needle-stick injury, unless there was evidence of direct nerve injury during the procedure.

Local infiltration provides sufficient anesthesia to place an implant with either flap or flapless techniques. Studies have shown there to be no statistically significant difference in patients' comfort having an implant placed under local infiltration versus regional block injection.[25,26] The reason for this is that implants are typically placed in poorly innervated healed or grafted extraction sockets, and the sensory innervations to the mandible are primarily from the periosteum. Marrow innervation is scant primarily in the venous sinuses. The profound pulpal anesthesia that is essential for restorative tooth preparation or tooth extractions is not necessary for implant placement.

Short Implants

Another strategy to avoid implant-related nerve injury is to use shorter implants in areas where the available vertical height is minimal superior to the IAN canal. The use of short implants has been studied and shown to have mixed outcomes. Some studies report an increased failure rate compared with standard-sized implants. Other investigators describe acceptable results when used in the appropriate situation and adhering to recommended technique. The use of short implants is a valid approach to place implants in the posterior mandible providing that the bone quality is suitable for primary stability. If multiple short implants are placed, splinting of the restorations should be considered.[27]

Bone Augmentation Techniques

In atrophic situations in which implant placement would encroach on the nerve canal, bone augmentation procedures may provide enough space for safe fixture placement. There are several procedures available to augment atrophic alveolar bone to provide the appropriate 2-mm safety zone from the IAN.[25] These procedures include distraction osteogenesis techniques, onlay bone grafting, interpositional sandwich grafting, and grafting using a barrier such as a titanium mesh. In addition, there are several bone sources that may be used with the procedures listed earlier. These sources include autologous bone, allogeneic bone, xenografts, alloplasts, and bone morphogenic protein. Discussion of the advantages or disadvantages of these procedures and materials is beyond the scope of this article. However, these procedures may provide enough bone to allow placement of an implant in an atrophic area, minimizing the risk of nerve injury. One important caveat about bone augmentation procedures is that they may only be used in situations in which there is sufficient interarch space for both the bone graft and a crown on the implant. It is common to have supereruption of the opposing arch limiting the interarch space. Bone augmentation in this instance limits or even precludes the placement of an abutment and crown on the implant. In this type of situation, a nerve lateralization procedure could be considered as alternative method of placing an implant without decreasing an already limited interarch space.

Nerve Lateralization Procedures

Nerve lateralization is a useful procedure to facilitate the placement of implants in atrophic posterior mandibles, especially in situations, described earlier, in which bone augmentation would encroach on the interarch space. This procedure makes available dense cortical bone inferior to the IAN canal for stable implant placement. Because thin knife-edge ridges can be removed and the implant can be placed more inferiorly, onlay bone grafting is rarely necessary.

Although useful, the procedure is more involved and requires skill and experience with manipulating nerves. This requirement likely limits its use in routine practice. Nerve lateralization involves decortication of the lateral cortex over the course of the inferior alveolar canal, and usually the mental foramen with anterior extension of the decorticated area to expose the incisive branch of the IAN (**Fig. 11**). The incisive branch is usually sectioned to permit mobility of the inferior alveolar trunk and mental branch, which allows the trunk and mental branch to be moved laterally. Once the nerve is repositioned, implants are placed in the center of the alveolus, medial to the repositioned nerve. The implants are placed as deep as necessary, including

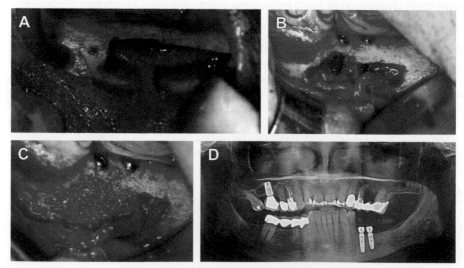

Fig. 11. Nerve lateralization. (*A*) Decortication around the mental foramen and IAN canal, (*B*) the incisive branch sectioned and nerve lateralized, with 2 implants placed into the inferior cortex. (*C*) The defect is then bone grafted. (*D*) Four-month postoperative radiograph after uncovering and placement of healing abutments.

into the inferior border as required for stability. The defect from the decortication can be grafted, and the nerve trunk replaced laterally. Some surgeons prefer to protect the nerve trunk with a type I/III collagen tube or polyglycolic acid tube.

After nerve lateralization surgery, patients experience neurosensory disturbance; however, it has been shown to be transient in most individuals. In a study by Hashemi,[28] the mean time to full recovery of sensory function was 37 ± 15 days. Only 3% of the patients studied had prolonged disturbance beyond 1 year. Although patients do have transient hypoesthesia following nerve lateralization, it remains a reliable procedure if other methods failed or are not an option because of limited interarch space.

Avoiding Implants in the Atrophic Mandibular Posterior by Cantilevering from the Anterior

Many patients have early loss of posterior mandibular teeth and wear a bilateral distal extension saddle partial denture. This situation is classified as a Kennedy class I. Over time, the posterior ridges become atrophic and denture wearing may become more difficult and uncomfortable. At this point the patient may be referred for implant consultation to replace the posterior teeth to remove the need for a partial denture. The same issues affecting partial denture stability, such as the atrophic ridges, also increase the complexity when planning implants in these regions.

When treatment planning atrophic mandibular cases, such as shown in **Fig. 12**, the aforementioned strategies may be used to carefully place implants in the posterior mandible. However, depending on the overall health of the remaining anterior teeth

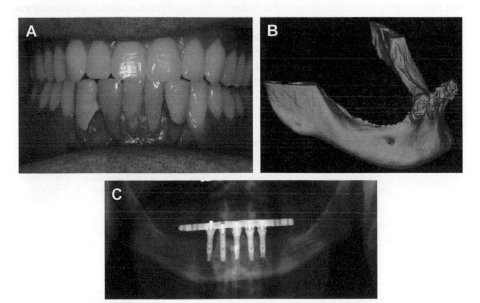

Fig. 12. (*A*) Bilateral free end distal extension partial denture. The patient has 5 remaining anterior teeth. The teeth have significant gingival recession and bone loss. (*B*) Three-dimensional model of the same patient showing bilateral atrophic alveolar ridges in the posterior regions. (*C*) Panorex showing completed treatment, after removal of the remaining anterior teeth and placement of 5 implants. The final prosthesis is cantilevered posteriorly to the first molar regions bilaterally to obviate implant placement in an atrophic mandible.

and the long-term prognosis of these teeth, another approach may be used. If the remaining anterior teeth have a poor long-term prognosis because of caries and or periodontal disease, the patient may benefit from removal of these teeth and placement of multiple implants anterior to the mental foramina with the intention a fabricating a fixed-hybrid appliance that cantilevers teeth to the posterior regions. The advantage of this treatment option is that it avoids other procedures in the posterior mandible that may cause injury to the IAN. Removal of teeth and placement of implants in the anterior mandible is more straightforward and involves less surgery than bone augmentation or nerve lateralization procedures. It may also provide more long-term stability than the use of short implants.

Removing teeth in order to replace other missing teeth may seem extreme. However, in a practical sense this treatment option is more conservative than performing multiple surgical procedures in the posterior mandible to facilitate posterior implants in the atrophic region only to have the natural anterior teeth fail later and have to be removed and also replaced with more implants. This treatment plan involves less time, less surgery, and fewer implants. For these reasons, it is a useful strategy to restore an atrophic posterior region and avoid potential nerve injuries.

MANAGEMENT OF IMPLANT-RELATED NERVE INJURIES

Even with careful planning and appropriate surgical technique, implant-related nerve injuries may occur.

In this situation, early identification and diagnosis of the problem is important. Not all implant-related nerve injuries are managed in exactly the same manner. An algorithm that summarizes the management of a patient who reports neurosensory disturbance following an implant procedure is provided in **Fig. 13**.

Suspected nerve injuries during implant placement follow a systematic approach as outlined in **Fig. 13**. Concern for nerve damage intraoperatively warrants prompt evaluation of the patient for numbness. If an IAN block was administered, a local anesthetic reversal agent (eg, phentolamine [OraVerse]), may be administered to

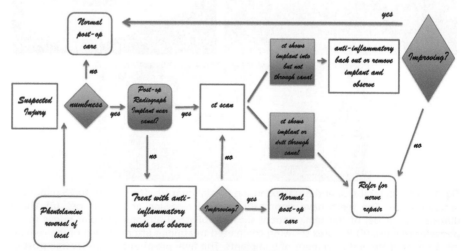

Fig. 13. Algorithm for suspected implant-related nerve injuries. (*Courtesy of* M.J. Steinberg, DDS, MD, Maywood, IL.)

expedite examination. A positive finding of numbness requires radiographic imaging to evaluate implant proximity to the inferior alveolar canal or mental foramen. If the implant is noted to be well away from vital structures and the patient reports numbness, a regimen of antiinflammatory medication (steroids or nonsteroidal medications)[17] is begun with continued observation for improvement. Radiographic evidence showing interruption of the canal demarcation or direct impingement on the nerve from either the implant or drill path necessitates further evaluation via CT scan.

CT review showing an implant impinging on, but not through, the canal should either be removed completely or backed out until the impingement has been alleviated. In addition, antiinflammatory medications may be started while observing for improvement. Patients showing progressive improvement can assume a normal postoperative course; however, no improvement within 3 months should be referred for nerve repair evaluation.[17] The ominous finding of drill path or implant placement through the canal warrants prompt referral to a specialist capable of nerve repair.

There is a significant difference in the way that injuries that just violate the superior aspect of the IAN canal and injuries that traverse the canal are managed. This important distinction is determined from a CT scan (**Fig. 14**). In situations in which the canal may be violated but not transected, the neurovascular bundle may be intact but probably has neuropraxia type injury. Edema of the tissues surrounding the nerve and intraneuronal edema may cause further ischemic axonal injury. In this situation decompression is important. Both mechanical decompression and medicinal decompression methods are usually used. Mechanical decompression includes either backing out the implant or removal of the implant. Medicinal decompression is accomplished by an antiinflammatory regimen. If CT shows that the canal has been transected, removing or backing out the implant will not undo or improve the situation. In many cases the IAN is able to be repaired with the implant still left in place. For this reason, early referral for evaluation and possible nerve repair is recommended.

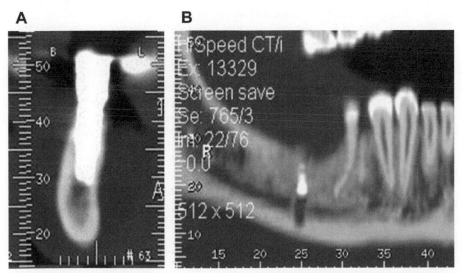

Fig. 14. (*A*) CT cross section showing the apex of an implant just at the superior cortex of the IAN canal. (*B*) CT scan showing the drill channel traversing the IAN canal.

SUMMARY

Implant application for the replacement of missing teeth is increasing and clinicians are using this therapy as the first-line replacement method. Knowledge of the local anatomy and available bone stock should be carefully assessed via both clinical examination and appropriate imaging to avoid injuries to important anatomic structures. In situations in which there may not be enough bone to safely place implants, advanced treatment planning strategies and preliminary procedures may be needed to facilitate implant application for tooth replacement. Should an implant-related nerve injury occur then a systematic approach to management should be used.

REFERENCES

1. Leung YY, Fung PP, Cheung LK. Treatment modalities of neurosensory deficit after lower third molar surgery: a systematic review. J Oral Maxillofac Surg 2012;70(4):768–78.
2. Kipp D, Goldstein B, Weiss W Jr. Dysesthesia after mandibular third molar surgery: a retrospective study and analysis of 1,377 surgical procedures. J Am Dent Assoc 1980;100(2):185–92.
3. Morris CD, Rasmussen J, Throckmorton GS, et al. The anatomic basis of lingual nerve trauma associated with inferior alveolar block injections. J Oral Maxillofac Surg 2010;68(11):2833–6.
4. Ahonen M, Tjäderhane L. Endodontic-related paresthesia: a case report and literature review. J Endod 2011;37(10):1460–4.
5. Kim J, Cha I, Kim S, et al. Which risk factors are associated with neurosensory deficits of inferior alveolar nerve after mandibular third molar extraction? J Oral Maxillofac Surg 2012;70(11):2508–14.
6. Kjølle GK, Bjørnland T. Low risk of neurosensory dysfunction after mandibular third molar surgery in patients less than 30 years of age. A prospective study following removal of 1220 mandibular third molars. Oral Surg Oral Med Oral Pathol Oral Radiol 2013;116(4):411–7.
7. Boffano P, Roccia F, Gallesio C. Lingual nerve deficit following mandibular third molar removal: Review of the literature and medicolegal considerations. Oral Surg Oral Med Oral Pathol Oral Radiol 2012;113(3):e10–8.
8. Juodzbalys G, Wang H, Sabalys G. Injury of the inferior alveolar nerve during implant placement: a literature review. J Oral Maxillofac Res 2011;2(1):e1.
9. Ellies L. The incidence of altered sensation of the mental nerve after mandibular implant placement. J Oral Maxillofac Surg 1999;57(12):1410–2.
10. Burstein J, Mastin C, Le B. Avoiding injury to the inferior alveolar nerve by routine use of intraoperative radiographs during implant placement. J Oral Implantol 2008;34(1):34–8.
11. Kiyak H, Beach B, Worthington P, et al. The psychological impact of osseointegrated dental implants. Int J Oral Maxillofac Implants 1990;5:272–81.
12. Libersa P, Savignat M, Tonnel A. Neurosensory disturbances of the inferior alveolar nerve: a retrospective study of complaints in a 10-year period. J Oral Maxillofac Surg 2007;65(8):1486–9.
13. Steed M. Peripheral nerve response to injury. Atlas Oral Maxillofac Surg Clin North Am 2011;19(1):1–13.
14. Ziccardi V, Zuniga J. Nerve injuries after third molar removal. Oral Maxillofac Surg Clin North Am 2007;19(1):105–15.

15. Marchiori ÉC, Barber JS, Williams WB, et al. Neuropathic pain following sagittal split ramus osteotomy of the mandible: prevalence, risk factors, and clinical course. J Oral Maxillofac Surg 2013;71(12):2115–22.
16. Worthington P. Injury to the inferior alveolar nerve during implant placement: a formula for protection of the patient and clinician. Int J Oral Maxillofac Implants 2004;19(5):731–4.
17. Misch C, Resnik R. Mandibular nerve neurosensory impairment after dental implant surgery: Management and protocol. Implant Dent 2010;19(5):378–86.
18. Lettry S, Seedhom BB, Berry E, et al. Quality assessment of the cortical bone of the human mandible. Bone 2003;32(1):35–44.
19. Alhassani A, AlGhamdi A. Inferior alveolar nerve injury in implant dentistry: diagnosis, causes, prevention, and management. J Oral Implantol 2010;36(5):401–7.
20. Greenstein G, Tarnow D. The mental foramen and nerve: clinical and anatomical factors related to dental implant placement: a literature review. J Periodontol 2006;77(12):1933–43.
21. Guo J, Su L, Zhao J, et al. Location of mental foramen based on soft- and hard-tissue landmarks in a Chinese population. J Craniofac Surg 2009;20(6):2235–7.
22. Mraiwa N, Jacobs R, Van Cleynenbreugel J, et al. The nasopalatine canal revisited using 2D and 3D CT imaging. Dentomaxillofac Radiol 2004;33(6):396–402.
23. Scher EL. Use of the incisive canal as a recipient site for root form implants: preliminary clinical reports. Implant Dent 1994;3(1):38–41.
24. Misch C. Premaxilla surgery: implant insertion, bone spreading, nasal floor elevation, and incisive foramen implants. In: Pendill J, editor. Contemporary implant dentistry. 3rd edition. St Louis (MO): Mosby Elsevier; 2008. p. 795–7.
25. Soydan S. Comparison of efficacy and safety of infiltration anesthesia and inferior alveolar nerve blockage for posterior mandibular implant insertion. J Oral Maxillofac Surg 2010;68(9 Suppl):e60–1.
26. Heller A, Shankland W. Alternative to the inferior alveolar nerve block anesthesia when placing mandibular dental implants posterior to the mental foramen. J Oral Implantol 2001;27:127–33.
27. Romeo E, Bivio A, Mosca D, et al. The use of short dental implants in clinical practice: literature review. Minerva Stomatol 2010;59(1–2):23–31.
28. Hashemi H. Neurosensory function following mandibular nerve lateralization for placement of implants. Int J Oral Maxillofac Surg 2010;39(5):452–6.

Maxillary Sinus Augmentation

Naveen Mohan, DDS[a],*, Joshua Wolf, DDS[a], Harry Dym, DDS[a,b,c,d,e]

KEYWORDS

- Sinus elevation • Lateral window • Lateral antrostomy • Transalveolar

KEY POINTS

- Atrophy of the posterior maxillary alveolar bone is commonly encountered after tooth loss.
- There are 2 main approaches to sinus augmentation in preparation for implant placement: transalveolar and lateral antrostomy.
- Knowledge of the complications associated with this procedure is essential for successful treatment.

HISTORY

The presence of the maxillary sinuses mystified scientists for several hundreds of years. Galen is credited as one of the first people to recognize the existence of the paranasal sinuses. He noted porosities in the bone that he thought made the head less heavy.[1]

Little scientific progress was made during the middle ages. During the Renaissance, Leonardo da Vinci and Andreas Vesalius both described the paranasal sinuses, including the maxillary sinus, in great detail. Fallopius recognized the enlargement of the sinuses with age. In the seventeenth century, Nathaniel Highmore recorded a case of odontogenic, purulent sinusitis.[2]

The American George Caldwell and the Frenchman Henry Luc separately described a procedure to access the maxillary sinus using a lateral window in 1893.[3] The procedure was used to treat disorders of the antrum.

In the 1970s, Tatum and colleagues[4] used the sinus cavity to increase available bone using graft material, which allowed greater implant-to-bone contact area once the bone graft matured.

Disclosure: The authors have nothing to disclose.
[a] Department of Dentistry/Oral Maxillofacial Surgery, The Brooklyn Hospital Center, 121 DeKalb Avenue, Brooklyn, NY 11201, USA; [b] Department of Dentistry/Oral and Maxillofacial Surgery, Columbia University College of Dental Medicine, 630 West 16th Street, New York, NY 10032, USA; [c] Oral and Maxillofacial Surgery, Residency Training Program, The Brooklyn Hospital Center, 121 Dekalb Avenue, Brooklyn, NY 11205, USA; [d] Woodhull Hospital, 760 Broadway, Brooklyn, NY 11206, USA; [e] New York Harbor Healthcare System, 423 East 23rd street, New York, NY 10010, USA
* Corresponding author.
E-mail address: ncm9001@nyp.org

PNEUMATIZATION OF THE SINUS

There has been a downward trend in rates of tooth loss in the United States. However, because of the growing elderly population, the absolute number of lost teeth is increasing. The department of health and human services (HHS) reported in the national health and nutrition examination survey (NHANES) study that 62% of Americans aged 35 to 44 years reported tooth loss caused by caries or periodontal disease. The prevalence of edentulism among seniors (aged 65 years and older) was 27%.[5] The American Academy of Implant Dentistry reports that 3 million people in the United States have dental implants. This number is expected to grow yearly by 500,000.[6]

Because of the presence of the maxillary sinuses, posterior maxillary alveolar bone loss creates a unique problem for implant placement after tooth extraction. The cause of this issue is increased pneumatization of the maxillary sinus (**Fig. 1**). Increased osteoclastic activity within the periosteum of the schneiderian membrane results in expansion of the maxillary sinuses. Also, increased positive pressure is thought to contribute to alveolar bone atrophy.[7] The soft, type IV bone in the posterior maxilla has low resistance to these processes. The end result is a decrease in vertical bone height (VBH) of the alveolus in the edentulous areas.

In a radiographic study, Sharan and Madjar[8] found that "sinus expansion was considerably larger in cases of extractions of teeth enveloped by a superiorly curving sinus floor… Sinus expansion was larger in cases of second molar extractions (in comparison to first molars) and in cases of extraction of 2 or more adjacent posterior teeth."

Davarpanah and colleagues[9] classified posterior maxillary bone loss into several categories:

- Vertical bone loss from within the sinus: a reduced distance from the floor of the sinus to the alveolar ridge crest. However, no loss of interocclusal distance.
- Vertical bone loss of the alveolar ridge: loss of alveolar ridge below the sinus. There is an increase in interocclusal distance.
- Horizontal bone loss of the alveolar ridge: a loss in buccopalatal width of alveolar bone.
- Combination subsinus loss: both vertical and horizontal bone loss.

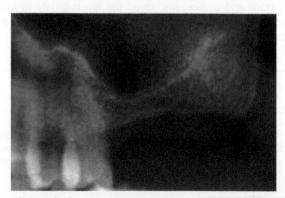

Fig. 1. Periapical radiograph showing pneumatization of the maxillary sinus secondary to loss of all molar teeth. (*From* Li J, Lee K, Chen H, et al. Piezoelectric surgery in the maxillary sinus floor elevation with hydraulic pressure for xenograft and simultaneous implant placement. J Prosthet Dent 2013;110(5):345; with permission.)

Other grafting techniques such as block grafting or guided bone regeneration are required to treat the different atrophy patterns. This article focuses on sinus augmentation to increase the VBH available for implant placement.

ANATOMY
Osteology

The largest of the paranasal sinuses, the maxillary sinuses are pyramidal in shape. The base of the pyramid is the lateral nasal wall with the apex pointing toward the zygomatic process of the maxillary bone. The average dimensions of the adult maxillary sinuses are 25 to 35 mm in width, 36 to 45 mm in height, and 38 to 45 mm in length. The inferior portion of the sinus is typically 1 cm below the nasal floor.[10] The average volume of the maxillary sinus is approximately 15 mL.[11] This volume tends to increase with partial and full edentulism.

The anterior wall of the sinus extends from the inferior orbital rim to the maxillary alveolar process. It is composed of thin bone and serves as the surgical site for the Caldwell-Luc (lateral antrostomy) approach. The superior wall is the floor of the orbit. The posterior wall separates the maxillary sinus from the infratemporal fossa. The medial wall is also the lateral wall of the nasal cavity. The medial wall houses the primary ostium, which serves as the main conduit for drainage of secretions. The primary ostium exits along the superomedial aspect of the medial wall. The superior positioning of the ostium allows placement of graft material without hindering drainage. It drains into the ethmoidal infundibulum, then into the middle meatus of the nasal cavity at the hiatus semilunaris (**Fig. 2**). Accessory ostia are found in approximately 15% to 40% of patients. They typically drain superior to the inferior turbinate, superior and posterior to the uncinate process.[12]

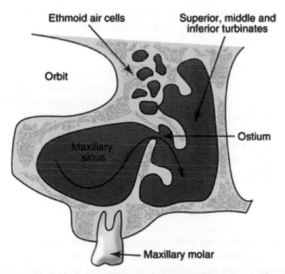

Fig. 2. The anatomy and drainage pathway of the maxillary sinus. The primary ostium is located along the superior medial aspect of the medial wall of the sinus. Fluids eventually drain into the middle meatus of the nasal cavity. (*From* Treadway AL, Bankston SA. Dental implant prosthetic rehabilitation: sinus grafting. In: Bagheri SC, Bell RB, Khan HA, editors. Current therapy in oral and maxillofacial surgery. 1st edition. St Louis (MO): Elsevier Saunders; 2012. p. 168; with permission.)

Vasculature and Innervation

The infraorbital and posterior superior alveolar arteries, both branches of the internal maxillary artery, supply the lateral aspect of the maxillary sinus. Traxler and colleagues[13] found that branches of these two vessels formed endosseous anastomoses in all specimens. In 44% of specimens there were also extraosseous anastomoses forming a double arterial arcade. The infraorbital artery, along with the nerve, runs along the superior wall of the antrum within the sinus mucosa. The artery gives off the middle and anterior superior alveolar arteries before exiting the skull. The infraorbital foramen is located on the anterior wall of the antrum. The medial aspect of the sinus receives blood supply from the posterior lateral nasal artery, a branch of the sphenopalatine artery. The high vascularity of this region results in a more favorable environment for graft integration.

Innervation is supplied by branches of the second division of the trigeminal nerve, which include the infraorbital, superior alveolar, and palatine nerves.

Schneiderian Membrane

The schneiderian membrane is composed of 3 layers. The first layer is periosteum, which covers the bone of the antrum. A layer of highly vascular connective tissue covers the periosteum. The last layer is pseudostratified columnar epithelium (respiratory epithelium) and is exposed to the sinus cavity.[11] The schneiderian membrane is continuous with the nasal mucosa as they connect at the ostia. The membrane is approximately 0.8 mm thick in the antrum.

Septa

Review of maxillary sinus anatomy cannot be complete without evaluation of septa. They can be divided into 2 groups: congenital and acquired. Congenital septa can be found anywhere in the maxillary sinus and develop as the midface grows. Acquired septa occur in areas where there is differential resorption of the maxillary alveolar bone along the sinus floor leading to bony crests. These septa are a result of tooth loss and eventual bone resorption.[14]

Relationship to Dentition

The maxillary premolars and molars have an intimate relationship with the inferior aspect of the maxillary sinus. As shown by oral-antral communications during tooth extraction, the bone separating the apices from the sinus cavity is often extremely thin. Eberhardt and colleagues[15] found that the mesiobuccal root apex of the second molar was closest to the sinus wall, with an average distance of 0.83 mm. The lingual root apex of the first premolar was the furthest from the sinus wall. In general, the molar roots were closer to the maxillary sinus than premolar roots.

PREOPERATIVE EVALUATION
Medical Evaluation

A thorough history and physical examination is required before the initiation of treatment. The patient's current medications as well as allergies should be reviewed. The patient evaluation may necessitate consultation with a primary care physician or specialist. Appropriate laboratory tests should be ordered as needed.

Dental Evaluation

A comprehensive dental evaluation determines whether the patient is an appropriate candidate for implant placement with sinus augmentation. Diagnostic models can be used to evaluate the proposed surgical site. The patient's occlusal scheme should be evaluated. In addition to horizontal measurements, the vertical dimension of the surgical site should be evaluated. An inadequate or excessive interarch distance can compromise the stability or esthetic outcome of the implants.[11] In addition, the transverse relationship of the maxilla and mandible should be evaluated.

Radiographic Evaluation

Panoramic imaging is useful for a preliminary evaluation of the maxillary sinuses. The amount of VBH at the proposed surgical site can be evaluated. Furthermore, the antra can be evaluated for any disorder.

The panoramic radiograph is limited because it is two-dimensional, often distorted, and is prone to ghost images or artifacts. As a result, measurements can be inaccurate or disorders can be hidden. With cone-beam computed tomography (CT) technology becoming more prevalent in dental offices, CT scanning is becoming the standard for evaluation of the sinuses. Accurate measurements can be made in 3 dimensions and the contents of the sinus can be evaluated accurately. A survey found that 58.7% of otolaryngologists in New York State recommended CT evaluation to rule out disorders before sinus lift procedures.[16]

Indications

The major indication for sinus augmentation is the atrophic posterior maxillary alveolus with loss of VBH. Pneumatization of the sinus results in insufficient bone to house an implant with adequate stability. There are 2 main approaches to sinus augmentation: transalveolar approach and lateral antrostomy (LA).

The decision as to which approach to use is largely based on the amount of residual maxillary alveolar bone remaining. Rosen and colleagues[17] found that implant survival decreases with the transalveolar technique when 4 mm or less of residual bone height is present: "When presurgical bone height beneath the sinus is compared to implant survival, the data demonstrate that in sites of 4mm or less, there was a survival rate of 85.7%, which improved to 96% in locations with more than 4 mm of initial bone height." Another study found that the transalveolar approach is indicated when greater than 6 mm of residual bone is present and 3 to 4 mm of bone height gain is planned. The LA approach was recommended for cases with less residual bone or if more bone height is needed.[18]

If the LA approach is used, the practitioner can opt to place implants immediately or to delay placement after graft maturation. This decision is based on several factors. The quality of the bone (ie, its density) should be assessed. The amount of residual alveolar bone should also be evaluated. Immediate placement can be considered if the clinician can achieve primary stability of the implant. Reports have been published showing implant success with as little as 3 mm of VBH before sinus augmentation.[19] However, it can be difficult to stabilize the implant with less than 3 mm of residual bone height. It is recommended that a minimum of 4 to 5 mm of residual bone height be present for immediate implant placement when using the LA technique (**Table 1**).[20]

Contraindications

Several factors can increase the risk of implant failure and other adverse sequelae. Implant placement in bone of poor quality should be avoided because of the decrease in primary stability. Local or systemic causes can compromise bone quality (**Box 1**).

Table 1 Transalveolar versus lateral antrostomy	
4 mm of residual bone height or less	Lateral antrostomy with delayed implant placement
4–5 mm of residual bone height	Lateral antrostomy, immediate implant placement if adequate stability can be achieved
6 mm of residual bone height or greater	Transalveolar technique

Before augmentation, the sinus should be evaluated for disorder. Contraindications include active sinus infection, recurrent chronic sinusitis, recurrent fungal sinusitis, uncontrolled diabetes, cystic fibrosis, maxillary sinus hypoplasia, neoplasms, and history of radiation therapy to the site.[20] Any findings of the previously described conditions require consultation with a specialist. Smoking has been linked to an increased risk of complications associated with implant integration and sinus augmentation. However, it is a relative contraindication because failure rates were only slightly higher compared with nonsmokers.[21]

TECHNIQUES
Transalveolar

The transalveolar sinus lift technique is more conservative than the LA approach. The sinus membrane is not directly instrumented. Also, the sinus cavity is not directly visualized and membrane perforations are more difficult to determine.[22]

There are several options for incision design. The midcrestal incision along the alveolar ridge in a mesiodistal direction can be used. Vertical releasing incisions can be made along the lateral aspect of the maxilla if necessary to gain more exposure. The alveolar bone is exposed using a full-thickness mucoperiosteal flap.

A round bur is used to mark the surgical site along the alveolar ridge. A pilot drill with a diameter 1 to 1.5 mm less than the final implant diameter is then used. The pilot hole is made to a depth approximately 2 mm from the sinus floor. Creation of a pilot hole is not necessary if 5 mm or less of VBH is remaining.[23]

Next, a mallet is used to drive successively larger osteotomes gradually to the final implant depth. Gradually increasing the depth decreases the potential for membrane tears.[20] The smallest (first) osteotome fractures the sinus floor. The area of fracture increases as larger osteotomes are used.[24] Single-site preparation is more prone to

Box 1 Absolute contraindications
Active sinus infection
Recurrent chronic sinusitis
Recurrent fungal sinusitis
Uncontrolled diabetes
Cystic fibrosis
Maxillary sinus hypoplasia
Neoplasms of the sinus
History of radiation therapy to maxilla

sinus perforation compared with multiple adjacent sites.[25] The final osteotome should have a diameter approximately 0.5 mm less than the planned implant diameter.[23]

Before implant placement, some investigators have proposed the introduction of bone graft into the osteotomy site. The rationale is to increase the amount of bone between the apex of the implant and the sinus floor. Si and colleagues[24] found similar implant survival rates and no advantage in grafted sites versus nongrafted sites.

Lateral Antrostomy

A midcrestal or palatally positioned incision is made in a mesiodistal direction, and vertically releasing incisions are made. A full-thickness mucoperiosteal flap is elevated exposing the lateral wall of the maxillary sinus.

The superoinferior and anteroposterior borders of the lateral window are determined by evaluating the CT radiograph. The inferior border of the window should be 2 to 5 mm superior to the sinus floor to prevent difficultly during infracturing. The anterior border is determined by the mesial extent of the sinus, whereas the distal border is in the area of the first molar.[20] The window is created with a low-speed drill with a diamond bur or a piezoelectric instrument. The window is prepared until a bluish hue is visible along the outline of the preparation. This indicates proximity to the schneiderian membrane. The corners should be rounded to prevent sharp edges, which can potentially perforate the membrane (**Fig. 3**).[26]

The bone window is then infractured into the sinus cavity and elevated in a superior direction along with the sinus membrane, which creates space inferior to the bone window for graft material. An alternative is to detach the bone window from the sinus membrane for use as an autologous graft.[25] With either technique, the sinus membrane is gently elevated superiorly with blunt dissection (**Fig. 4**).

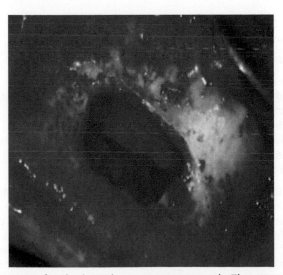

Fig. 3. Access osteotome for the lateral antrostomy approach. The corners of the window are rounded to prevent perforation of the membrane. (*From* Treadway AL, Bankston SA. Dental implant prosthetic rehabilitation: sinus grafting. In: Bagheri SC, Bell RB, Khan HA, editors. Current therapy in oral and maxillofacial surgery. 1st edition. St Louis (MO): Elsevier Saunders; 2012. p. 171; with permission.)

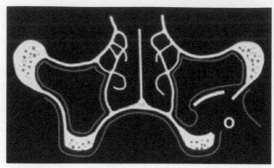

Fig. 4. A coronal section through the maxillary sinuses. The lateral window is infractured and elevated superiorly. A space is created inferior to the elevated bone window. (*From* Boyne PJ. Augmentation of the posterior maxilla by way of sinus grafting procedures: recent research and clinical observations. Oral Maxillofac Surg Clin North Am 2004;16(1):24; with permission.)

Graft material is introduced into the space created inferior to the sinus membrane. Graft should fill the cavity loosely. Overpacking the site can compromise angiogenesis into the graft or obstruct the primary ostium.[3,20] As stated previously, sufficient VBH should be present if the decision is made to place implants at the time of sinus augmentation.

The decision to place a membrane over the antrostomy site is based on provider preference. If a larger window is created, it is recommended that a barrier membrane be placed before closure.[27] However, Torres García-Denche and colleagues[28] found no significant difference if a membrane was used versus not used. The mucoperiosteal flap is then sutured tension free.

POSTOPERATIVE CARE
Patient Instructions

Postoperative instructions are similar to those for other oral surgical procedures:

- Avoid strenuous activity and smoking.
- Place a cold compress superficially on the skin overlying the surgical site for the first 24 hours.
- Maintain a soft diet to avoid trauma to the surgical site.[23,26]
- A removable prosthesis can be used if the surface contacting the surgical site is relieved. Several adjustments must be made postoperatively because remodeling of bone and swelling are expected.

Patients must also maintain good oral hygiene to facilitate healing and reduce infection risk. Rigorous rinsing can disrupt the surgical site and should be avoided initially. After 24 hours patients can use warm saline or chlorhexidine rinses daily.

Patients should adhere strictly to sinus precautions to reduce the chance of graft failure (**Box 2**).[20,26] It is important to avoid excessive positive and negative pressure to create an ideal environment for graft maturation and membrane healing.

Follow-up

The patient should be evaluated postoperatively at 1, 3, and 4 weeks. The graft should be allowed to mature for 3 to 6 months postoperatively for delayed

---
Box 2
Sinus precautions

No blowing nose

No using straws or smoking

No exhalation against pressure, such as inflating balloons or blowing into instruments

No bending over

Sneeze and cough with mouth open

---

implantation.[20,26,28] If healing is uneventful, the practitioner can proceed with the routine protocol for implant placement.

MEDICATIONS
Antimicrobials

The sinus flora, oral flora, and introduction of foreign material make the risk of infection greater in sinus augmentation compared with other oral surgical procedures.[20] Many antibiotic regimens are used. Recommendations for antibiotic prophylaxis range from 1 day to 1 hour before surgery.[3,19,20] Postoperative antibiotics are almost universally recommended. Between 7 and 10 days of antibiotics are typically used.[3,23] Various antibiotics are used, including amoxicillin, Augmentin, and clindamycin.

An oral chlorhexidine rinse for 1 minute before initiation of the procedure is also recommended to decrease the oral bacterial concentration. Some investigators advocate daily rinses for 2 weeks postoperatively.[19,23]

Other Medications

Use of steroids to reduce swelling, pain, and inflammation is common. Some texts suggest a tapering dose of dexamethasone,[20] whereas others recommend methylprednisolone.[26] Opioids with acetaminophen or ibuprofen are routinely prescribed for pain control.

Systemic and topical decongestants are useful to prevent blockage of the ostia postoperatively.[11] Medications used include phenylephrine or oxymetazoline. The practitioner must be cautious in order to avoid rebound congestion after discontinuation of a decongestant.[20]

COMPLICATIONS

Membrane perforation, presence of septa, and infection are the most frequent sinus-related complications during augmentation.[21,29]

Schneiderian Membrane Perforation

The most common complication of sinus augmentation is perforation of the schneiderian membrane, especially if the LA technique is used. The most frequently cited cause for membrane tears is vigorous elevation. Vlassis and Fugazatto[30,31] proposed a classification system for evaluation and treatment (**Box 3**).

For class I and II perforations, elevation of the remaining membrane often produces folds that prevent graft material from entering the sinus cavity. Collagen tape can also be placed over the perforation if there is concern for ingress of graft material into the sinus. If necessary, the perforation can be sutured with resorbable material. Treatment

---

Box 3
Classification of sinus perforations: Vlassis and Fugazatto

Class I

Perforation is adjacent to the osteotomy site. Class I perforations are often sealed off as a result of the membrane folding on itself following completion of elevation. Treatment should be considered when the perforation is still evident after membrane reflection.

Class II

A class II perforation is located in the midsuperior aspect of the osteotomy, extending mesio-distally for two-thirds of the dimension of total osteotomy site. A class II perforation occurs most frequently when infracture design of the osteotomy is used. Repair and treatment are similar to those for class I.

Class III

A class III perforation is located at the inferior border of the osteotomy at its mesial or distal sixth. This class is the most common perforation and is almost always the result of inadequacy of osteotomy or improper execution of membrane reflection. Completion of membrane refraction rarely results in covering a class III perforation and treatment is needed.

Class IV

A class IV perforation is located in the central two-thirds of the inferior border of the osteotomy site. Such a perforation is rare, is almost always caused by lack of care when preparing the osteotomy site, and represents a considerable clinical challenge.

---

modalities for class III and IV perforations include suturing or placement of a lamellar bone sheet. Extension of the osteotomy may be necessary to access the margins of the perforations.[30]

Hernández-Alfaro and colleagues[32] found that implants placed under reconstructed sinus membranes have a higher failure rate. They concluded that implant failure rates increase proportionately with the size of the perforation. Sinus perforation also increased rates of postoperative sinusitis, infection, and graft failure.[33]

Septa

Septa are commonly encountered in the maxillary sinus. They should be identified pre-operatively in order to plan the procedure appropriately. The most common location is the middle region of the antrum.[20,29] It is more difficult or even impossible to elevate the bony window and bluntly dissect the membrane in the presence of septa. Several methods have been suggested to address this issue.

If anteriorly located, 2 lateral windows can be created on both sides of the septum. Both windows are infractured and the membrane is gently elevated. The septum is reduced with a rongeur to remove the sharp edge. The procedure then continues as previously described.[34]

If both sides of the septum cannot be accessed, the base of the septum can be cut and removed. The membrane is simultaneously torn. The membrane must be repaired in accordance with the previously mentioned protocol.[3]

Infection

If a postoperative infection is limited to the area outside the sinus cavity, a simple incision and drainage with irrigation/curettage can be performed. However, if the infection spreads into the sinus, infected graft material must be removed. Infected graft has been described as loose, mobile, and gray as opposed to confined and immobile.[35] Culture and sensitivity testing should be obtained. Systemic antibiotics are to be adjusted accordingly.[3,11]

OUTCOMES

Sinus augmentation of the atrophic posterior maxilla has high success rates. In a meta-analysis of the transalveolar technique, Tan and colleagues[22] found a 3-year implant success rate of 92.8%. In a related meta-analysis, Pjetursson and colleagues[36] found an overall 3-year implant survival rate of 90.1% using the LA technique.

Del Fabbro and colleagues[37] found implant survival rates of 92.17% and 92.93% for simultaneous and delayed procedures respectively. All sinus augmentations were performed by LA in their systematic review. A systematic review for the transalveolar sinus lift was performed by the same group. They found an overall implant success rate of 92.7% for implants placed in bone with less than 5 mm of VBH. The success rate increased to 96.9% if greater than 5 mm of VBH was present.[38]

ALTERNATIVE METHODS
Dentium Advanced Sinus Kit

There now exists a new surgical instrument kit, the Dentium Advanced Sinus Kit (DASK) system, developed exclusively for maxillary sinus lift augmentation procedures. Whether the classic LA approach or the transalveolar procedure is used, it is the opinion of the senior author (HD) that the system has greatly improved surgical outcomes. This procedure has also significantly reduced the surgical time associated with sinus lift procedures as well as decreasing associated morbidity such as membrane perforations and tears.

The traditional approach to creating a lateral sinus bone window in order to access and lift the maxillary sinus membrane before grafting the maxillary sinus included the use of a carbide or diamond bur. Sinus membrane tears (both large and small) are sometimes outcomes of this approach. An alternative technique such as the use of the piezo system has resulted in fewer membrane perforations; however, the piezo technique is time consuming and requires much patience by the treating practitioner.

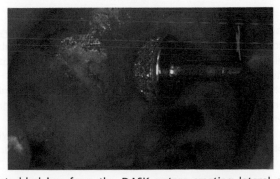

Fig. 5. Diamond-studded bur from the DASK system creating lateral antrostomy access window. (*From* Wallace SS, Tarnow DP, Froum SJ, et al. Maxillary sinus elevation by lateral window approach: evolution of technology and technique. J Evid Base Dent Pract 2012;12(Suppl 3):168; with permission.)

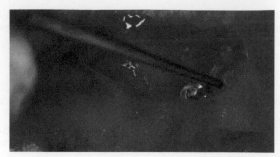

Fig. 6. Instrument from DASK system used for initial elevation of sinus. (*From* Wallace SS, Tarnow DP, Froum SJ, et al. Maxillary sinus elevation by lateral window approach: evolution of technology and technique. J Evid Base Dent Pract 2012;12(Suppl 3):169; with permission.)

The DASK system consists of a series of diamond-studded concave burns (**Fig. 5**) along with a series of hand instruments that is easy to learn, simple to use, and quick to master (**Fig. 6**). Because of its fast learning curve, it has quickly become the surgical approach of choice in the senior author's residency program. The ease of the DASK procedure coupled with the quick learning curve and the predictability of obtaining a perforation-free sinus membrane makes this surgical system, in the opinion of the senior author HD, the ideal surgical approach for use by general dentists.

Balloon Antral Elevation

The use of balloons to elevate the sinus membrane was first introduced in 2006. The technique is intended to be less technique sensitive and reduce the incidence of membrane perforations. Rao and colleagues[39] had a sinus perforation rate of 3% compared with the reported 7% to 35% perforation rate for traditional techniques.

The initial access of the sinus cavity is similar to the LA technique. Rather than elevating the membrane with hand instruments, a balloon is introduced to the sinus membrane. Up to 5 mL of saline are slowly delivered into the balloon. The amount of saline injected into the balloon depends on the amount of elevation necessary. The standard LA approach is then resumed. Petruzzi and colleagues[40] achieved a mean VBH gain of 6.66 mm using this technique.

SUMMARY

Pneumatization of the maxillary sinus secondary to posterior maxillary tooth loss is an extremely common finding. Significant atrophy of the maxilla prevents implant placement in this region. For several decades, sinus augmentation has been used to develop these sites for dental implant placement.

The 2 main techniques for increasing the VBH of the posterior maxilla are the transalveolar and lateral antrostomy approaches. The clinical and radiographic examinations dictate which method is appropriate for each clinical situation. Both techniques have been shown to have high success rates. However, practitioners must be aware of potential complications and how to address them.

REFERENCES

1. Blanton PL, Biggs NL. Eighteen hundred years of controversy: the paranasal sinuses. Am J Anat 1969;124:135–47.

2. Helidonis ES. The history of otolaryngology from ancient to modern times. Am J Otol 1993;14(6):382–93.
3. Fonseca RJ, Marciani RD, Turvey TA. Oral and maxillofacial surgery. 2nd edition. St Louis (MO): Saunders; 2008.
4. Tatum H. Maxillary and sinus implant reconstructions. Dent Clin North Am 1986; 30(2):207–29.
5. Dye BA, Tan S, Smith V, et al. Trends in oral health status: United States, 1988–1994 and 1999–2004. Vital Health Stat 11 2007;(248):1–92 National Center for Health Statistics.
6. Dental implants facts and figures. American Academy of Implant Dentistry. Available at: http://www.aaid.com/about/Press_Room/Dental_Implants_FAQ.html.
7. Raja SV. Management of the posterior maxilla with sinus lift: review of techniques. J Oral Maxillofac Surg 2009;67(8):1730–4.
8. Sharan A, Madjar M. Maxillary sinus pneumatization following extractions: a radiographic study. Int J Oral Maxillofac Implants 2008;23(1):48–56.
9. Davarpanah M, Martinez H, Tecucianu JF, et al. The modified osteotome technique. Int J Periodontics Restorative Dent 2001;21(6):599–607.
10. Van Den Bergh JP, ten Bruggenkate CM, Disch FJ, et al. Anatomical aspects of sinus floor elevations. Clin Oral Implants Res 2000;11(3):256–65.
11. Kaufman F. Maxillary sinus elevation surgery: an overview. J Esthet Restor Dent 2003;15(5):272–83.
12. Johnson J. Bailey's head and neck surgery: otolaryngology. 5th edition. Philadelphia: Lippincott Williams & Wilkins; 2013.
13. Traxler H, Windisch A, Geyerhofer U, et al. Arterial blood supply of the maxillary sinus. Clin Anat 1999;12(6):417–21.
14. Krennmair G, Ulm CW, Lugmayr H, et al. The incidence, location, and height of maxillary sinus septa in the edentulous and dentate maxilla. J Oral Maxillofac Surg 1999;57(6):667–71.
15. Eberhardt JA, Torabinejad M, Christiansen EL. A computed tomographic study of the distances between the maxillary sinus floor and the apices of the maxillary posterior teeth. Oral Surg Oral Med Oral Pathol 1992;73(3):345–6.
16. Cote MT, Segelnick SL, Rastogi A, et al. New York state ear, nose, and throat specialists' views on pre-sinus lift referral. J Periodontol 2011;82(2):227–33.
17. Rosen PS, Summers R, Mellado JR, et al. The bone-added osteotome sinus floor elevation technique: multicenter retrospective report of consecutively treated patients. Int J Oral Maxillofac Implants 1999;14(6):853–8.
18. Zitzmann NU, Schärer P. Sinus elevation procedures in the resorbed posterior maxilla: comparison of the crestal and lateral approaches. Oral Surg Oral Med Oral Pathol Oral Radiol Endod 1998;85(1):8–17.
19. Felice P, Pistilli R, Piattelli M, et al. 1-stage versus 2-stage lateral sinus lift procedures: 1-year post-loading results of a multicentre randomised controlled trial. Eur J Oral Implantol 2014;7(1):65–75.
20. Misch CE. Contemporary implant dentistry. 3rd edition. St Louis (MO): Mosby Elsevier; 2008.
21. Moreno Vazquez JC, Gonzalez de Rivera AS, Gil HS, et al. Complication rate in 200 consecutive sinus lift procedures: guidelines for prevention and treatment. J Oral Maxillofac Surg 2014;72(5):892–901.
22. Tan WC, Lang NP, Zwahlen M, et al. A systematic review of the success of sinus floor elevation and survival of implants inserted in combination with sinus floor elevation part II: transalveolar technique. J Clin Periodontol 2008;35(Suppl 8): 241–54.

23. Lindhe J. Clinical periodontology and implant dentistry. 5th edition. Oxford: Blackwell Publishing; 2008.
24. Si MS, Zhuang LF, Gu YX, et al. Osteotome sinus floor elevation with or without grafting: a 3-year randomized controlled clinical trial. J Clin Periodontol 2013; 40(4):396–403.
25. Andersson L, Kahnberg KE, Porgrel MA. Oral and maxillofacial surgery. Oxford: Blackwell Publishing; 2010.
26. Farhat FF, Kinaia B, Gross HB. Sinus bone augmentation: a review of the common techniques. Compend Contin Educ Dent 2008;29(7):388–92, 394–7.
27. Miloro M, Ghali GE, Larsen P, et al. Peterson's principles of oral and maxillofacial surgery. 2nd edition. Shelton (CT): People's Medical Publishing House; 2004.
28. Torres García-Denche J, Wu X, Martinez PP, et al. Membranes over the lateral window in sinus augmentation procedures: a two-arm and split-mouth randomized clinical trials. J Clin Periodontol 2013;40(11):1043–51.
29. Maestre-Ferrín L, Carrillo-García C, Galán-Gil S, et al. Prevalence, location, and size of maxillary sinus septa: panoramic radiograph versus computed tomography scan. J Oral Maxillofac Surg 2011;69(2):507–11.
30. Vlassis J, Fugazzotto PA. A classification system for sinus membrane perforations during augmentation procedures with options for repair. J Periodontol 1999;70(6): 692–9.
31. Ardekian L, Oved-Peleg E, Mactei EE, et al. The clinical significance of sinus membrane perforation during augmentation of the maxillary sinus. J Oral Maxillofac Surg 2006;64(2):277–82.
32. Hernández-Alfaro F, Torradeflot MM, Marti C, et al. Prevalence and management of schneiderian membrane perforations during sinus-lift procedures. Clin Oral Implants Res 2008;19(1):91–8.
33. Nolan PJ, Freeman K, Kraut RA, et al. Correlation between schneiderian membrane perforation and sinus lift graft outcome: a retrospective evaluation of 359 augmented sinus. J Oral Maxillofac Surg 2014;72(1):47–52.
34. Betts NJ, Miloro M. Modification of the sinus lift procedure for septa in the maxillary antrum. J Oral Maxillofac Surg 1994;52(3):332–3.
35. Urban IA, Nagursky H, Church C, et al. Incidence, diagnosis, and treatment of sinus graft infection after sinus floor elevation: a clinical study. Int J Oral Maxillofac Implants 2012;27(2):449–57.
36. Pjetursson BE, Tan WC, Zwahlen M, et al. A systematic review of the success of sinus floor elevation and survival of implants inserted in combination with sinus floor elevation. J Clin Periodontol 2008;35(Suppl 8):216–40.
37. Del Fabbro M, Testori T, Francetti L, et al. Systematic review of survival rates for implants placed in the grafted maxillary sinus. Int J Periodontics Restorative Dent 2004;24(6):565–77.
38. Del Fabbro M, Corbella S, Weinstein T, et al. Implant survival rates after osteotome-mediated maxillary sinus augmentation: a systematic review. Clin Implant Dent Relat Res 2012;14(Suppl 1):e159–68.
39. Rao GS, Reddy SK. Antral balloon sinus elevation and grafting prior to dental implant placement: review of 34 cases. Int J Oral Maxillofac Implants 2014; 29(2):414–8.
40. Petruzzi M, Ceccarelli R, Testori T, et al. Sinus floor augmentation with a hydropneumatic technique: a retrospective study in 40 patients. Int J Periodontics Restorative Dent 2012;32(2):205–10.

Surgical Techniques for Augmentation in the Horizontally and Vertically Compromised Alveolus

 CrossMark

Ladi Doonquah, MD, DDS[a],*, Ryan Lodenquai, BSc, MBBS[b], Anika D. Mitchell, BSc, MBBS[b]

KEYWORDS

- Alveolar • Bone graft • Onlay • Block • Regeneration

KEY POINTS

- Optimum wound healing is achieved with gentle manipulation of the mucoperiosteal envelope.
- In vertical augmentation the inverted L shaped block graft is most suited.
- Appropriate vector control of the transport segment is critical.
- Correct surgical technique is enhanced by the use of adjuncts such as bone morphogenic protein.

INTRODUCTION

Remarkable advances in dentistry have occurred in the twenty-first century, and the achievements are many. However, partial and complete edentulism is still a significant health care problem today, and this has major negative ramifications, both for the individuals afflicted and the wider society. The situation is even worse in a large segment of the developing world, where public dental health care is grossly inadequate or nonexistent. Despite this, patients worldwide still expect the best solutions for their problems, hence the greater utilization of implant solutions in dental health care.

This development has been driven by several factors, the major ones being improvements in technology, cost reductions, increased simplicity of the procedure,

Disclosures: The authors have nothing to disclose.
[a] Department of Surgery, Faculty of Medical Sciences, University Hospital of the West Indies, University of the West Indies - Mona, Kingston, Jamaica; [b] Department of Surgery, Faculty of Medical Sciences, University of the West Indies - Mona, Kingston, Jamaica
* Corresponding author.
E-mail address: ldoonquah@hotmail.com

Dent Clin N Am 59 (2015) 389–407
http://dx.doi.org/10.1016/j.cden.2014.10.004
0011-8532/15/$ – see front matter © 2015 Elsevier Inc. All rights reserved.

dental.theclinics.com

and greater demand from patients. However, one of the major scientific factors that have contributed to this growth is our understanding and, by extension, use of bone-grafting techniques to provide implant options to patients who previously were not candidates for this treatment modality because of inadequate bone. This article seeks to explore this realm of implant surgery, and suggests guidelines in the management of patients with deficient alveolar bone.

BIOLOGICAL PRINCIPLES

To use bone grafts efficiently, it is important to have a complete understanding of the physiology underlying bone grafting. The biological principles of autogenous bone grafting are similar to those that apply to how long bone fractures heal. The sequence of events starts with the immediate phase, followed by the development of osteogenic tissue and, finally, remodeling.

During the immediate phase, hemostasis occurs with clot formation and inflammation. Following the immediate phase, with the appropriate chemical signals, osteogenic tissue then lays down new bone material that will eventually become remodeled. These events are not distinct but actually overlap.[1]

Specific to bone grafting are 3 important terms: osteogenesis, osteoconduction, and osteoinduction.

When a graft is positioned in a donor site, it carries with it osteogenic cells, some of which survive and are able to contribute to osteoid formation. These osteogenic cells are believed to come from the periosteum (especially the cambium layer), endosteum, marrow, and intracortical structures of the graft.[1,2]

As the bone graft sits in the recipient site, it is surrounded by an inflammatory milieu, and partial bone necrosis of the graft occurs via osteoclasts. The extent and duration of osteoclastic activity depends on the nature of the bone graft (cortical vs cancellous) and, by extension, the density of the graft. Once the graft has undergone some amount of necrosis and resorption, it then acts as a scaffold for neoangiogenesis to occur within the graft. This vessel penetration of the graft allows osteogenic cells to invade the graft and create new bone formation. This series of events is termed osteoconduction (creeping substitution). During the proliferative phase of the graft take, certain molecules induce significant amounts of mitosis of osteoprogenitor cells and then direct these cells to be committed into differentiated osteoblasts. This phenomenon is called osteoinduction, and of these molecules bone morphogenic protein (BMP) is one that has been extensively studied and has been shown to have significant impact on new bone formation, particularly BMP-2, BMP-4, and BMP-7.[1–6]

Within autogenous bone grafts, the biological environment varies somewhat between cancellous and cortical graft. Cancellous grafts are less dense and, as such, the amount of necrosis and osteoclastic bone resorption necessary for vascular invasion is less. Osteoprogenitor cells are brought into and penetrate further into the graft, allowing for a more complete revascularization and replacement of bone. Owing to their dense organization, cortical grafts have to undergo more necrosis and osteoclastic activity for new vessels to permeate them. As a result of this, the extent of vascularization is less thorough, hence there is less new bone formation.

Other factors that affect bone graft survival include surgical and recipient site factors.

Surgical factors, such as graft orientation in the recipient site, are important. Having the graft's cancellous portion abutting the recipient site's cancellous segment is called orthotopic adaptation, and aids in increasing graft survival. The preservation of the periosteum of the graft is also crucial, as the cambium layer harbors significant amounts of osteoprogenitor cells.

Recipient site factors include presence of infection, previous irradiation, and whether the graft is fixed or not. Both infection and previous irradiation provide a hostile environment for the graft, which decreases the likelihood of graft take. Graft fixation is of greater importance when performing block grafting.

TYPES OF BONE GRAFTS

Bone grafts are generally categorized into autogenous and nonautogenous grafts. These 2 broad categories can then be further subdivided. The difference between them is the actual source of graft material. Autogenous bone is obtained from the individual, whereas nonautogenous is either allogenic (ie, obtained from another human being) or xenogeneic (ie, from another species).

Autogenous bone grafts are considered the gold standard for bone grafting. However, there are several factors that have driven greater consideration for the use allogenic and xenogeneic bone grafts. These issues are primarily donor site morbidity, the quantity of graft material available, and the ease of procurement in an outpatient setting.

Bone grafts can be used in the form of blocks, which may be cortical or corticocancellous, or particulate, which also can be cortical, cancellous, or a mixture of both (**Table 1**).

Block corticocancellous grafts have the advantage of bringing both cancellous and cortical bone into the recipient site. This combination gives rise to immediate structural support via its cortical component, and the cancellous part brings in tissue that allows for faster neoangiogenesis of the graft and results in a more complete revascularization, thus limiting the amount of graft resorption. Moreover, block grafts can be used to fill larger defects without requiring the use of membranes.

Cortical grafts, as mentioned earlier, provide immediate support to the recipient site without the need for a membrane to protect it. The shortcoming of cortical grafts is that they eventually undergo more resorption and tend to revascularize less thoroughly.[7]

Table 1 Predominant nature of donor bone	
Donor Site	Type
Mandibular symphysis	Corticocancellous
Mandibular ramus	Corticocancellous
Coronoid process	Cortical
Zygomatic buttress	Cortical
Maxillary tuberosity	Cancellocortical
Maxillary tori	Corticocancellous
Mandibular tori	Corticocancellous
Calvarium	Cortical
Clavicle	Cortical
Ilium	Corticocancellous
Tibia	Cancellocortical
Rib	Cancellocortical

Cancellous and corticocancellous particulate grafts can act as fillers, but generally need a barrier membrane to hold the graft in situ. Cancellous grafts have the advantage, in the setting where there is already adequate stability, of bringing material that becomes rapidly revascularized and is almost fully ossified. Particulate grafts can represent several different types of grafts; mineralized and demineralized cortical bone and mineralized and demineralized corticocancellous bone are a few examples. These types of grafts require barrier membranes to be used during grafting. In autogenous and some allogenic particulate grafts, BMPs are retained and assist in bone formation via osteoinduction.[3]

The use of allogenic bone grafts in implantology has been steadily increasing, and studies are demonstrating its consistent efficacious use. One of the major concerns about allogenic grafts is their antigenicity and the possibility of human immunodeficiency virus (HIV) transmission.[2] One particular study demonstrated no significant antigenicity in an allograft transplantation present for 30 years.[8] Some studies state that after processing an allogenic bone graft, because of better screening of donors, there is a 1 in 8,000,000 chance of the graft being infected with HIV[8,9] and that the effective rate of transmission is approximately 1 in 1,600,000 grafts, rendering the risk extremely low.[2]

Xenografts, like allografts, have been in use for some time and, like allografts, the main reasons for their use are to reduce donor site morbidity, increase the available quantity, and provide greater simplicity of procurement and use. The major type used to date is bovine bone. There has also been increased interest in the use of equine bone.[10] Several studies are emerging to indicate that xenografts can be just as successful in grafting as autogenous grafts.[11,12]

Alloplasts are natural or synthetic materials that consist of block or particulate forms of calcium-derived inorganic materials, primarily calcium phosphates, calcium sulfates, and bioactive glass. Alloplasts are used as fillers, most often combined with autogenous or allogenic bone. In more recent times, various growth factors and platelet-rich plasma (PRP) have been added to the proverbial soup. These materials provide a scaffold for the ingress of native bone-forming tissue and autogenous bone-forming cells to aid in bone production. At present their efficacy as standalone bone graft materials has not been proven.

EVALUATION OF ALVEOLAR BONE AND ADJACENT SOFT TISSUE

The magnitude and nature of the residual bone is the major determinant in deciding on the type of graft material used and from where it is obtained. The height and width of the ridge together with the inherent quality of the bone can be readily assessed with clinical examination and radiographic studies. More detailed information about the quantity and quality of the bone is readily available with the use of cone-beam computed tomography (CBCT) scanning technology. Gulsahi[13] classified the different types of alveolar bone as types 1 to 4, with type 1 being the most compact and type 4 the least dense.[13]

CHOICES OF GRAFT MATERIAL

The decision on what type of graft material to use depends on several factors. Recipient-site defect location, the extent of the size of the defect, the medical status of the patient, the patient's desires, and prosthodontic considerations are a few of the variables to consider. Autogenous donor-site harvesting can be from local, regional, or distant sites.[14]

For small to moderate size defects, local donor sites include posterior mandibular ramus, mandibular symphysis, coronoid process, and zygomatic buttress, to name a few.[15] Maxillary tuberosities and maxillary and mandibular tori can also be used.[16,17] The advantages of using these local grafts are that they can be performed as office procedures and produce minimal morbidity. A list of donor graft sites are outlined in **Table 2**.[16] The main disadvantage of using these local sites is the limited supply (see **Table 1**; **Table 2**).

Table 2 Bone donor sites		
Local	**Regional**	**Distant**
Symphysis	Clavicle	Rib
Mandibular ramus	Calvarium	Radius
Coronoid process		Tibia
Maxillary tuberosity		Ilium
Maxilla and mandibular tori		
Zygoma buttress		

There are many distant donor sites. The selection depends on the type of graft that needs to be harvested (block or particulate, cortical, corticocancellous, or cancellous) and the amount required. When large blocks are needed, most surgeons prefer the ilium. Several studies have documented that harvesting bone from the anterior ilium has a lower morbidity than was previously thought.[7] A significant amount of cancellous bone can also be obtained from the tibia with a limited amount of cortical bone and minimal side effects. It also does not require general anesthesia and can be obtained in an outpatient setting.[16] The calvarium has been used to provide long strips of cortical bone when necessary. However, harvesting of cranial bone is usually performed under general anesthesia. Smaller amounts can be obtained as an office procedure with minimal morbidity.[16] Other sites used for bone grafting include the rib and fibula.

As stated earlier, allografts and xenografts are now being used with increasing frequency, often combined with BMP and other bone growth–promoting factors. Many reports in the literature studying their use have documented their efficacy in a variety of clinical situations. Some actually show results comparable with those for autogenous grafts.[18] Further ongoing evaluation of their antigenicity and the risk of disease transmission will help to dispel some of the fears of both patients and clinicians.

SURGICAL TECHNIQUES
Suggested Bone-Grafting Protocol

There is a plethora of techniques currently used to address alveolar ridge deficiencies. The current gold standard for the type of graft material remains autogenous bone. However, other materials by themselves or in combination with autogenous bone are currently used with varying degrees of success. Several studies have even suggested that materials other than autogenous bone have a significantly greater implant success rate. Al-Nawas and Schiegnitz[18] have suggested the same in a recent European-based retrospective analysis that compared autogenous bone grafts with other materials used in sinus grafting and alveolar ridge block grafting. The reality is that with the inclusion of BMP, PRP, and other growth-promoting factors, there is greater choice for graft materials that do not involve a second surgical site, which are especially appropriate for small defects.

Achieving bone formation in defects via the innate ability of local tissues such as periosteum and the schneiderian membrane without introduction of a graft has been documented since early 2000. Lundgren and colleagues[19] described the formation of new bone in the sinus simply by doing a sinus lift. No graft material or exogenous bone growth–promoting factors were placed in the wound. A recent article by Altintas and colleagues,[20] in which a double-blind prospective study was done comparing bone formation after sinus lift with and without grafting, showed no significant difference in the amount and quality of the bone 3 months after surgery. In fact, the 6-month follow-up evaluation showed greater density of bone in the nongrafted sinus. This finding is important, not just because of the implication that clinicians may induce bone formation now and in the future without the introduction of graft material or growth-promoting factors, but also because it reinforces the need to treat the adjacent tissues gently and to preserve the potential bone-inducing areas even when graft material is being placed, as this will improve success rates.

Some grafting methods may be site specific while others can be used in most situations. However, procedures such as guided bone regeneration and especially the ridge-splitting technique do not produce predictable results in vertical defects, and are therefore restricted to horizontal defects.

Vertical augmentation remains the most challenging scenario.[16,17] Guided bone regeneration with a titanium-reinforced membrane or titanium mesh, vertical onlay block grafts, subnasal grafting, sinus lifts, LeFort I with horizontal interpositional grafts, and isolated horizontal interpositional grafts are all used to increase the height of the alveolar bone, with different degrees of success. Distraction osteogenesis however a more reliable and predictable technique to effectuate changes in the vertical dimension (**Table 3**).

The more common surgical methods used at the authors' center are: guided bone regeneration with particulate matter; ridge splitting with interpositional bone graft; onlay block bone grafting; distraction osteogenesis; LeFort maxillary downfracture with interpositional graft; subnasal graft; and mandibular sandwich osteotomy (**Fig. 1**).

The focus here is on the more frequently performed procedures. Radiographic studies, including a CBCT scan to assess the dimensions of the defect and to plan for possible donor sites, should be done. A thorough physical examination with a review of the medical history is also performed.

Table 3
Types of defects and suggested management

Horizontal Defects	Horizontal/Vertical Defects	Vertical Defects
Guided bone regeneration (GBR) with graft	GBR with graft	GBR with graft and tented membrane
Horizontal onlay corticocancellous blocks with or without membrane	Horizontal/vertical onlay block bone graft	Onlay block bone grafts
Split vertical alveolar ridge with interpositional graft	Distraction osteogenesis	Distraction osteogenesis
	Titanium mesh crib with particulate bone graft	Le Fort I with horizontal interpositional bone graft
		Titanium mesh crib with particulate bone graft

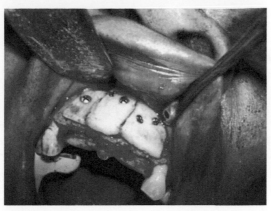

Fig. 1. Block grafts.

Implant therapy is restorative driven. Therefore, a thorough restorative workup by the restorative dentist is vital before surgery. This workup should include mounted study models and waxups of the desired location of the final restoration. This model will help in deciding the reconstructive method of choice and the graft materials to be used.

Guided bone regeneration

This technique consists of creating a mucoperiosteal envelope that will contain the graft material. A variety of incisional designs are used. The authors' standard approach is to use a crestal incision with extension around the gingival sulcus where teeth are adjacent to the defect. The vertical leg of the incision is made 1 or 2 teeth away from the defect, depending on the quality and disease status of the gingiva. The incision is limited to 1 vertical leg if possible. Extensive mobilization of the flap is then done after periosteal release incisions are made (**Figs. 2** and **3**).

The recipient bone site is slightly roughened with a large burr, then multiple small holes are made in the cancellous area. This approach serves to allow quicker and more complete integration of the donor graft material. The cavity is maintained by the graft material.

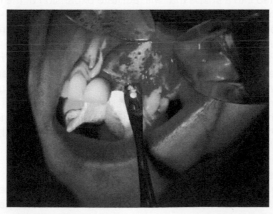

Fig. 2. Preparation of bone recipient site.

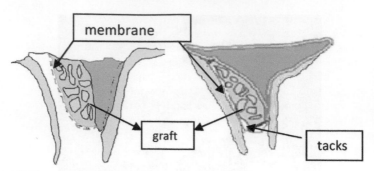

Fig. 3. Guided bone regeneration with absorbable membrane.

A membrane is fashioned to fit over the grafted bone and extend on to the native bone. It can be laid passively over the graft or fixated onto the recipient bone with tacks. The membrane most commonly used is a resorbable one. Nonresorbable membranes maintain their shape to some extent. However, they have a greater rate of dehiscence of the wound with subsequent membrane exposure, and are also more prone to infection.[21] Nonetheless, nonresorbable membranes are required if the vertical dimension of the defect needs to be increased.

The membrane serves to prevent epithelial downgrowth into the wound. This part of the process is critical, as the migration of the epithelium and connective tissue significantly decreases the amount of bony regeneration that can occur. The prevention of this migration allows the graft material along with other factors including BMP, native osteoblasts, and pluripotent cells to combine and produce new bone. The membrane also helps to maintain the soft-tissue closure above the wound and to limit bacterial entry into the wound site. Dehiscence of the wound above the membrane is also well tolerated, provided it is recognized and wound-management measures are started quickly. Several studies have documented the efficacy of these barriers to effectuate bone formation when used properly.[21]

The choice of membrane is based on the surgeon's preference, as most of them are equally efficacious. The authors use Bio-Gide (Geistlich Pharma North America Inc, Princeton, NJ, USA) or RCM6 (Collagen Matrix Inc, Oakland, NJ, USA). The graft material of choice combined with BMP, PRP, or other growth-promoting factors is placed and then compacted into a shape that will facilitate expansion of the ridge. The membrane is placed and closure of the wound is done with either 4-0 or 5-0 undyed Vicryl. Closure is achieved using a watertight technique with horizontal mattress suture and a running continuous locking suture.

For situations in which vertical enhancement is needed, titanium reinforced membranes are used, as this upholds the overlying architecture. These membranes require removal and are more prone to wound dehiscence, exposure, and subsequent infection of the overlying graft. The prosthesis is then adjusted to prevent pressure points being placed on the wound, especially in the region of the incision and graft area. Implants placed in the new grafted bone function as well as implants that are placed in native bone.[22,23]

Onlay block grafts
The flap development is similar to the one used for guided bone regeneration except that the vertical part of the incision is 3 cm away from the defect in partially dentulous patients or 2 cm from the recipient site in areas where there are no teeth. Adequate

mobilization of the overlying mucoperiosteal flap is important, because the blocks are rigid and are fixated with screws, both factors that can lead to dehiscence if there is tension in the wound envelope. The recipient osseous site is then prepared as described earlier, and two 1.5-mm screws are used to fixate each bony segment. The screws are placed via a lag-screw technique, which serves to compress the donor segment of bone onto the recipient area. It is important to place a larger width than is required, as there is some degree of resorption. However, a substantial portion of the thickness obtained is maintained at the time of reentry. The closure procedure is as stated earlier (**Figs. 4** and **5**).

When vertical or combined horizontal and vertical augmentation is required using the onlay block-grafting method, the donor bone segment is designed differently. The shape required is an inverse L, with the horizontal segment of the L placed superiorly on the ridge to facilitate greater height increase, the vertical portion lying parallel with the native bone. This positioning facilitates the holding screws being placed laterally instead of superiorly, decreasing the possibility of dehiscence over the superior portion of the wound.

Onlay block grafting is a predictable, relatively straightforward procedure that yields consistently good results. Even the lateral maxillary wall in conjunction with growth factors can be used for onlay grafting.[24] It is important to pay attention to the small details, particularly in relation to developing the overlying flap and closing the wound site.

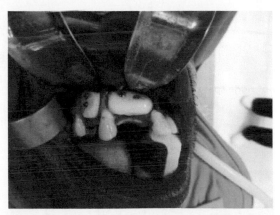

Fig. 4. Block grafting.

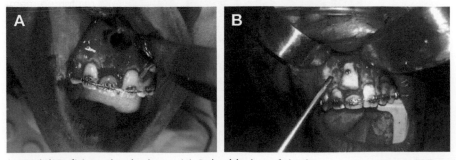

Fig. 5. (*A*) Deficient alveolar bone. (*B*) Onlay block graft in situ.

Ridge split with interpositional graft

This technique is primarily suited for smaller defects that have a minimum crestal width of 3 mm and located in the maxilla. When it was first introduced by Tatum,[25] like many new interventions the expectation for widespread use was high. Experience, however, has shown greater limitations in its applicability (**Fig. 6**).

The basic approach is a crestal incision with limited elevation of the mucoperiosteum over the area of the intended osteotomy. The rest of the periosteum is left undisturbed to provide vascularity to the expanded osseous segments. A crestal osteotomy with a very thin oscillating saw to provide initial access for the osteotomes is performed. Some clinicians prefer using piezoelectric surgery to do the osteotomy, although the authors found no difference in the outcome and the procedure took longer.[26] Sequential introduction of osteotomes starting with the smallest is then done (**Fig. 7**).

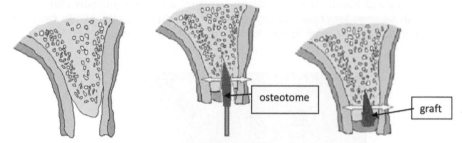

Fig. 6. Lateral view of ridge split of maxillary alveolus.

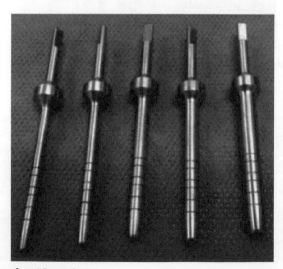

Fig. 7. Osteotomes for ridge splitting.

When adequate width is attained, a suitably sized implant can be placed and graft material placed in the adjacent defect. The authors tend to place a mixture of particulate autogenous bone and Bio-Oss (Geistlich Pharma) into the space adjacent to the implant. If the implant cannot be placed, properly shaped segments of bone are fitted into the defect and fixated with obliquely placed screws. In the authors' experience, placing particulate graft in this situation does not maintain the expanded ridge width. A split mucosal flap that leaves the periosteum intact is advanced to close the surgical site. Most studies document the importance of leaving the periosteum attached to the underlying bone. In a comparison of 3 flap types, Jensen and colleagues[27] noted significant bone loss on the buccal aspect when a full-thickness flap was raised.

Even though it is a relatively simple technique that allows for immediate placement of the implant while widening the ridge, it has limitations, especially in that the implant angulation reduces the areas where it can be used.[28]

Titanium mesh crib

A predictable, ideally shaped alveolar ridge form is a consistent desire among reconstructive surgeons. Alveolar ridge reconstruction of the severely atrophic edentulous mandible and maxilla with preformed titanium mesh trays is a method designed to achieve this result. It is a more extensive and costly intervention, however, with a high rate of dehiscence over the tray (**Fig. 8**).

This method is not new, and actually has been around for 3 decades. Boyne and colleagues[29] described utilizing a more rigid mesh tray with autogenous bone, and reported problems with dehiscence and mesh exposure. Louis and colleagues[30] used thinner, more malleable mesh trays that were tailored to the defect. Different access incisions and soft-tissue closure were suggested in a later article by Louis,[31] ostensibly to combat the tendency for mesh exposure while allowing for greater vertical and horizontal enhancement. This approach has helped to provide better outcomes.

The basic approach is outlined herein for completely edentulous maxilla and mandible. A circumvestibular incision in the mandible from the retromolar trigone to the contralateral side is performed. In the maxilla it would start from the tuberosity region, where an oblique vertical limb angled posteriorly is placed to allow greater flexibility in closing over large grafts. A mucoperiosteal flap with a wide base is raised. Care should be exercised with the lingual flap on the mandible, as the mucosa tends to be very thin and less robust in elderly patients.

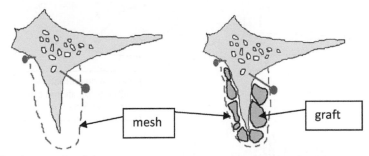

Fig. 8. Titanium mesh crib/tray.

In the maxilla it is elevated at least 1.5 to 2.0 cm above where the superior aspect of the mesh is fixated. This action also facilitates intrasinus grafting if desired. The recipient bone is prepared as previously described. The mesh tray is contoured to fit the defect, and the bone graft is compacted in the tray. The tray is then secured with screws high up on the facial aspect of the maxilla. Screws are also placed on the palatal side closer to the horizontal part. The wound is then closed as described earlier.

In the mandible the situation is a little more complicated, because the usual decreased height of the mandible and the more superior position of the mental foramen demands greater flexibility in the design and fixation of the tray. If the foramen is high, the nerve is repositioned. The recipient osseous segment is prepared, and the tray is contoured to fit the segment. The graft is compacted into the tray and fixated with screws low on the facial aspect of the mandible. Screws are also placed on the lingual side.

Le Fort I osteotomy with interpositional bone graft

Patients with long-standing edentulous maxilla are prone to develop severe atrophy with a highly pneumatized maxillary sinus, especially when the maxilla occludes with natural teeth in the mandible; this also results in a pseudo–class III occlusal relationship. For these patients The Le Fort I advancement osteotomy with interpositional bone graft augments the maxilla and corrects the jaw malocclusion in one setting. BMP and other growth factors can be added to the interpositional graft.[4]

A standard maxillary circumvestibular incision is made and a mucoperiosteal flap is elevated. A Le Fort I osteotomy with a step laterally is done. The maxilla is grafted with autogenous bone and advanced if necessary, and fixated to the superior maxilla. The ilium is the preferred donor site, as these patients require significant amounts of bone. The incision is then closed. Implants are placed in 6 months (**Fig. 9**).

Newer studies documenting minimally invasive grafting procedures using BMP in a collagen carrier are constantly stretching the boundaries to supplant these procedures now and in the near future (**Figs. 10** and **11**).[32]

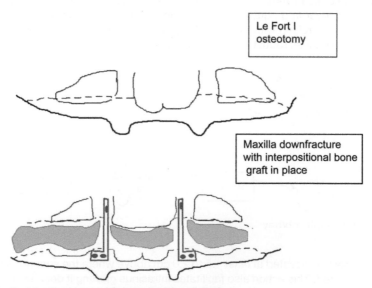

Le Fort I osteotomy

Maxilla downfracture with interpositional bone graft in place

Fig. 9. Le Fort I osteotomy with interpositional graft.

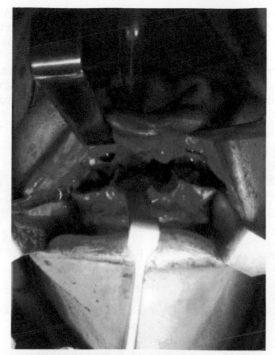

Fig. 10. Maxillary osteotomy in preparation for grafting.

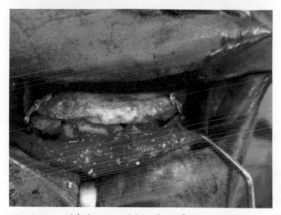

Fig. 11. Maxillary osteotomy with interpositional graft.

Distraction osteogenesis

The most reliable and long-term sustainable method to increase bone height is vertical distraction osteogenesis. McCarthy and colleagues[33] performed distraction in the facial skeleton to correct a case of hemifacial microsomia. With the experience gained, other reports surfaced illustrating the extension of this technique to smaller segments of bone, specifically alveolar bone.[34] This procedure, however, requires greater patient cooperation.

For experienced surgeons the method is predictable, reliable, and versatile, to the extent that it is being applied to nontraditional areas. Several reports in the literature have shown where bone grafts and free vascularized osseous flaps have been successfully distracted and restored with implants. Novel solutions to traditional problems such as reconstruction of the mandibular condyle have also been successfully addressed using distraction therapy **(Fig. 12)**.[35,36]

The design of the access incision depends on many factors, chief among which are the type of distractor, the segment of bone that is being distracted, and the location of the defect. Limited dissection of the mucosa overlying the segment to be distracted is performed.

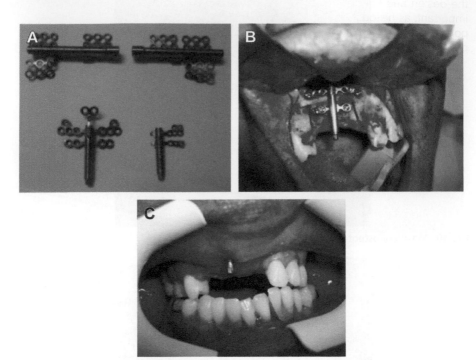

Fig. 12. (*A*) Types of distractors (to be put in place separately). (*B*) Distractor in place before activation. (*C*) Distracted segment.

The osteotomies are outlined, after which the distractor is oriented to facilitate distraction along the proper vector and the fixation holes are placed. The geometry of the vertical limbs of the transport segment must be slightly divergent as it approaches the crest, to facilitate movement of the segment. The osteotomy is then performed using very thin saw blades. The segment is then fractured from the basal bone. The distractor arm is reapplied and the segment is distracted to make sure there is no impediment to transport.

A recurring challenge for the surgeon is to have the distractor limb positioned to be effective but to not impede any prosthesis that the patient is wearing. It is also necessary to camouflage the distractor limb when it is in the anterior maxilla.

There is a period of latency of approximately 5 to 7 days during which the callous is allowed to form before distraction. Various suggestions exist in the literature as to the rhythm and frequency of moving the segment.[37–39] At the authors' center the protocol is 0.5 mm twice daily. When the result has been reached the distractor is kept in place for 12 weeks, after which it is removed and the implants placed.

The distraction appliances are becoming smaller, with removable arms and other innovations. Some researchers are investigating appliances that are activated via electronic sensors and that change angulation to adjust vector direction on command.

Management of the soft-tissue envelope is crucial to the favorable outcome of alveolar ridge reconstruction regardless of which technique is used. This aspect refers to the design of the access incision and the various release incisions used to expand the mucoperiosteal envelope. Delicate handling of the tissue intraoperatively is also crucial. Vertical distraction osteogenesis, in particular, demands greater attention to detail in the design and handling of the overlying mucoperiosteum. This factor is especially important, as histogenesis is occurring simultaneously with osteogenesis. The egress points where the distractor limbs exit the soft-tissue space also have to be placed to prevent exposure of the callus and underlying transport segment (**Figs. 13** and **14**).

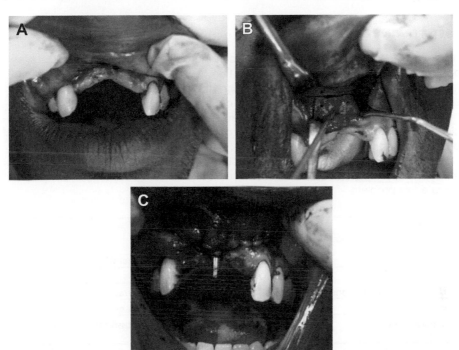

Fig. 13. (*A*) Vertical defect of maxilla. (*B*) Osteotomy in preparation for distraction. (*C*) Distractor in place and wound closed.

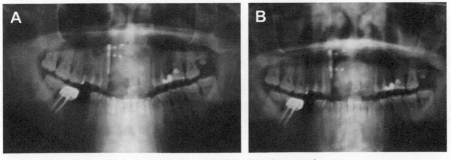

Fig. 14. (*A*) Distractor before activation. (*B*) Segment distracted.

COMPLICATIONS

The predictability and reliability of bone graft procedures has increased significantly in recent times, although unforeseen results still occur. Prompt recognition and early intervention is critical for successful management of complications. There are 3 main categories: intraoperative, early postoperative, and late postoperative complications.

OPERATIVE COMPLICATIONS

Once the complication has been recognized, early decisive treatment should be initiated. Managing some of the problems can be tricky and may require more watching and waiting than operative intervention, and experience helps to guide this decision (**Table 4**).

POSTOPERATIVE CARE

A successful surgical reconstruction can be compromised by poor postsurgical management. Several factors can contribute to this. Wound dehiscence, recipient-site hematoma, trauma to the tissue overlying the graft, improper choice of sutures, and poor suturing techniques are some of the more common considerations.

Wound dehiscence, a frequent but preventable occurrence, is due primarily to closure under tension, injudicious handling of the overlying flap, and pressure exerted by an overlying prosthesis.

Hematomas are a death knell for particulate grafts and must be evacuated in a timely fashion. Proper hemostatic measures before closing the wound will help to obviate this problem.

Table 4
Major operative complications

Intraoperative	Early Postoperative	Late Postoperative
Bleeding	Hematoma	Infection
Fracture of recipient bone	Bleeding	Soft-tissue trauma
Damage to soft tissues	Wound dehiscence	Exposure of graft
Damage to nerves	Damage to soft tissues	Premature ossification of distracted callus
	Distractor malfunction	Resorption of transport segment
		Distractor malfunction
		Vector malalignment

DISCUSSION

The decision to rebuild deficient bone requires a clear knowledge of the likely outcome. Dealing with isolated horizontal defects affords greater choices. Combined defects are more problematic. Vertical deficiencies represent the most challenging alveolar reconstruction scenario. Several procedures have been outlined for the management of such defects. The choices are guided by local factors related to the amount and type of the defect, systemic factors such as the medical status of the patient, and regional factors such as the location of the donor site. It is important to realize that each treatment decision has to be tailored to the particular individual situation. Often the suggested treatment options are based on the clinician's skills or lack thereof, which compromises the results that can be obtained. Simple solutions that are evidence based must be the guiding principle, but the ability to offer and perform complicated procedures when they are needed is a requirement to providing the full spectrum of solutions for patients.

FUTURE DIRECTIONS

The fields of biotechnology and tissue engineering are undergoing rapid advances that will make complex bone-grafting reconstructive surgery a thing of the past. Even now, innovative procedures using BMP and other bone growth factors, minimally invasive techniques, and newer implant placement methods are decreasing the number of invasive procedures being performed.[40] Studies involving 3-dimensional printing of defect subunits, and collagen scaffolds that are impregnated with more efficacious bone growth–stimulating factors, are currently under way. Regenerative science is undergoing tremendous advances that in the not too distant future will allow us to regrow missing anatomic segments from our own stem cells. These advances will only continue to accelerate in the future, and augur well for the successful management of our patients.

SUMMARY

Reconstruction of dental alveolar bone is a cornerstone of dental implantology that has allowed almost any patient to be a candidate for implants. The methods and materials available continue to increase exponentially. The science is continually evolving and allowing for greater simplicity even as it explores new frontiers. The dental community must continue to embrace this direction, and with a team approach will ensure that no patient who needs dental implants is left behind.

REFERENCES

1. McKibbin B. The biology of fracture healing in long bones. J Bone Joint Surg Br 1978;60-B(2):150–62.
2. Oppenheimer AJ, Tong L, Buchman SR. Craniofacial bone grafting: Wolff's law revisited. Craniomaxillofac Trauma Reconstr 2008;1(1):49–61.
3. Dimitriou R, Jones E, McGonagle D, et al. Bone regeneration: current concepts and future directions. BMC Med 2011;9:66.
4. Jensen OT, Cottam JR, Ringeman JL, et al. Experience with bone morphogenetic protein-2 and interpositional grafting of edentulous maxillae: a comparison of Le Fort I downfracture to full-arch (horseshoe) segmental osteotomy done in conjunction with sinus floor grafting. Int J Oral Maxillofac Implants 2013;28(6):e331–48.
5. Jensen OT, Cottam J, Ringeman J, et al. Trans-sinus dental implants, bone morphogenetic protein 2, and immediate function for all-on-4 treatment of severe maxillary atrophy. J Oral Maxillofac Surg 2012;70(1):141–8.
6. Urist MR. Bone: formation by autoinduction. Science 1965;150(3698):893–9.
7. Rawashdeh MA, Telfah H. Secondary alveolar bone grafting: the dilemma of donor site selection and morbidity. Br J Oral Maxillofac Surg 2008;46(8):665–70.
8. Acocella A, Bertolai R, Ellis E 3rd, et al. Maxillary alveolar ridge reconstruction with monocortical fresh-frozen bone blocks: a clinical, histological and histomorphometric study. J Craniomaxillofac Surg 2012;40(6):525–33.
9. Boyce T, Edwards J, Scarborough N. Allograft bone. The influence of processing on safety and performance. Orthop Clin North Am 1999;30(4):571–81.

10. Kim TI, Chung CP, Heo MS, et al. Periodontal regeneration capacity of equine particulate bone in canine alveolar bone defects. J Periodontal Implant Sci 2010;40(5):220–6.

11. Benlidayi ME, Tatli U, Kurkcu M, et al. Comparison of bovine-derived hydroxyapatite and autogenous bone for secondary alveolar bone grafting in patients with alveolar clefts. J Oral Maxillofac Surg 2012;70(1):e95–102.

12. Block MS, Ducote CW, Mercante DE. Horizontal augmentation of thin maxillary ridge with bovine particulate xenograft is stable during 500 days of follow-up: preliminary results of 12 consecutive patients. J Oral Maxillofac Surg 2012; 70(6):1321–30.

13. Gulsahi A. Bone quality assessment for dental implants. In: Implant dentistry. 2011.

14. Lekholm U. Patient selection and preparation. In: Tissue-integrated prosthesis: osseointegration in clinical dentistry. 1985. p. 199–209.

15. De Riu G, Meloni MS, Pisano M, et al. Mandibular coronoid process grafting for alveolar ridge defects. Oral Surg Oral Med Oral Pathol Oral Radiol 2012;114(4): 430–6.

16. Louis PJ. Bone grafting the mandible. Dent Clin North Am 2011;55(4):673–95.

17. Misch CM. Maxillary autogenous bone grafting. Dent Clin North Am 2011;55(4): 697–713.

18. Al-Nawas B, Schiegnitz E. Augmentation procedures using bone substitute materials or autogenous bone—a systematic review and meta-analysis. Eur J Oral Implantol 2014;7(2):219–34.

19. Lundgren S, Andersson S, Gualini F, et al. Bone reformation with sinus membrane elevation: a new surgical technique for maxillary sinus floor augmentation. Clin Implant Dent Relat Res 2004;6(3):165–73.

20. Altintas NY, Senel FC, Kayipmaz S, et al. Comparative radiologic analyses of newly formed bone after maxillary sinus augmentation with and without bone grafting. J Oral Maxillofac Surg 2013;71(9):1520–30.

21. Wang HL, Carroll MJ. Guided bone regeneration using bone grafts and collagen membranes. Quintessence Int 2001;32(7):504–15.

22. Al-Khaldi N, Sleeman D, Allen F. Stability of dental implants in grafted bone in the anterior maxilla: longitudinal study. Br J Oral Maxillofac Surg 2011;49(4): 319–23.

23. Clementini M, Morlupi A, Agrestini C, et al. Immediate versus delayed positioning of dental implants in guided bone regeneration or onlay graft regenerated areas: a systematic review. Int J Oral Maxillofac Surg 2013;42(5):643–50.

24. Anitua E, Alkhraisat MH, Miguel-Sanchez A, et al. Surgical correction of horizontal bone defect using the lateral maxillary wall: outcomes of a retrospective study. J Oral Maxillofac Surg 2014;72(4):683–93.

25. Tatum H Jr. Maxillary and sinus implant reconstructions. Dent Clin North Am 1986; 30(2):207–29.

26. Danza M, Guidi R, Carinci F. Comparison between implants inserted into piezo split and unsplit alveolar crests. J Oral Maxillofac Surg 2009;67(11):2460–5.

27. Jensen OT, Cullum DR, Baer D. Marginal bone stability using 3 different flap approaches for alveolar split expansion for dental implants: a 1-year clinical study. J Oral Maxillofac Surg 2009;67(9):1921–30.

28. Misch CM. Implant site development using ridge splitting techniques. Oral Maxillofac Surg Clin North Am 2004;16(1):65–74, vi.

29. Boyne PJ, Cole MD, Stringer D, et al. A technique for osseous restoration of deficient edentulous maxillary ridges. J Oral Maxillofac Surg 1985;43(2):87–91.

30. Louis PJ, Gutta R, Said-Al-Naief N, et al. Reconstruction of the maxilla and mandible with particulate bone graft and titanium mesh for implant placement. J Oral Maxillofac Surg 2008;66(2):235–45.
31. Louis PJ. Vertical ridge augmentation using titanium mesh. Oral Maxillofac Surg Clin North Am 2010;22(3):353–68, v.
32. Urban IA, Jovanovic SA, Lozada JL. Vertical ridge augmentation using guided bone regeneration (GBR) in three clinical scenarios prior to implant placement: a retrospective study of 35 patients 12 to 72 months after loading. Int J Oral Maxillofac Implants 2009;24(3):502–10.
33. McCarthy JG, Schreiber J, Karp N, et al. Lengthening the human mandible by gradual distraction. Plast Reconstr Surg 1992;89(1):1–8 [discussion: 9–10].
34. Chin M, Toth BA. Distraction osteogenesis in maxillofacial surgery using internal devices: review of five cases. J Oral Maxillofac Surg 1996;54(1):45–53 [discussion: 54].
35. Stucki-McCormick SU, Fox RM, Mizrahi RD. Reconstruction of a neocondyle using transport distraction osteogenesis. Semin Orthod 1999;5(1):59–63.
36. Schwartz HC. Transport distraction osteogenesis for reconstruction of the ramus-condyle unit of the temporomandibular joint: surgical technique. J Oral Maxillofac Surg 2009;67(10):2197–200.
37. White SH, Kenwright J. The timing of distraction of an osteotomy. J Bone Joint Surg Br 1990;72(3):356–61.
38. Kessler PA, Merten HA, Neukam FW, et al. The effects of magnitude and frequency of distraction forces on tissue regeneration in distraction osteogenesis of the mandible. Plast Reconstr Surg 2002;109(1):171–80.
39. Batal HS, Cottrell DA. Alveolar distraction osteogenesis for implant site development. Oral Maxillofac Surg Clin North Am 2004;16(1):91–109, vii.
40. Boyne PJ, Marx RE, Nevins M, et al. A feasibility study evaluating rhBMP-2/absorbable collagen sponge for maxillary sinus floor augmentation. Int J Periodontics Restorative Dent 1997;17(1):11–25.

Autogenous Bone Harvest for Implant Reconstruction

Avichai Stern, DDS, Golaleh Barzani, DMD*

KEYWORDS

- Autogenous bone harvest • Intra-oral donor sites • Extra oral donor sites
- Anterior iliac crest bone harvest • Comparison of intra-oral harvest sites
- Autogenous bone • Xenograft • Allograft

KEY POINTS

- Autogenous bone harvest is the gold standard for restoring deficiencies of the recipient site.
- A deficient site requires adequate grafting before placement of implants; therefore, proper understanding of grafting options is a key to successfully planned implant dentistry.
- General dentists require an understanding of autogenous bone harvest and variety of techniques available to provide the best outcomes for the patient.

INTRODUCTION

Bone volume deficit in completely edentulous and partially edentulous patients creates both surgical and prosthetic challenges in implant dentistry. Placement of endosseous implants in a location with inadequate alveolar bone leads commonly to disappointing results for both the patient and the provider. In severe atrophic cases, compromised bony structure prevents placement of endosseous implants. The cosmetic and functional success of dental implant reconstruction depends on proper and adequate restoration of bony structure contour, continuity, and volume. In this article, we introduce the reader to basic concepts in alveolar bone reconstruction using autogenous bone, including biology, donor sites, technique, risks, and common complications.[1,2]

Autogenous Bone Versus Other Sources (Xenograft, Allograft, Alloplast)

The ideal bone graft should possess 3 qualities: osteoconductivity, osteoinductivity, and existing osteogenic cells. The presence of an osteoconductive matrix allows for vascular ingrowth and migration of osteoprogenitor cells into the graft site. This matrix can be composed of biologic or nonbiologic material and often is resorbed during the

The authors have nothing to disclose.
Oral and Maxillofacial Surgery Training Program, The Brooklyn Hospital Center, 121 Dekalb ave, Brooklyn, NY 11201, USA
* Corresponding author.
E-mail address: gbarzani@gmail.com

bone maturation process. Osteoinductivity speaks to the ability of graft components to stimulate native tissues to produce and/or recruit osteogenic cells. The presence of existing osteogenic cells in the grafted tissue allows for earlier de novo bone formation in the grafted tissue than if those cells were not present.[1,2]

There are several possible sources for obtaining graft material for bone reconstruction. Allogeneic bone is donated cadaveric human bone. Potential donors are pre-screened for communicable diseases and all bone that is ultimately donated is heat sterilized and freeze dried to remove all biologic components. This process, although it minimizes the potential for disease transmission and graft rejection, also eliminates the bone's osteoinductive capacity and osteogenic cells. The graft retains its utility by functioning as an osteogenic scaffold. Xenograft material obtained from another species behaves similarly because all biologic material is eliminated during processing. A xenograft may be indicated over allogeneic bone in certain circumstances owing to its greater longevity. Alloplastic materials such as calcium sulfate, calcium phosphate and hydroxyapatite (S + A coral) are nonbiologic and have no intrinsic osteoinductive properties or osteogenic potential; however, they are biocompatible and function as an osteoconductive scaffold. Recombinant human bone morphogenic protein (BMP) 2 is a bioengineered version of a potent osteoinductive cytokine generally produced during normal bone healing. After reconstitution, the protein is delivered via a sponge to the proposed graft site. Although recombinant human BMP 2 is powerfully osteoinductive, the delivery medium has no bulk and therefore has no osteoconductive properties.[1,2]

Autogenous bone is the gold standard material for bone grafting. Autogenous bone is the only graft material that contains intrinsic osteogenic potential through the always present osteoprogenitor cells. Naturally present BMP is the source of osteoinduction in living bone grafts. Of course, regardless of whether the graft used is cortical or cancellous, the solid nature of the graft provides an osteoconductive medium through which vascular ingrowth can occur and over which new bone growth can take place. The cellular and molecular elements that accompany autogenous bone graft serve multiple purposes. The first advantage is that the osteoconductive scaffolding recruits osteoprogenitor cells. This osteoconduction makes the autogenous graft more reliable and predictable. The second advantage of the autogenous bone graft is owing to its osteoinductive qualities derived from the molecular growth factors embedded in the autogenous graft. These factors include fibroblasts growth factors, transforming growth factor beta 1, vascular endothelial growth factor, and the BMP. These factors play an important role in new bone formation. This article discusses some of the most common autogenous sites for bone graft harvest and provides a guide for general practitioners. Each option carries its own limitations, such as volume constraints, donor site morbidity, and patient comfort.[1,2]

To review, alloplasts, xenografts, and autografts all have osteoconductive properties; recombinant human BMP has osteoinductive properties. However, only autogenous bone grafts possess osteogenic potential and osteconductive and osteoinductive properties.[1,2]

CORTICAL BONE: INDICATIONS AND DONOR SITES

Cortical bone grafts contain a rigid lamellar architecture that does not deform with compression or tension. This unique feature allows rigid fixation of the graft in high stress areas. Owing to its high concentration of BMP, it enhances osteoinductive properties of the graft. However, owing to the lamellar architecture of the cortical bone, it does not possess a high concentration of osteocompetent cells; therefore, maintenance of viable osteoblasts or osteoprogenitor cells becomes difficult. Cortical bone, owing to its high lamellar concentration, has little surface area and is more susceptible to infection. It is absolutely crucial to maintain the soft tissue coverage over the graft. In the event that soft tissue cover is compromised, graft viability will be lost.[2]

Onlay

Cortical blocks of bone are the most common form of onlay graft. Cortical blocks offer the benefit of the onlay autogenous bone grafting, a simple and well-used method that is successful and predictable if basic concepts are used and followed properly. Onlay grafts can be segmental or arched. These grafts can be used to restore both height and width of an atrophic and deficient area. These grafts are routinely used in maxilla and mandible in preparation of the site for implant placement. Indications for using the onlay cortical graft is as follows[2]:

1. Inadequate residual alveolar ridge height and width to provide support for a functional prosthesis
2. Contour defects that compromise implant support, function, and esthetics
3. Segmental alveolar bone loss.

Graft healing

The most crucial operator-dependent steps in the survival of the graft are achieving graft stability and obtaining primary closure over the graft. It is not recommended to place the implant in the graft alone, because this is associated with a high failure rate. Therefore, a staged procedure is recommended to achieve better implant positioning after graft consolidation.

Management of graft tissue, preparation, and placement

The mucoperiosteal flap is designed in a way to adequately expose the underlying, deficient recipient site and maintain a base for vascular support and a tension-free primary closure. Usually, a midcrestal incision is preferred because it maximizes the vascularity to the margins of the flap and will minimize the ischemia. Labial vertical releases are made as needed for access. After exposing the entire alveolar process, gross bony irregularities should be made smooth to allow for maximum adaptation to the underlying alveolus. It is important that the size and contour of the graft be limited to what is needed to support the implants. Oversized or undersized grafts complicate soft tissue closure and interfere with planned prosthetic reconstruction. Upon completion of the grafting procedure, all voids and defects should be filled with particulate cancellous bone and marrow to provide good contour and to eliminate the dead space between the graft and recipient site. A primary, tension-free closure must be achieved to prevent wound breakdown and graft exposure, which will cause graft failure.[2]

Risks, common complications, and management

1. Graft exposure owing to poor primary closure
2. Graft mobility
3. Donor site morbidity
4. Oversized or undersized graft
5. Infection
6. Poor osseous contact between graft and the recipient site[2]

Cancellous Bone: Indications and Donor Sites

Cancellous bones have a wide scope of use because they can be placed within variety of alloplastic and allogenic materials, as well as reconstructive plates without any special instrumentation, long hospitalization, or high costs. Survival of harvested cancellous cellular bone allows the surgeon to transplant viable osteocompetent cells in to a well-vascularized tissue bed, ultimately resulting in a well-consolidated bone graft. Cancellous bone grafts respond favorably and predictably to transplantation as long as the recipient tissue bed is able to provide the metabolic needs of the implanted graft placed. Cancellous bone can be used in variety of procedures, such as socket preservation and sinus floor elevation grafting.[2,3]

Socket Preservation

Cancellous bone can be used to preserve extraction sockets after an extraction in preparation for future implant placement. Extraction socket can be preserved and grafted by packing a mixture of alloplastic, allogenic, and/or xenograft bone. Gel foam or collaplug can be placed over the extraction socket to secure the graft material. One figure-of-8 suture can be placed with a 3.0 silk suture to secure the graft material. The extraction socket can be revisited in 3 to 4 months for placement of an endousseous implant.

Sinus Floor Elevation Graft

Cancellous bone can routinely be used for sinus floor augmentation. Mixture of autogenous cancellous, allogenic, and/or alloplastic bone could be used for sinus augmentation. After grafting, and average of 4 to 6 months is needed for proper graft maturation before implant placement.

a. *Onlay.* Cancellous bone can be used to fill in the osseous gaps in onlay grafting.
b. *Ridge split.* Cancellous bone can be used to fill in the osseous gaps in a split ridge.

Graft healing

In the late 19th and early 20th centuries, 2 conflicting theories of cancellous cellular bone healing existed. One was the osteoblastic theory, which originated with Ollier in 1867 and Axhausen in 1909. This theory was based on the belief that bone marrow and the periosteum survived implantation and produced bone. The induction theory originally by Phemister's creeping substitution theory in 1914, which was expanded by Urist in 1953, held that transplanted bone did not survive the trauma of harvest. This theory proposed that the entire graft underwent an aseptic necrosis and was replaced by bone produced the connective tissue stem cells of the host–recipient bed or host–bone ends. Bone necrosis was linked with new bone formation. It is now known that the osteoblastic and induction theories of cancellous bone are not mutually exclusive. Current concept of cancellous cellular bone graft healing involves a 2-phased theory.[3]

MANAGEMENT OF GRAFT TISSUE, PREPARATION, AND PLACEMENT

Preparation of the recipient tissue bed to optimize quantity and quality, milling the bone and compacting it into the recipient tissue bed to increase cellular density in the graft, and precise stabilization of the graft can improve the quantity of bone produced by the graft, as well as the length of time it lasts.[3]

Donor Sites

Oral donor sites

Intraoral autogenous bone has been commonly used for reconstruction of maxillofacial defects in preparation for implant placement. Intraoral donor sites have multiple advantages compared with distant donor sites: these sites are easily accessible, have a low cost, and are associated with low morbidity. The amount of harvested bone varies among each intraoral donor site. This article discusses each site in detail.

Ramus

Bone type
Ramus is 100% cortical bone. Ramus grafts can be used for horizontal or vertical ridge augmentation in maxilla or mandible and, less commonly, for sinus lifts or for osteotomy separations in orthognathic surgery (**Fig. 1**).[4,5]

Potential yield
Ramus can augment an atrophic bone by 3 to 4 mm in horizontal and vertical dimensions. Up to 3 to 4 tooth edentulous sites can be augmented with a thickness of 2 to 4.5 mm, with an average augmentation of 3 to 4 mm. Ramus provides a thin cortical block of cortical bone approximately 3 × 5 cm for onlay grafting with maximum size of 0.4 × 3 × 5 cm. Ramus provides the greatest average surface area and volume (×2) compared with symphysis or other intraoral harvest sites.[4,5]

Risks and benefits
The benefit of this procedure is that the donor site is close to the recipient site and harvest can be performed in an outpatient setting. The area of retrievable cortical bone is typically sufficient to reconstruct a 3- to 4-cm alveolar segment or multiple smaller areas. Ramus graft provides the greatest average surface area; its volume is almost double compared with symphysis or other intraoral harvest sites.

Risks associated with the ramus graft include, but are not limited to, inferior alveolar nerve and/or lingual nerve injury, hematoma, infection, fracture, and trismus. It is important to exercise caution if impacted mandibular third molars are located directly in the harvest site or if there is a previous history of ramus injury, bisphosphonate use, or radiation therapy.[4,5]

Techniques
Various techniques have been proposed to reduce the risk of injury to the inferior alveolar nerve or the mandibular structure. The osteotomy dimensions are: a superior cut is made on the external oblique along the anterior border of the ramus approximately one third of the width of the mandible. Anteriorly, the cut is made on the distal half of the first molar. In the posterior dimension, it extends to the extent of the lingual. Inferior cut should be made 4 mm above the border of mandible. The medial cut is made through the lateral cortex. Once the border of the osteotomy is outlined, it can be completed with use of chisel and mallet (**Fig. 2**). The clinician should take care to avoid

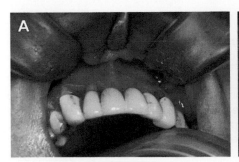 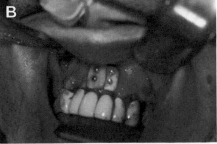

Fig. 1. (*A*) Hypoplastic maxilla. (*B*) Onlay block graft to deficient maxilla.

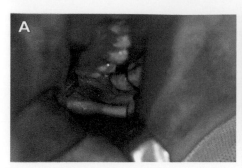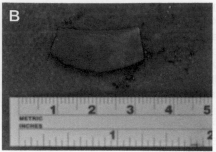

Fig. 2. (*A*) Lateral ramus bone harvest. (*B*) Cortical block graft.

injury to inferior alveolar nerve by angling the chisel toward buccal surface. Postoperative management includes precautions of soft food and ice to the harvest site for the first 24 to 48 hours, as well as use of antibiotics and no heavy or strenuous activity for 2 to 3 weeks.[1,4,5]

Piezo versus rotary versus osteotome

I. Piezosurgery offers the benefits of lower risk to the inferior alveolar nerve.
II. A combination of high speed, rear vented rotary used to score the cortical bone and an osteotome is another common technique. This technique is intended to protect the nerve as well, at a much lower cost. Osteotomes are variably tolerated by patients and patient anxiety may be a relative contraindication to its use.
III. Regardless of technique, after harvest the margins of the site should be debrided of sharp edges and bone splinters. The site should be irrigated with copious normal saline and local hemostatic measures should be applied if necessary. Neurotoxic hemostatic materials should be avoided.
IV. Recipient site management is the same as discussed in the Ramus section.

Tuberosity

Bone type
The tuberosity is an autogenous cancellous marrow graft suitable for small defects.

Yield
The tuberosity is good for socket grafting, small sinus lift, and to fill in small osteotomy gaps. It contains limited amount of bone (between 1 and 3 mL). In patients older than 50 years of age, the tuberosity becomes very fatty and therefore does not provide a good source of osteogenic cells.[6]

Piezo versus rotary versus osteotome
Either osteotome could be used for the harvest, although the piezo osteotome provides a much safer instrument for harvest of the maxillary tuberosity.

Risks and benefits
One of the complications associated with this procedure is entry to maxillary sinus resulting in a oroantral communication. Bleeding from the posterior superior alveolar artery or the sphenopalatine is another potential complication resulting from this intraoral harvest site. Another postoperative complication, although rare, is periostitis, which can result from sharp edges of the harvest site causing injury to the periosteum.[2,6]

Technique and donor site management
Access can be achieved by a midcrest incision made in the humular notch extended to second molar area. A rongeur is used to remove bone from the tuberosity, allowing for a 2-mm clearance from the sinus. The site can then be closed using primary closure with a resorbable suture. In the event of oroantral communication, a buccal sliding flap, buccal fat pad, or palatal finger flap can be used to obtain closure. No dressing is necessary.[2,6]

Symphysis

Bone type
The symphysis provides primarily cortical bone, but soft cortical and cancellous bone are also found.

Yield
The symphysis provides the thickest portion of mandible and the greatest amount of cancellous bone among the other intraoral harvest sites. A corticocancellous block of approximately 1.5 × 6 cm can be harvested from the midline. If it is harvested from each side of the midline, paramedian harvest can yield two 1.5 × 3-cm corticocancellous blocks with maximum amount available recorded as 0.7 × 1.5 × 6 cm. In block form, it can be used for horizontal and or vertical ridge augmentation or for osteotomy gaps during orthognathic surgery. If it is used as a source of cancellous bone, harvested from this site can be used for sinus augmentation.

Risks and benefits
The symphysis has lower associated morbidity compared with ramus and provides the largest intraoral source of cancellous bone. Morbidity associated with bone harvest from the symphysis region includes altered sensation to lower anterior teeth, periapical defects, altered sensation to lower lip and chin, and defects in chin contour. Review of literature shows that 30% of patients experienced symptoms 1 week postoperatively, but most resolved within 1 month after the surgery. Based on the study by Deatherage and colleagues,[1] only 13% of patients had continued altered sensation and the most common persistent symptoms were paresthesia of lower lip and chin followed by anesthesia of lower anterior teeth.

Technique and donor site management
An incision is made through the labial mucosa 1 cm apical to the junction between the attached gingiva and unattached mucosa, from canine to canine. The incision should extend from posterior aspect of 1 canine to the other. Care should be taken to avoid injury to the labial branch of the mental nerve. When the nerve is identified, the incision is then deepened through the mentalis muscle. It is important to not strip mentalis muscle to prevent the postoperative complication of chin ptosis. At this time and with direct visualization of the buccal cortex, osteotomies can be made. The dimensions of the osteotomy are as follows: in dentate mandible, the superior dimension of the osteotomy is 5 mm apical to the root apices. In edentulous mandible, a superior osteotomy can be made 5 mm from the crest of alveolar ridge. An inferior osteotomy can be made 4 mm superior to the inferior border of mandible. The lateral extension should not be closer than 5 mm anterior to the mental foramen. After the harvest is complete, special care must be taken to reposition and close the mentalis muscle as accurately as possible. Resorbable sutures, such as 3.0 chromic or 3.0 Vicryl sutures, can be used. A chin dressing needs to be applied postoperatively with fluffed spunges over the chin prominence followed by elastic tape with crossover slits. This dressing prevents hematoma formation and help readapt the soft tissues.[1]

Miscellaneous sources of autogenous bone

a. *Lateral maxilla.* The lateral maxilla could be used to obtain morselized cortical bone. The site can be scraped by using a bone scraper. There is no literature on the amount of bone obtained from lateral maxilla, but it varies depending on patient's native bone and the clinician. Different instruments could be used to remove the bone from lateral maxilla. A simple bone scraper or piezo drill could be used to scrape the bone from lateral maxilla. There are minimal risks associated with this procedure. Risks involved are those associated with every surgical procedure and include but are not limited to bleeding, infection, and edema at the surgical site. Bone harvest from the lateral maxilla involves minimal risk for the donor site and could be used more frequently for grafting extraction sockets in preparation for implant placement.

b. *Implant osteotomy* sites can also be used as a source for cortical bone graft. Implant drill or trephine bur can be used to remove a block of bone from the osteotomy site. This bone can be used for grafting of dehiscence or perforation on placement of implants or as socket preservation for future implant placement. There are minimal risks associated with this procedure. Risks involved are those associated implant placement including but not limited to bleeding, infection, edema, injury to the nerve, and sinus perforation. Bone harvest from an implant osteotomy site involves minimal risk for the donor site and could be used more frequently.

COMPARISON OF INTRAORAL SITES

Intraoral harvest sites are a good source of autogenous bone with low donor morbidity, good patient satisfaction, and very good clinical results. Multiple papers compare the volume of bone obtained from each of these intraoral sites and they collectively agree that ramus provides the greatest volume of bone and the greatest amount of cortical bone compared with other intraoral sites.

The symphysis provides the second largest intraoral harvest site and it has much less associated morbidity compared with ramus. The symphysis provides the largest cancellous source among the intraoral sites.

The lateral maxilla and the implant osteotomy provide minimal bone.[1,5]

DISTANT DONOR SITES
Anterior Iliac Crest

Bone type

Bone harvested from the anterior iliac crest has been shown to contain the greatest concentration of osteogenic cells compared with other autogenous sites. The total volume of osteoprogenitor cells present is inversely proportional to the age of the patient. This autogenous source provides both cortical and cancellous bone. The anterior iliac crest has a marrow compartment that begins 1 cm posterior to the anterior superior iliac spine.[1,7]

Yield

An anterior iliac crest bone graft will yield about 50 mL of uncompressed particulate cancellous bone or up to a 2 × 6-cm piece (average of 13.5 cm^3) of corticocancellous block graft (**Fig. 3**).[1,7]

Risks and benefits

Anterior iliac crest harvesting can be performed potentially in an outpatient setting. The anterior iliac crest often requires a second surgical team or site and it provides

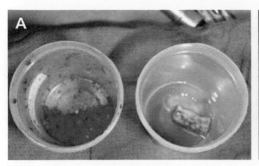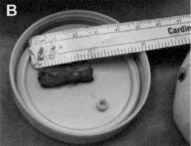

Fig. 3. (*A*) Cortical and cancellous bone harvested from anterior iliac crest. (*B*) Cortical bone harvested from the anterior iliac crest.

less bone than the posterior iliac crest. Potential complications of autogenous iliac crest bone graft are gait disturbances, instability of sacroiliac joints, infection, blood loss, nerve injury (painful neuropathy of the lateral femoral cutaneous nerve), peritoneal perforation, adynamic ileus, hematoma, ureteral injury, and pelvic fracture.[1,7]

Technique
The surgical site is prepped and draped in sterile fashion, leaving the anterior part of the crest and the anterior superior iliac spine accessible. The skin is stretched medially over the iliac crest before the incision is made. This maneuver avoids possible irritation of the scar from tight-fitting clothes and provides a more esthetic scar. The incision is started 1 cm behind the anterior superior iliac spine and continued posteriorly, following the iliac crest. The medial cortical plate of the ilium is then exposed by reflecting the iliac muscle subperiosteally. A corticocancellous bone block is then harvested by making vertical and horizontal cuts with an osteotome. Cancellous bone can be harvested using bone currettes. Harvested bone should be kept in cold saline until it is ready for use. The cartilaginous cap is reapproximated with resorbable sutures, a microfibrillar collagen (eg, Aviten) is placed in the bony cavity for hemostatic purposes, and the site is closed in layers. A Jackson–Pratt drain may be placed through a separate incision superficial to the perieosteol closure if needed (**Fig. 4**).[1,7]

Postoperative and donor site management
Patients are immobilized for 24 hours postoperatively and then guided in their rehabilitation by a physiotherapist. Patients are advised to walk with 2 crutches during the first 2 weeks and 1 crutch during the next 2 weeks. All patients undergoing anterior iliac crest bone harvest should receive routine antibiotics and steroids postoperatively.

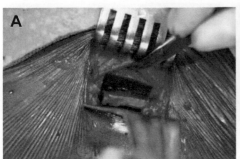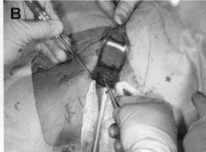

Fig. 4. (*A*) Autogenous iliac crest bone graft osteotomy. (*B*) Cancellous bone harvest.

It is also recommended that patients receive thrombosis prophylaxis. The average length of hospitalization depends on how quickly patients are able to return to function and it varies between 0-2 days.[1,7]

Tibial Plateau

Bone type
The tibial plateau provides cancellous bone that is adequate bone for grafting with a low incidence of complications. None of the complications of tibial bone graft are considered long term.[8]

Yield
Use of tibia as a donor site can obtain up to 42 mL of uncompressed cancellous bone (**Fig. 5**D).[8]

Risks and benefits
Tibial bone graft sites heal exceptionally well; however, the radiographic defect at the donor site may remain indefinitely. Tibial bone grafting cannot be used in young, growing patients because of the risk of disturbances to growth centers. Tibial bone can be used successfully in a variety of operative procedures, such as mandibular reconstruction, sinus lifts, maxillary reconstruction, and or orthognatic surgery.[8]

Technique
The graft is usually harvested with patient in the supine position. Some authors suggest that the graft can also be obtained with patient in the prone position. Surgical access is a 3-cm longitudinal incision made through skin overlying Gerdy's tubercle. Sharp dissection is used to expose Gerdy's tubercle and obtain cortical bone; the cortical window is made and measures 1 × 1 cm. The window should incorporate the crest of tubercle at the superior portion of the window. The crest represents a

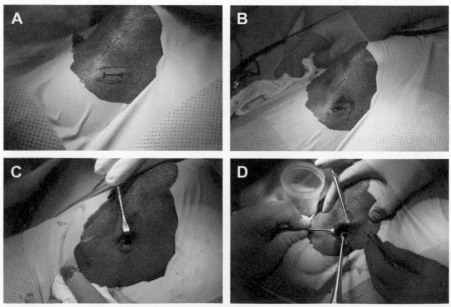

Fig. 5. (*A*) Tibia bone harvest outline. (*B*) Incision. (*C*) Osteotomy. (*D*) Cancellous bone harvest.

crucial landmark to avoid the articular surface of the tibia and the joint space. It is recommended to keep at least a 2-cm distance from the articular surface of the tibia to avoid damage. It has also been suggested to obtain the graft via a medial approach to avoid insertion of the iliotibial tract and other anatomic structures. Two important landmarks exist in the medial approach; the first is a vertical line drawn through the patella and tibial tuberosity and the second is drawn perpendicular to the first, through the tibial tuberosity. It is recommended that an oblique incision be made centered over a point 15 mm superior to the horizontal line and 15 mm medial to the vertical line. The bony window is made to gain access to cancellous bone. Regardless of the approach used, both yield a sufficient amount of cancellous bone for reconstruction. It is also suggested that, if a small amount of bone needed (<15 mL), the bone can be obtained with a stab incision and by using bone trephine and curettes (see **Fig. 5A–C**).[8]

Postoperative and donor site management
The donor site can be closed with layer closures; no drains are needed. Both tibial donor sites can be used if a greater amount of bone is required. If both tibial donor sites are used, the patient should be made aware of possible problems with early ambulation.[8]

Proximal Ulna

Bone type and yield
The proximal humeral metaphysis provides a useful site for harvesting both autogenous cortical and cancellous bone. The metaphyseal diaphyseal junction, distal to the coronoid process, is the ideal site for this harvest. This graft provides both viable cells and metabolic activity from cancellous bone, as well as stability and density through the cortical component.[9]

Risks and benefits
The proximal humeral metaphysis provides a useful site for harvesting autogenous corticocancellous bone with minimal postoperative patient discomfort, such as pain, edema, hematoma, ecchymosis, or limitations in range of motion. The biologic properties, levels of BMP, and mechanical properties of this graft are consistent with other grafts from more commonly used sites. Considering the minimal amount of dissection required, ease of harvest, and minimal donor site morbidity, this graft provides a viable option for autogenous bone harvest.[9]

Technique
Optimal patient positioning is supine, with the arm containing the selected donor site excluded for preparation. Antibiotics are given intravenously at the time of the general anesthesia induction and before inflation of the tourniquet. The donor site is prepped from the band to the axilla with betadine and draped in sterile fashion. The operator is best positioned for graft harvest by standing or sitting between the patient's head and arm, facilitating the surgical approach from lateral to medial. The arm is flexed for the remainder of the procedure. The proximal ulna is marked with a sterile pen, and the lateral extent of ulna is palpated and marked medially and laterally. The key anatomic landmark for this harvest site is palpating the radial head, which corresponds with the coronoid process of the ulna in the transverse plane. The clinician should make sure that the landmark marked is distal to the coronoid process of the ulna in a transverse plane. This ensures that there is less of a chance to penetrate the ulnohumeral joint. Infiltration of 2 mL of 1% to 2% lidocaine with 1:100,000 epinephrine is infiltrated into the area of incision into the periosteum for management of pain and bleeding at the donor surgical site.[9]

A 2-cm incision line is made on the skin fold 3 cm from the most proximal portion of the olecranon tip, directed mediolaterally through skin and subcutaneous tissue directly over the dorsum of proximal ulna. Drill bits are used to outline the area of approximately 1 cm^2. A window of dense cortical bone measuring approximately 1 cm^2 is then harvested from the site. The cortical window then is transported to the recipient site. At this time, the entire cancellous bone of the olecranon process is available to collect. Two-layer closure with periosteum and skin is made, with a pressure dressing applied and removed 1 day postoperatively.[9]

Postoperative and donor site management

For the most part, this graft is well tolerated by patients postoperatively. There is reported minimal postoperative pain, hematoma, or range of mobility limitations for this harvest site. The pressure dressing has to be applied postoperatively and removed 24 hours after the surgery. Surgical site wound care applies.[9]

REFERENCES

1. Deatherage J. Bone materials available for alveolar grafting. Oral Maxillofacial Surg Clin N Am 2010;22:347–52.
2. Triplet RG, Schow SR. Autologous bone grafts and endosseous implants: complementary techniques. J Oral Maxillofac Surg 1996;54:486–94.
3. Carlson ER, Marx RE. Mandibular reconstruction using cancellous cellular bone grafts. J Oral Maxillofac Surg 1996;54:689–897.
4. Felice P, Iezzi G, Lizio G, et al. Reconstruction of atrophied posterior mandible with inlay technique and mandibular ramus block graft for implant prosthetic rehabilitation. J Oral Maxillofac Surg 2009;67:372–80.
5. Yates DM, Brockhoff HC II, Finn R, et al. Comparison of intraoral harvest sites for corticocancellous bone grafts. J Oral Maxillofac Surg 2013;71:497–504.
6. Tolstunov L. Maxillary tuberosity block bone graft: innovative technique and case report. J Oral Maxillofac Surg 2009;67:1723–9.
7. Abramowicz S, Katsnelson A, Forbes W, et al. Anterior versus posterior approach to iliac crest for alveolar cleft bone grafting, 2012 American Association of Oral and Maxillofacial Surgeons. J Oral Maxillofac Surg 2012;70:211–5.
8. Hernández-Alfaro F, Martí C, José Biosca M, et al. Minimally invasive tibial bone, harvesting under intravenous sedation. J Oral Maxillofac Surg 2005;63:464–70.
9. Madsen MJ, Mauffrey C, Bowles N, et al. Using the proximal ulna as a novel site for autogenous bone graft harvesting. J Oral Maxillofac Surg 2011;69:1930–3.

Contemporary "All-on-4" Concept

Michael H. Chan, DDS[a,b,*], Curtis Holmes, DDS[b]

KEYWORDS

- All-on-4 concept • Implants • Prosthetic • Atrophic maxilla & mandible
- Edentulous maxillary & mandible • Immediate function restoration

KEY POINTS

- Two angled posterior implants when combined with 2 straight implants can have similar rates as traditional straight implants when splinted together using only anterior jaws.
- Splinted implants along with full arch prosthesis are biomechanically sound with marginal bone height maintained with these implants.
- Immediate load is possible when implants are torqued > 35 Ncm with full arch provisional prosthesis with one tooth cantilever maximum.
- Final restoration can have 10–12 teeth for proper esthetics and function.
- Medium (3–5 years) and long term data (5–10 years) have high degree of predictability (92%–100% success rate) utilizing the "All-on-4" concept by various authors.

INTRODUCTION: NATURE OF PROBLEM

The "All-on-4" concept is founded on the principle that 4 implants, a combination of 2 straight anterior and 2 tilted posterior, placed within the premaxilla or anterior mandible, would provide enough support to maintain a full-arch fixed prosthesis. The skepticism of this design has many clinicians shy away from this procedure. If 2 implants support a 3-unit bridge, how could 4 implants ever support a full-arch prosthesis, especially when some are tilted? The answer lies within the biomechanics of how these implants are strategically placed coupled with the prosthetic design.

THE EVOLUTION OF THE "ALL-ON-4" CONCEPT AND BIOMECHANICS

The "All-on-4" technique has evolved from original work of Branemark and colleagues[1] in 1977, whereby they utilized 4 to 6 vertical implants placed within the

[a] Oral & Maxillofacial Surgery/Dental Service, Department of Veterans Affairs, New York Harbor Healthcare System (Brooklyn Campus), 800 Poly Place (Bk-160), Brooklyn, NY 11209, USA; [b] Department Dentistry/Oral and Maxillofacial Surgery, The Brooklyn Hospital Center, 121 DeKalb Avenue, Box 187, Brooklyn, NY 11201, USA
* Corresponding author. Oral & Maxillofacial Surgery/Dental Service, Department of Veterans Affairs, New York Harbor Healthcare System (Brooklyn Campus), 800 Poly Place (Bk-160), Brooklyn, NY 11209.
E-mail address: chanoms@yahoo.com

Dent Clin N Am 59 (2015) 421–470
http://dx.doi.org/10.1016/j.cden.2014.12.001
0011-8532/15/$ – see front matter Published by Elsevier Inc.
dental.theclinics.com

anterior segment of the edentulous maxilla and mandible cantilevered to accommodate a full-arch fixed prosthesis. Although there is good success from their 10-year study (78.3%–80.3% for the maxilla and 88.4%–93.2% for the mandible), the cantilever remains too long and problematic, having to extend and provide adequate posterior dentition. Posterior bone grafting, sinus or ridge augmentation for atrophic jaws, before implant placement can be an alternative; however, additional surgeries, cost, extended length of treatment, and comorbidities precluded others to become innovative to circumvent these procedures and problems. Inferior alveolar nerve lateralization has been tried with an extremely high rate of parasthesia, and so many have abandoned this surgery. In an effort to improve implant position and decrease the cantilever length, the concept of angled distal implants was studied.

One of the early designs of the "All-on-4" style concept can be traced back to Mattsson and colleagues[2] in 1999 whereby they treated 15 patients (68 implants) with severely resorbed edentulous maxilla by inserting 4 to 6 implants in the premaxilla to avoid sinus augmentation (**Fig. 1**). They selected alveolar ridge heights 10 mm or less with 4 mm in horizontal width and successfully restored them with fixed prosthesis with 12 teeth supported by superstructure. Mattsson and colleagues[2] reported only one failed implant with 100% prosthesis stability in a 3 to 4.5 year period.

Angulation of distal implants provides numerous biomechanical and clinical advantages for fixed restorations with less invasive techniques when compared with grafted procedures with traditional axial implants (**Box 1**).[3–12] In 2000, Krekmanov and colleagues[3] were also able to demonstrate posterior tilted implant-supported prosthesis was possible. Simply by increasing the anterior-posterior (A-P) spread, shortening the cantilever, coupled with cross-arch stabilization, the implant/prosthetic outcome would be similar to traditional axial loaded cases.[8,9] The angulation also provides the opportunity for longer implants to be placed while moving the implant support posteriorly and enhancing load distribution. Furthermore, the forces on the implants are reduced with a rigid prosthesis.[3] The rigidity of the prosthesis along with improved load distribution helps minimize any significant movement and negates coronal stress at the marginal bone level.[3,6,11,12] Angulation of distal implants in a 30° to 45° position relative to the occlusal plane allows the final prosthesis to have 10 to 12 teeth per arch.[13] Last, these 4 implants could spread out in a more favorable distance for cleanability and hygiene.[14]

"All-on-4"

The design of the "All-on-4" immediate-function concept was developed in 2003 by Malo and colleagues.[15] The approach to rehabilitate the fully edentulous mandibular jaw by placing only 4 implants in the following combination: 2 anterior implants placed axially and 2 posterior implants placed distally tilted within the mandibular parasymphyseal region (**Fig. 2**).[16] These implants were immediately loaded with a full fixed acrylic prosthesis within 2 hours of surgery.

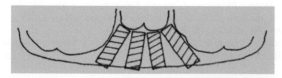

Fig. 1. Mesial-distal angulation of the implants, permitting longer implants posteriorly. (*From* Mattsson T, Konsell P, Gynther G, et al. Implant treatment without bone grafting in severely resorbed edentoulous maxillae. J Oral Maxillofac Surg 1999;57:282; with permission.)

Box 1
Biomechanical advantages of "All-on-4" design

1. Implants follow a dense bone structure

2. Longer implants can be placed by tilting them posteriorly

3. Tilting improves A-P spread of implants

4. A-P spread enhances load distribution for prosthesis

5. Shorten cantilever (maximum of 7 mm for maxilla and 1.5–2.0 × A-P spread for mandible) reduces prosthetic fracture/instability and marginal bone height stability[52]

6. Marginal bone height of implants is maintained with rigid prosthesis

7. Tilted implants have similar success rate as traditional implants when splinted together

Data from Refs.[3–12]

Building on the mandibular "All-on-4" success, Malo and colleagues replicated the same design for the maxilla in 2005.[4] Similar successes have been duplicated by other authors[11,17,18]; however, most would advocate the use of additional 2 maxillary implants for patients when encountered with certain risk factors (ie, poor bone quality, opposing natural dentition, and men with parafunctional habits).

"All-on-4" Variations

All-on-4: zygoma implants and quad zygoma

Branemark initially developed zygoma implants for 3 primary reasons as his treatment modality for (1) maxillary defect with post cancer (CA) resection, (2) trauma, (3) severe maxillary atrophy. The concept of the zygoma implants is to use available bone at a distant site when locally insufficient. The apex of the implant gets engaged to the body of the zygoma, transversing the maxillary sinus and emerging from the first molar position at a 45° angle.[19]

Bedrossian categorizes the maxilla into 3 zones radiographically: zone 1 = premaxilla, zone 2 = premolar, zone 3 = molar (**Fig. 3**).[20] The zygoma implants are indicated where there is insufficient bone in the premolar and molar regions, leaving only the anterior premaxilla available. The implant configuration will be 2 axial implants in the anterior position and 2 zygoma implants in the posterior region (**Fig. 4**).[20]

If there is absolutely no available bone in the maxilla, the Quad Zygoma uses 4 zygomatic implants to support a full-arch prosthesis (**Fig. 5**).[20]

All-on-4 "V-4"

In 2009, Jensen and Adams[21] described 2 case reports of an "All-on-4" concept called "V-4" and how these implants are primarily placed in such a formation in the anterior mandible. All-on-4 "V-4"is indicated for patients with severe mandibular atrophy

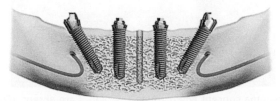

Fig. 2. Schematic picture of mandibular "All-on-4." (*From* Bedrossian E. Implant treatment planning for the edentulous patients, a graftless approach to immediate loading. St Louis (MO): Mosby, an imprint of Elsevier; 2011. Fig. 8-33B; with permission.)

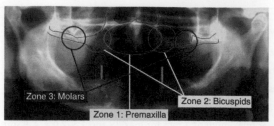

Fig. 3. The zones of the maxilla. (*From* Bedrossian E, Sullivan RM, Fortin Y, et al. Fixed-prosthetic implant restoration of the edentulous maxilla: a systematic pretreatment evaluation method. J Oral Maxillofac Surg 2008;66(1):112–22; with permission.)

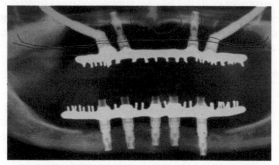

Fig. 4. The zygomatic concept when zone 1 is present. (*From* Bedrossian E. Chapter 15: graftless solution for atrophic maxilla. In: Babbush C, Hahn J, Krauser J, et al, editors. Dental implants, the arts and science, 2nd edition. St. Louis (MO): Saunders, an imprint of Elsevier; 2011. p. 258, Fig. 15-15; with permission.)

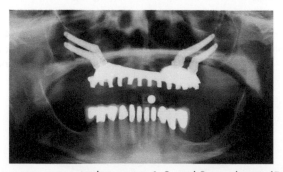

Fig. 5. The quad-zygoma concept when zones 1, 2, and 3 are absent. (*From* Bedrossian E. Chapter 15: graftless solution for atrophic maxilla. In: Babbush C, Hahn J, Krauser J, et al, editors. Dental implants, the arts and science, 2nd edition. St. Louis (MO): Saunders, an imprint of Elsevier; 2011. p. 258, Fig. 15-17; with permission.)

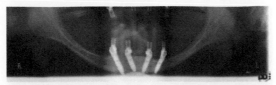

Fig. 6. Placement of 2 anterior implants angled at 30° to midline created a V shape for "all-on-4" placement, designated V-4. (*From* Jensen OT, Adams MW. All-on-4 treatment of highly atrophic mandible with mandibular V-4: report of 2 cases. J Oral Maxillofac Surg 2009;67:1503–9; with permission.)

typically with 5 to 7 mm of remaining native bone. These 4 implants are placed at a 30° angle to help support a full-arch prosthesis (**Fig. 6**).

All-on-4 shelf: Maxilla

The All-on-4 Shelf: Maxilla can be a treatment option for mild, moderate, and severe maxillary resorption cases. In 2010, Jensen and colleagues[22] described a variation of the "All-on-4" technique called the All-on-4 Shelf: Maxilla, whereby the alveolus topography is re-created by bony reduction, allowing implants to be placed strategically within the premaxilla in an "M" configuration when viewed from the frontal aspect (**Fig. 7**). The reduction of thin crestal bone helps uncover thicker basal bone. Moreover, it allows for proper interocclusal distance of 22 mm required for the final prosthesis (**Fig. 8**). The anterior and posterior implants converge apically in a 30° angulation using the native bone for maximal anchorage. The posterior site "S point" denotes the most anterior point of the anterior wall of maxillary sinus, and the "M point" denotes the maximum bone available at the pyriform rim just above the nasal floor (**Fig. 9**).[22] The divergence of these implants toward the alveolus ridge helps increase the A-P spread for better prosthetic load distribution. The only contraindication for the All-on-4 Shelf: Maxilla is if there is an indistinction between the nasal fossa and the maxillary sinus, making it 1 continuous cavity in which zygomatic implants can be the alternative treatment option.[22]

All-on-4 shelf: Mandible

Jensen and colleagues[23] in 2011 followed with their previous All-on-4 Shelf: Maxilla with the All-on-4 Shelf: Mandible with the same strategy in which bone reduction rather than bone augmentation is used to rehabilitate the edentulous arch. Flat alveolus ridge and proper interarch space, a minimum of 20 mm, are required for the

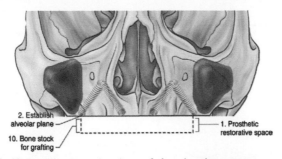

Fig. 7. All-on-4 Shelf; Maxilla. Bone leveling of the alveolus creates a new alveolar plane that functions as a "shelf" on which to place dental implants. The All-on-4 technique must take advantage of available bone, which is best observed using the All-on-4 Shelf approach, for which angled implants and compensating angled abutments are placed. (*From* Jensen OT, Adams M, Cottam J, et al. The All-on-4: shelf. J Oral Maxillofac Surg 2010;68:2520–7; with permission.)

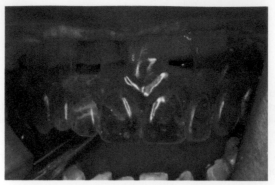

Fig. 8. A clear acrylic bone reduction guide ensures there is adequate restorative space for abutments and titanium bar housed within the prosthesis. (*From* Jensen OT, Adams M, Cottam J, et al. The All-on-4: shelf. J Oral Maxillofac Surg 2010;68:2520–7; with permission.)

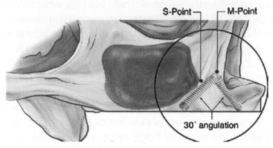

Fig. 9. When the shelf is well away from the sinus, the most anterior sinus deflection (S point) is identified using a lateral antrostomy burr hole. The space from this point to the shelf is measured. This same distance posterior of the S point perpendicular should be the entrance location of the posterior implant site (when placed at 30°) to avoid the sinus. (*From* Jensen OT, Adams M, Cottam J, et al. The All-on-4: shelf. J Oral Maxillofac Surg 2010;68:2520–7; with permission.)

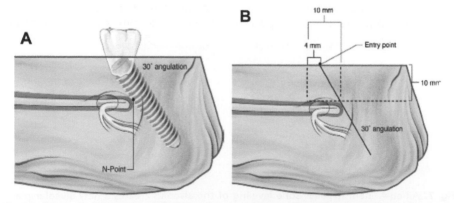

Fig. 10. (*A*) The most anterior deflection of the intraosseous nerve is termed N point. (*B*). A 10-mm vertical height measured from N point to the All-on-4 shelf allows for a 10-mm distalization on the shelf when an implant is placed at 30°. This usually allows for an increased anterior posterior spread of implants of 1 full bicuspid tooth. (*From* Jensen OT, Adams M, Cottam J, et al. The All on 4 Shelf: mandible. J Oral Maxillofac Surg 2011;69:175–81; with permission.)

mandibular arch. The implant configuration is identical to Malo's "All-on-4" design, with 2 exceptions in regards to the posterior implants. First, the 1:1 ratio represents the available bone height from alveolar bone to mental nerve (N point) and the number of millimeters of distance gained by tilting the posterior implant in a 30° angle (**Fig. 10**). The second key point is that the posterior implant can be positioned behind the mental foramen when sufficient bone is present, unspecified by the authors, above the inferior alveolar nerve via a transalveolus fashion from buccal to lingual with engagement to the lingual cortex for better A-P spread (**Fig. 11**).[23]

All-on-4 transsinus technique

In 2012, Jensen and colleagues[24] described an alternative surgical technique to zygomatic implants using a combination of sinus floor grafting bone morphogenic protein ((BMP)-2) with simultaneous transsinus implant placement and immediate function. The indication for this type of procedure is for patients with either atrophic maxilla, post-All-on-4 Shelf: Maxilla horizontal bone reduction, or pneumatized sinus traversing the canine/lateral and sometimes the central incisor region (**Fig. 12**).[25] These implants are placed in an "M" configuration with engagement to the "M point," where the pyriform rim has good-quality bone.[24] Jensen and colleagues[24] used 15 mm to 18 mm

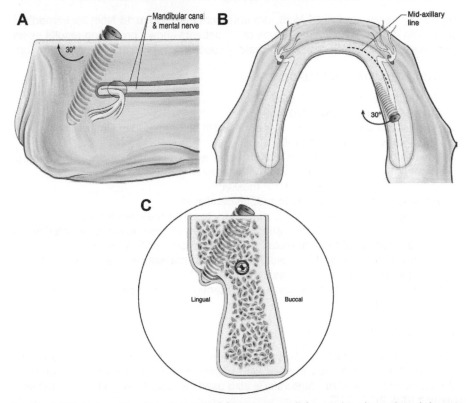

Fig. 11. (A) Occasionally, when the mental foraman is well forward in the arch and there is adequate height of bone over the nerve, implants can be placed transalveolarly, buccal to lingual. (B) This technique allows implant placement without nerve manipulation. (C) The implant is placed at a 30° angle from the axis of the alveolus at a 30° flared angle engaging the lingual plate when viewed occultly. (*From* Jensen OT, Adams M, Cottam J, et al. The All on 4 Shelf: mandible. J Oral Maxillofac Surg 2011;69:175–81; with permission.)

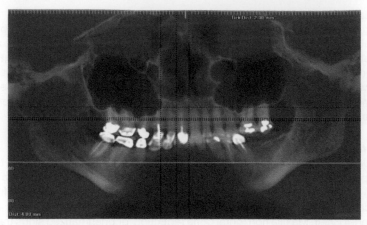

Fig. 12. Panoramic radiograph of sinus extending forward below nasal fossa into canine lateral region. (*From* Jensen OT, Cottam J, Ringeman J, et al. Trans-sinus dental implants, bone morphogenic protein 2, and immediate function for All-on-4 treatment of severe maxillary atrophy. J Oral Maxillofac Surg 2012;70:141–8; with permission.)

length implants torqued to 35 Ncm with abutment insertion at 15 Ncm for immediate load criteria (**Fig. 13**). Preliminary study of 19 patients shows promising results as an alternative to zygomatic implants with a rate of success at 94.8% after 1-year follow-up.

INCLUSION CRITERIA FOR "ALL-ON-4"[25]

1. No severe parafunctional habits
2. Standard mouth opening (40 mm)
3. Edentulous maxilla with minimum bone width of 5 mm and minimum bone height of 10 mm within the premaxilla
4. Edentulous mandible with minimum bone width of 5 mm and minimum bone height of 8 mm within the intraforamen region[13]
5. Minimal 10 mm implant length for maxilla[26]
6. Tilt implant at 45° maximally to reduce cantilever
7. If angulation is 30° or more, it is necessary to splint the tilted implants
8. For posterior tilted implants, plan the distal screw access hole to be located at the occlusal surface of the first molar, second premolar, or first premolar
9. Can accommodate 10 to 12 teeth as a fixed prosthesis with a maximum 1 to 2 teeth cantilever in final prosthesis (**Fig. 14**).[13,20]
10. If planned extraction cases, clean sites thoroughly and place implants in between extraction sites

PATIENT WORKUP

"All-on-4" workup consists of clinical evaluations, radiographic evaluations, and laboratory analysis of mounted models with duplicate clear denture(s) for composite defect detection. This clear denture(s) is also used clinically to aid in future prosthetic selection (**Box 2**).

　　Vertical dimension of occlusion (VDO) is one of the most important factors to verify (**Fig. 15**)[16] and can be confirmed with the patient's existing denture or natural dentition if full-mouth edentulation is planned. An interim prosthesis can be fabricated by the laboratory technician or by computer-aided design (CAD)/ computer-aided manufacturing (CAM) technology with the correct VDO before immediate load. For

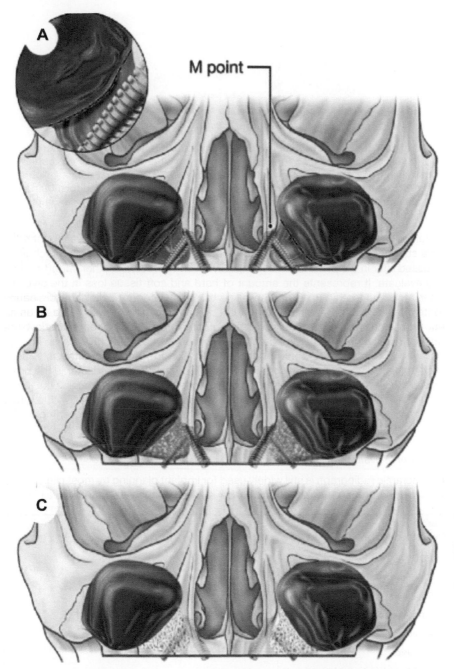

Fig. 13. (*A–C*) Once the sinus is elevated and the membrane reflected posteriorly, the trans-sinus implant can be placed, engaging lateral nasal bone. (*From* Jensen OT, Cottam J, Ringeman J, et al. Trans-sinus dental implants, bone morphogenic protein 2, and immediate function for All-on-4 treatment of severe maxillary atrophy. J Oral Maxillofac Surg 2012;70:141–8; with permission.)

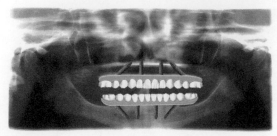

Fig. 14. All-on-4 concept clinical rationale. Four immediate function implants supporting a fixed bridge with a minimum of 10 teeth in the provisional prosthesis (with no cantilevers) and a maximum of 2 cantilever teeth in the final prosthesis. (*From* Malo P, Lopes I, Nobre M. Chapter 27: The All-on-4 concept. In: Babbush C, Hahn J, Krauser J, et al, editors. Dental implants, the arts and science, 2nd edition. Maryland Heights (MO): Saunders, an imprint of Elsevier; 2011. p. 436. Fig. 27-1; with permission.)

edentulous patients who do not have a set of dentures, a new set is recommended before starting the "All-on-4" surgery for immediate prosthetic conversion technique (discussed later in the prosthetic section). Composite defect is another important factor to evaluate. It represents the amount of hard and soft tissue loss in the alveolus proper, including teeth (**Fig. 16**).[16] Smile line is also an important clinical examination to determine (**Fig. 17**).[16] A mixture of natural and artificial gingiva will create an unesthetic transition, leading to a disastrous outcome (**Fig. 18**).[16] Preprosthetic bone reduction may be needed to remedy this situation for fixed-hybrid prosthesis. For patients who opt not to have bone reduction, then a fixed-removal prosthesis (Marius Bridge) can mask the alveolus ridge. The Marius Bridge is discussed later in the prosthetic section. Proper lip support should be inspected as well as determining the future maxillary A-P tooth position. A flat alveolar ridge is necessary and will allow the future implant and prosthetic connections to emerge at the same level. Proper centric occlusion should be examined for proper canine and protrusive guidance.[13,16]

Radiographic Evaluation

The panoramic radiograph is still widely used for implant planning by most clinicians. It allows pertinent anatomic structures to be surveyed, such as anterior wall of the

---

Box 2
Clinical evaluation for "All-on-4"

1. VDO

2. Composite defect detection (hard and soft tissue loss)

3. Smile line

4. Lip support and A-P tooth position of maxilla

5. Alveolus ridge plateau

6. Occlusion

7. Sufficient keratinized tissue

Data from Malo P, Lopes I, Nobre M. Chapter 27: the All-on-4 concept. In: Babbush C, Hahn J, Krauser J, et al, editors. Dental implants, the arts and science. 2nd edition. Maryland Heights (MO): Saunders, an imprint of Elsevier; 2011. p. 435–447; and Bedrossian E. Implant treatment planning for the edentulous patients, a graftless approach to immediate loading. St Louis (MO): Mosby, an imprint of Elsevier; 2011.

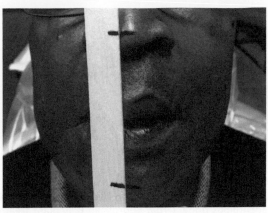

Fig. 15. Vertical dimension of rest (VDO).

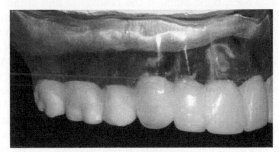

Fig. 16. Composite defect: patient missing teeth, soft tissue, and hard tissue mass. (*From* Bedrossian E. Implant treatment planning for the edentulous patients, a graftless approach to immediate loading. St Louis (MO): Mosby, an imprint of Elsevier; 2011. Fig. 5-4; with permission.)

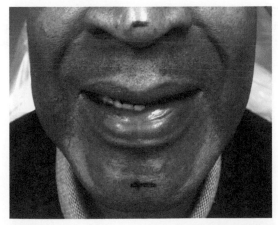

Fig. 17. Smile line detection. The hidden transition line (without visible alveolus ridge) allows for an esthetic outcome with a profile prosthesis.

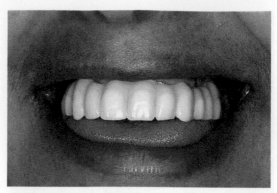

Fig. 18. A visible transition line during animation results in an unesthetic exposure of the prosthesis and the edentulous ridge. (*From* Bedrossian E. Implant treatment planning for the edentulous patients, a graftless approach to immediate loading. St Louis (MO): Mosby, an imprint of Elsevier; 2011. Fig. 5-11; with permission.)

maxillary sinus, nasal floor, bone stock in the premaxilla and anterior mandible, the inferior alveolar nerve, and mental foramen and its loop. Preoperative planning can predict the amount of hard and soft tissue defect, number of teeth to be replaced, and location of the implants. The panoramic film could only show the length and spacing of the predicted implants, thus limiting its usefulness (**Fig. 19**). Cone-beam computed tomography (CT) has been commercially available since the early 1990s to allow clinicians to see the maxilla and mandible in a 3-dimensional view (height, width, and volume). It also shows the quality of bone expressed in Hounsfield Units (HU). A study by Parel and Phillips[18] suggested bone quality less than 100 HU units reflects poor quality bone and will result in high failure rates. Virtual implant planning could be performed by using the "prosthetic driven approach." The prosthesis, abutment, and implants can be designed to ensure proper emergence of the implant to prosthetic interface (**Fig. 20**).[19] Moreover, these implants can be seen in multiple views (ie, axial and sagittal) for bony support. For guided surgery cases, this information can be transferred to the laboratory technician for surgical guide fabrication. This topic is discussed in detail in the guided surgery section.

Laboratory Workup

After completing the above evaluations, a denture wax-up in proper VDO should be mounted in an articulator. To further evaluate the composite defect, the patient's

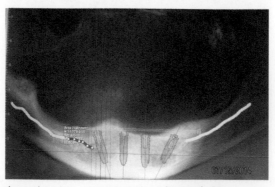

Fig. 19. Virtual implant planning on panoramic radiograph 2D.

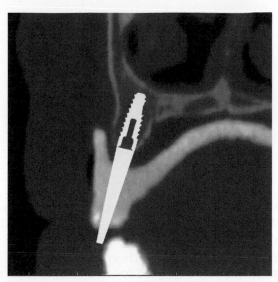

Fig. 20. The cross-sectional view allows for inspection of the alveolus process in relation to the proposed tooth position. (*From* Ganz, Scott D. Chapter 10: The use of CT/CBCT and interactive virtual treatment planning and the triangle bone: Defining new paradigms for assessment of implant receptor sites. In: Babbush C, Hahn J, Krauser J, et al, editors. Dental implants, the arts and science, 2nd edition. Maryland Heights (MO): Saunders, an imprint of Elsevier; 2011. p. 163. Fig. 10-26 C; with permission.)

denture should be duplicated in a Lang duplicator with clear resin (**Fig. 21**).[16] This clear denture should be reseated either in the patient's mouth or on the cast and the extent of hard and soft tissue loss determined (**Fig. 22**).[16] The amount of tissue loss would allow the restorative clinician to select the type of prosthesis to restore.

If tooth-only defect is present, then standard ceramo-metal restoration is indicated. There are 2 basic options that clinicians can offer patients when both hard and soft tissue deficiencies are identified.[16] Fixed-hybrid (profile prosthesis) would be suited

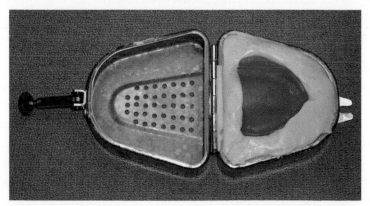

Fig. 21. Lang duplicator to reproduce an existing denture. (*From* Bedrossian E. Implant treatment planning for the edentulous patients, a graftless approach to immediate loading. St Louis (MO): Mosby, an imprint of Elsevier; 2011. Fig. 5-5; with permission.)

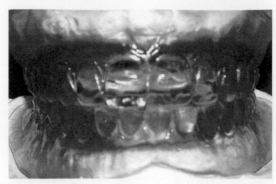

Fig. 22. Reseat the clear stent on cast or patient and note the moderate composite defect between the teeth and alveolus ridge. (*From* Bedrossian E. Implant treatment planning for the edentulous patients, a graftless approach to immediate loading. St Louis (MO): Mosby, an imprint of Elsevier; 2011. Fig. 5-7; with permission.)

when the transitional line is *not visible* during high smile line, whereas fixed-removable prosthesis (Marius Bridge) would be good for visible ridges during high smile line assessment because the flange can extend into the vestibule and mask the transition line. More details are discussed later in the prosthetic section.

TREATMENT OPTIONS

Treatment option is based on degree of bone resorption in the edentulous arches (**Box 3**).

SURGICAL APPROACH: "ALL-ON-4"

The clinician can offer the "All-on-4" treatment concept for edentulous patients with the opportunity to receive a provisional prosthesis within the same day of surgery if sufficient torque is achieved after implant placement or as an immediate implant placement for planned extraction case for immediate load. The extraction sites

---

Box 3
"All-on-4" maxilla and mandibular resorption treatment options

Mild	Moderately	Severe
Maxilla Resorption Treatment Options		
1. "All-on-4"	1. "All-on-4"	1. Zygoma
2. All-on-4: Shelf	2. All-on-4: Shelf	2. Quad zygoma
		3. All-on-4: Shelf
		4. Transsinus technique
Mandibular Resorption Treatment Options		
1. "All-on-4"	1. "All-on-4"	1. All-on-4: "V-4"
2. All-on-4: Shelf	2. All-on-4: Shelf	

Data from Refs.[15,16,19,22,24]

need to be thoroughly debrided and the alveolar ridge plateaued before implant installation.

The following surgical protocol described later is for regular platform (RP): 4.3 mm × 13 mm tapered implants (ie, NobelReplace Tapered Groovy, Replace Select Tapered, and Replace Select Tapered PMC, NobelReplace Conical Connection, and NobelReplace Conical Connection PMC) for both maxilla and mandible (**Boxes 4–6**).[27,28] Please refer to Nobel Biocare's drill protocol for other implants within this "All-on-4" list. Nobel Biocare's straight implant line has a variety of drill sizes that will allow the clinician to be more precise when performing the osteotomy in different bone densities. Undersizing the osteotomy will help implant stability when soft bone is encountered.

Maxillary Approach "All-on-4"

An incision is made from first molar to first molar with bilateral buccal releasing incisions distally. A full-thickness mucoperiosteal flap reflection is performed. Next, take a round bur and locate and perforate through the anterior wall of the maxillary sinus at the most anterior aspect (**Fig. 23**).[16] The exact location of the anterior wall is important because it allows the posterior implants to be placed distally while maximizing the implant length in this highly dense cortical region. Outline the anterior wall of the maxillary sinus with a surgical marker. Next, an All-on-4 Guide (Nobel Biocare AB, Gothenborg, Sweden) is placed in the midline after an osteotomy is made with a 2-mm twist drill going to 10-mm depth (**Fig. 24**). If possible, the contour of the guide should be situated so it follows the opposing arch; this allows implants to be directed against the opposing arch for proper inclination. Starting with the posterior implant sites, the drill should be angulated distally with 30° to 45° with respect to the guide (**Fig. 25**). Start the osteotomy with a precision drill (starter drill) at least 4.5 to 5 mm from the previously outlined anterior wall of the maxillary sinus and repeat the same for the contralateral side. Using the same precision drill for the anterior sites, place the osteotomy in either the central or the lateral position with 0° tilt. Take an intraoperative radiograph to verify the depth and angulation of these 4 drills. Next, sequentially enlarge it to 2.0 mm twist drill, then Narrow Platform (NP) tapered drill × 13 mm drill, and finally, RP tapered drill × 13 mm drill. When inserting these implants, do not exceed greater than 45 Ncm because bone necrosis and implant fracture can occur, in which bone tapping is recommended when resistance is met during implant insertion (**Fig. 26**). A measure of 4.3 mm is the smallest diameter recommended for the posterior sites and 3.5 mm for the anterior sites. For the internal trichannel design, make sure one of the lobes of the posterior implant is facing distally or buccally, whereas the flat side of the internal conical connection should be parallel to the buccal surface (**Box 7, Fig. 27**).[27] The internal conical implant driver has

---

Box 4
Armamentarium for "All-on-4" surgery

1. Preoperative planning for implants on radiographs

2. Implant motor and handpiece

3. Nobel Biocare Surgical Kit with "All-on-4" Guide

4. Nobel Biocare Implants

5. Nobel Prosthetic Kit with related components

6. Impression materials

7. Provisional prosthesis

Box 5
Nobel Biocare Implants for "All-on-4"

Internal conical connection

1. NobelActive (excluding 3.0) = Straight
2. NobelReplace Conical Connection = Tapered
3. NobelReplace Conical Connection PMC = Tapered

Internal trichannel connection

1. NobelReplace Straight = Straight
2. Replace Select Straight = Straight
3. NobleSpeedy Replace = Straight
4. Replace Select TC = Straight
5. NobelReplace Tapered Groovy = Tapered
6. Replace Select Tapered = Tapered
7. NobelReplace Platform Shift = Tapered
8. Replace Select Tapered PMC = Tapered

External hex connection

1. NobelSpeedy Groovy = Straight and most studied
2. Branemark System Mk III Groovy = Straight
3. Branemark System Mk III TiUnite = Straight
4. Branemark System Mk IV TiUnite = Straight
5. Branemark System Zygoma TiUnite and Machine Surface = Straight

Data from Nobel Biocare product catalog 2013/2014, Zurich (Switzerland): 2013.

Box 6
Drill sequence for "All-on-4" (RP) 4.3 mm × 13 mm tapered implants

1. Place "All-on-4" guide in the midline of the arch
2. Start with posterior sites, angle drill 30–45° distally
3. Precision drill (Starter Drill) for initial osteotomy (Max. 800 rpm)
4. 2.0 mm Twist Drill (Max. 800 rpm)
5. NP Tapered Drill (Max. 800 rpm)
6. RP Tapered Drill (Max. 800 rpm)
7. RP Dense Bone Drill for 13-mm to 16-mm length implants or dense bone regions (Max. 800 rpm)
8. (Optional) Screw tap tapered drill for dense bone regions (Max. 45 Ncm)
9. Insert implant with handpiece at maximum 45 Ncm
10. Repeat steps 3 to 8 for anterior implants with 0° tilt

Data from Nobel Biocare product catalog 2013/2014, Zurich (Switzerland): 2013.

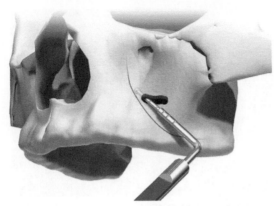

Fig. 23. A small opening is created to allow the clinician to feel the most anterior aspect of the anterior wall of the maxillary sinus. (*From* Bedrossian E. Implant treatment planning for the edentulous patients, a graftless approach to immediate loading. St Louis (MO): Mosby, an imprint of Elsevier; 2011. Fig. 6-20; with permission.)

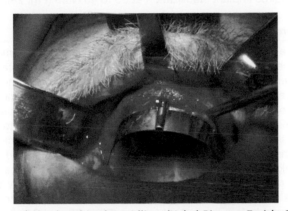

Fig. 24. All-on-4 guide is placed in the midline. (Nobel Biocare, Zurich, Switzerland; with permission.)

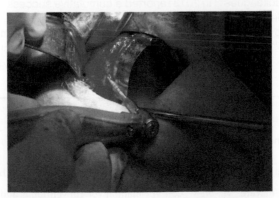

Fig. 25. Starter drill is 30–45° to the guide. Note the hole into the anterior wall of the maxillary sinus.

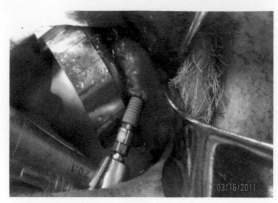

Fig. 26. Insertion of posterior implant at 45°.

demarcated lines or a color-coded dot to represent the flat surface of internal hex. This demarcation will aid the clinician when fine tuning the implant placement. Immediate load protocol requires implant stabilization at 35 to 45 Ncm (**Fig. 28**).

Mandibular Approach

A bilateral oblique releasing incision is made at the second molar positions; this is then connected to the crestal incision.[24] A full-thickness mucoperiosteal reflection is created with attention to locate and avoid damaging the mental nerve (**Fig. 29**).[13] The clinician must know the exact location of the mental nerve and anticipate the loop to course approximately 5 mm anterior to the foramen.[16,29] Again, starting with the posterior implant site, angle the precision drill distally at a 30° to 45° angle with respect to the guide and drill to a planned depth (**Fig. 30**). The precision drill is also used in the anterior implant site and is usually placed along the solid vertical lines at 0° next to the midline (**Fig. 31**). Again, verify the angulation of these precision drills with an intraoperative radiograph (**Fig. 32**). Enlarge the osteotomy and adjust the angulation to the desired implant size. Tapping the osteotomy is necessary if dense bone is encountered before implant placement (**Figs. 33** and **34**). It is imperative to keep the drill centered within the bone marrow and be cognizant not to perforate the lingual or buccal cortices during the osteotomies.

Babbush and colleagues[30] in 2013 reported a cumulative success rate of 98.7% after 3 years of using NP NobelActive implants with a minimum of 10 mm in length for severely atrophic maxilla and mandibles. This success rate is similar to the well-studied "All-on-4" cases by numerous authors. Babbush owed the success of NobelActive implants to the aggressive thread design to aid binding to soft bone;

Box 7
Special considerations for placement of implant

1. Internal trichannel implants, make sure (posterior implant) one lobe is pointing distally or buccally

2. Internal conical connection, make sure one of the flat sides is parallel to buccal surface

Data from Nobel Biocare "All-on-4" Concept manual for conventional and guided surgery 2012, Zurich (Switzerland): 2012.

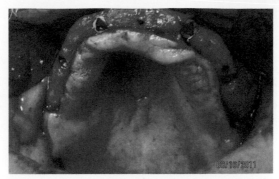

Fig. 27. Placement of 4 maxillary implants. Note the triangular portion lobe of the implant should be facing the buccal aspect.

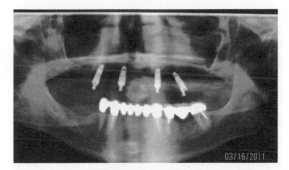

Fig. 28. Postoperative panoramic radiograph of "All-on-4" maxilla.

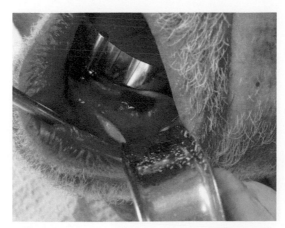

Fig. 29. Mental nerve isolated.

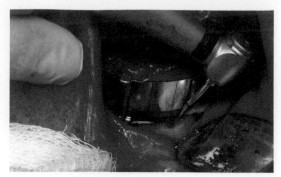

Fig. 30. The drill is 30° to 45° positioned to the guide for posterior osteotomy.

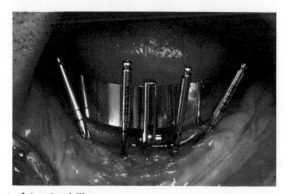

Fig. 31. Placement of 4 twist drills.

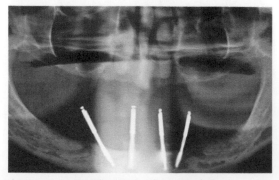

Fig. 32. Intraoperative panoramic radiograph of 4 twist drills.

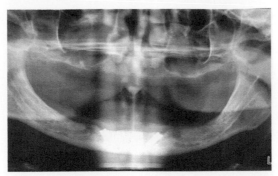

Fig. 33. Postoperative panoramic radiograph of four mandibular implants.

furthermore, the tapered collar helps maintain alveolar bone height and peri-implant soft tissue stability.[30]

PROSTHETIC PROCEDURE: "ALL-ON-4"
Provisional Prosthesis Conversion with Existing Mandibular Denture for Immediate Load

1. Confirm implant torque to greater than 35 Ncm (**Fig. 35**)[16]
2. Take a bite registration[16]
3. Place 30° or 17° multiunit abutments at posterior sites and place 0° or 17° multiunit abutments at the anterior sites so they emerge toward the occlusal surface of the denture (**Fig. 36**).[16]
4. Confirm seating with a radiograph and then torque the posterior abutments to 15 Ncm and 30 Ncm for the anterior abutments[16]
5. Place a protective healing cap on these abutments and suture the surgical site with resorbable sutures (ie, 3-0 or 4-0 chromic gut) (**Fig. 37**)[16]
6. Index the denture with impression material (ie, polyvinylsiloxane [PVS]) (**Fig. 38**)[16]
7. Create adequate space with an acrylic bur in the denture where index markings are present (**Figs. 39** and **40**)[16]
8. Remove the protective healing cap and place temporary coping (multiunit) onto the multiunit abutments[16]
9. Adequate clearance is needed for temporary coping (multiunit) and denture (**Fig. 41**)[16]

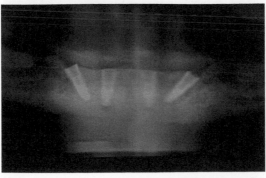

Fig. 34. Close-up of postoperative panoramic radiograph of 4 mandibular implants in "All-on-4" configuration.

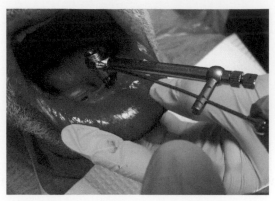

Fig. 35. Confirm implant torque to 35 Ncm.

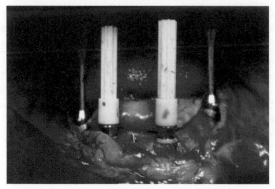

Fig. 36. Placement of multiunit abutments onto posterior and anterior implants. Note the emergence of abutment toward the occlusal surface.

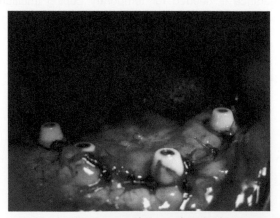

Fig. 37. Place the protective healing cap on these multiunit abutments and suture the surgical sites.

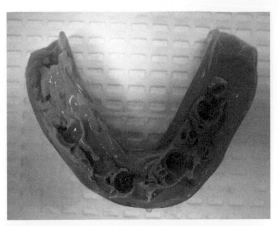

Fig. 38. Index the denture with PVS to locate the multiunit abutments.

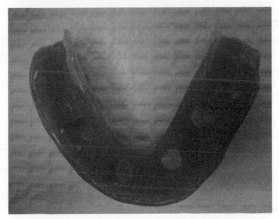

Fig. 39. Tissue surface view. Create adequate space with an acrylic bur in the denture where index markings are present.

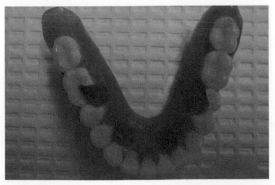

Fig. 40. Occlusal view. Create adequate space with an acrylic bur in the denture where index markings are present. Note adequate thickness of acrylic is needed to prevent fracture.

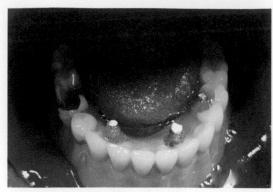

Fig. 41. Adequate room is need circumferentially around the temporary coping (multiunit).

10. Recheck occlusion to be coincident before luting with acrylic[16]
11. Lute the temporary coping (multiunit) with acrylic material (**Fig. 42**)[16]
12. Lute the tissue-baring surface of the denture to the temporary coping (multiunit) with acrylic (**Fig. 43**)[16]
13. Reduce excess temporary coping (multiunit) flush with denture level (**Fig. 44**)[16]
14. Provisional prosthesis is inserted with prosthesis screws at 15 Ncm[16]
15. Seal access hole with material (ie, thread seal tape and cavit or PVS)[16]
16. Bilateral group function occlusion with one-tooth cantilever maximum (**Fig. 45**)[16]
17. Soft diet recommended[16]

Alternatively, if a provisional is not available after completion of the surgical procedure, mucoperiosteal flaps are sutured and multiunit abutments are placed and torqued to the same specifications (**Box 8**).[16,27] Next, place the impression copings closed tray onto the multiunit abutments and take an impression using either polyether or PVS material (**Figs. 46** and **47**). Both open-tray and closed-tray techniques are acceptable with the closed-tray technique demonstrated here. The impression is removed, inspected, and sent to the dental laboratory for soft tissue model and fabrication of provisional prosthesis. Protective healing caps are placed over the multiunit abutments while the provisional is being fabricated. A full-arch interim acrylic prosthesis is placed and secured with prosthetic screws torqued to 15 Ncm; this is completed within 2 to 3 hours of surgery (**Fig. 48**).

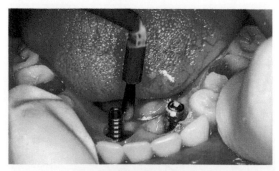

Fig. 42. Lute the temporary coping (multiunit) with acrylic material. (*From* Bedrossian E: Implant treatment planning for the edentulous patients, a graftless approach to immediate loading. St Louis (MO): Mosby an imprint of Elsevier; 2011. Fig. 8-41B; with permission.)

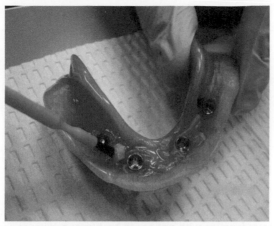

Fig. 43. Lute the tissue-baring surface of the denture to the temporary coping.

Final Prosthetic Options: "All-on-4" (4 to 6 Months After Initial Implant Placement)

Again, if there is no composite defect and tooth-only loss is identified, then a ceramo-metal restoration is indicated (**Box 9, Fig. 49**).[20] The clinician can offer 2 fundamental prosthetic options to their patients based on degree of composite defect and the visibility of the alveolar ridge during high smile assessment.[20,27] Fixed-hybrid (profile prosthesis) is suitable for a nonvisible alveolar ridge (**Fig. 50**), although a fixed-removable prosthesis (Marius Bridge) is warranted when the ridge is visible (**Box 10, Fig. 51**).[20,27]

Nobel Biocare has 3 lines of NobelProcera Implant Bridges with titanium and Zirconia framework available as their fixed-hybrid option. The Basic option is a titanium implant bridge with acrylic teeth and acrylic gingival.[27] Their Medium option is

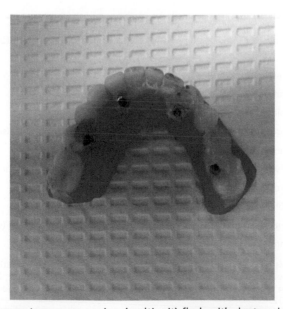

Fig. 44. Reduce excess temporary coping (multiunit) flush with denture level.

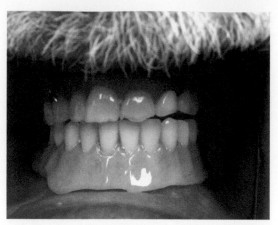

Fig. 45. Bilateral group function with one-tooth cantilever maximum.

a titanium implant bridge veneered with composite teeth, porcelain, or E-Max crowns.[27] Last, the Premium option is a bridge with either individualized NobelProcera's alumina or zirconia crowns, each cemented to NobelProcera's framework.[27] Canine and anterior guidance are incorporated into this final occlusion and the prosthetic-mucosal surface places slight pressure against soft tissue. Fixed-removable restoration is an acrylic prosthesis that can accommodate the following type of bars: Dolder, Hader, Round, Paris, and or Free Form Milled Bar to the final prosthesis as an overdenture option. There are many different attachments clinicians can choose based on level of comfort (ie, locators, balls, clips). Bilateral group function is incorporated into the final occlusion and the final prosthesis should have at least 12 teeth for proper esthetics and function.

Box 8
Impression technique for provisional prosthesis fabrication day of surgery (2–3 hours after surgery)

1. Confirm implant torque to greater than 35 Ncm

2. Place multiunit abutments on implants as previously described

3. Suture flaps closed

4. Place the impression copings closed tray onto the multiunit abutments (see **Fig. 46**)

5. Take an impression and send to laboratory (see **Fig. 47**)

6. Place protective healing caps on abutments while provisional is being made

7. Provisional prosthesis is torqued to 15 Ncm

8. Seal access hole

9. Bilateral Group Function Occlusion with one tooth cantilever maximum (see **Fig. 48**)

10. Soft diet recommended

Data from Bedrossian E. Implant treatment planning for the edentulous patients, a graftless approach to immediate loading. St Louis (MO): Mosby, an imprint of Elsevier; 2011; and Nobel Biocare "All-on-4" Concept manual for conventional and guided surgery 2012, Zurich (Switzerland): 2012.

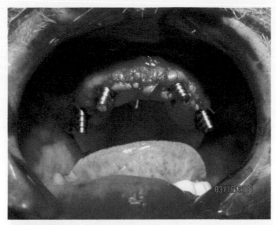

Fig. 46. Place the impression copings closed tray onto the multiunit abutments.

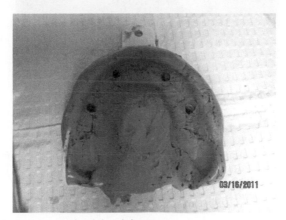

Fig. 47. Take an impression and send to laboratory.

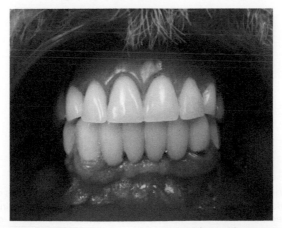

Fig. 48. Bilateral group function occlusion with one-tooth cantilever maximum.

Box 9
High smile line assessment flow chart

No Composite Defect		Composite Defect
Visible Ridge (Ceramo-metal)	Nonvisible ridge (fixed-hybrid)	Visible ridge (fixed-removable)

Data from Bedrossian E. Implant treatment planning for the edentulous patients, a graftless approach to immediate loading. St Louis (MO): Mosby, an imprint of Elsevier; 2011.

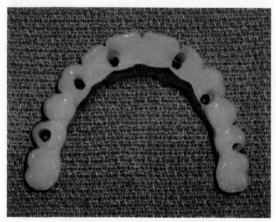

Fig. 49. Ceramo-metal restoration. (*From* Bedrossian E. Chapter 15: graftless solution for atrophic maxilla. In: Babbush C, Hahn J, Krauser J, et al, editors. Dental implants, the arts and science, 2nd edition. Maryland Heights (MO): Saunders, an imprint of Elsevier; 2011. p. 253. Fig. 15-3; with permission.)

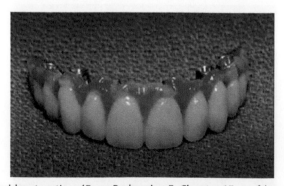

Fig. 50. Fixed-hybrid restoration. (*From* Bedrossian E. Chapter 15: graftless solution for atrophic maxilla. In: Babbush C, Hahn J, Krauser J, et al, editors. Dental implants, the arts and science, 2nd edition. Maryland Heights (MO): Saunders, an imprint of Elsevier; 2011. p. 254. Fig. 15-4; with permission.)

Box 10	
Nobel Biocare's prosthetic flow chart options with composite defect	
Fixed-Hybrid (Profile Prosthesis) Ridge is *NOT visible* during high smile assessment	**Fixed-Removable (Marius Bridge)** Ridge is *visible* during high smile assessment
1. Basic option = Titanium framework (with acrylic teeth and acrylic gingiva)	Bars available
	1. Dolder Bar
2. Medium option = Titanium framework (with veneered composite, porcelain, or E-Max)	2. Hader Bar
	3. Round Bar
3. Premium option = Titanium/Ziconia framework (with individual alumina or ziconia crowns cemented)	4. Paris Bar
	5. Free Form Milled Bar

Data from Nobel Biocare "All-on-4" Concept manual for conventional and guided surgery 2012, Zurich (Switzerland): 2012.

Final prosthesis fabrication can commence after 4 to 6 months of healing (**Box 11**).[16] The provisional prosthesis is removed, and implant stability and abutment torque need to be reconfirmed to be equivalent to immediate function specifications. Replace the provisional prosthesis in the patient's mouth and take a bite registration.[16] After which, remove the provisional prosthesis and place multiunit laboratory analogs to the denture and mount it against a counter model on an articulator (see **Figs. 52** and **53**).[16] A putty index is performed on the prosthesis that provides information to the laboratory technician the length of the future resin pattern framework (see **Fig. 54**).[16] This resin pattern is fabricated in the laboratory in multiple sections that are transferred to the

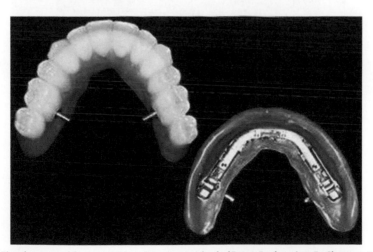

Fig. 51. Fixed-removable restoration (Marius Bridge). (*From* Bedrossian E. Chapter 15: graftless solution for atrophic maxilla. In: Babbush C, Hahn J, Krauser J, et al, editors. Dental implants, the arts and science, 2nd edition. Maryland Heights (MO): Saunders, an imprint of Elsevier; 2011. p. 254. Fig. 15-5; with permission.)

Box 11
Final prosthesis: "All-on-4" (4–6 months after initial implant placement)

1. (*Visit 1*) Remove provisional and confirm torque of implant greater than 35 Ncm
2. (*Visit 1*) Replace provisional and take bite registration
3. Remove provisional and place multiunit laboratory analog to denture and mount on articulator against a counter model (**Figs. 52** and **53**)
4. Index the prosthesis with putty (**Fig. 54**)
5. (*Laboratory procedure*) Resin pattern is fabricated in sections (**Fig. 55**)
6. (*Visit 2*) Transfer the sectioned resin pattern to patient's mouth and lute the sections together with resin (**Figs. 56** and **57**)
7. (*Laboratory procedure*) This resin pattern gets scanned and framework is made by CAD/CAM technology (**Fig. 58**)
8. (*Visit 3*) Try-in framework (passive fit) in patient's mouth (**Fig. 59**)
9. (*Visit 3*) Soft tissue index of framework and intaglio's surface (**Fig. 60**)
10. (*Visit 4*) Wax try-in with teeth
11. (*Visit 5*) Final delivery of prosthesis (**Fig. 61**)

Data from Bedrossian E. Implant treatment planning for the edentulous patients, a graftless approach to immediate loading. St Louis (MO): Mosby, an imprint of Elsevier; 2011.

patient's mouth and luted with more autopolymerizing resin to ensure an accurate fit (see **Figs. 55** and **57**).[16] The completed pattern gets transferred back onto the cast and a framework is fabricated with CAD/CAM technology and returned to the patient's mouth for try-in (see **Figs. 58** and **59**).[16] A passive fit is paramount to ensure accuracy and not to translate undue strain onto the implants. Soft tissue index is performed and

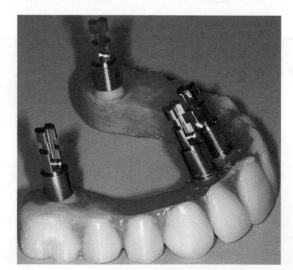

Fig. 52. Remove provisional and place multiunit laboratory analog to denture. (*From* Bedrossian E. Implant treatment planning for the edentulous patients, a graftless approach to immediate loading. St Louis (MO): Mosby, an imprint of Elsevier; 2011. Fig. 13-60B; with permission.)

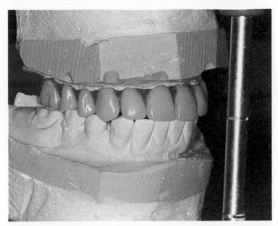

Fig. 53. Mount the denture with the multiunit analog against a counter model. (*From* Bedrossian E. Implant treatment planning for the edentulous patients, a graftless approach to immediate loading. St Louis (MO): Mosby, an imprint of Elsevier; 2011. Fig. 13-60D; with permission.)

sent back to the laboratory for a set up (see **Fig. 60**).[16] This relationship of soft tissue and the tissue-baring surface of the future prosthesis is determined so an intimate adaptation can be fabricated from this index. Wax try-in is performed with framework, and the final prosthesis is seated in the patient's mouth (see **Fig. 61**).[16]

"ALL-ON-4" GUIDED SURGERY: NOBELGUIDE

Guided Surgery enables the clinician to place implants with a high degree of accuracy and confidence.[31–35] The flexibility of guided surgery allows the clinician to choose either an open flap, a mini flap, or a flapless approach (**Box 12**).[27] Flapless surgery is indicated for patients who have sufficient keratinized gingival tissue, good interarch opening (around 40 mm), and edentulous arches that do not require preprosthetic surgery. An advantage of the flawless approach is that it requires less surgical time

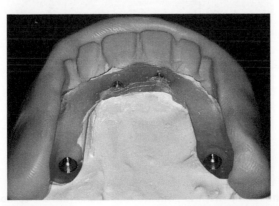

Fig. 54. Index the prosthesis with putty. (*From* Bedrossian E. Implant treatment planning for the edentulous patients, a graftless approach to immediate loading. St Louis (MO): Mosby, an imprint of Elsevier; 2011. Fig. 13-61A; with permission.)

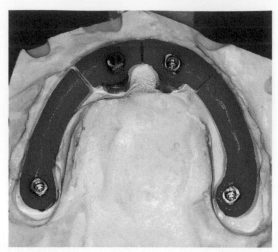

Fig. 55. Resin pattern is fabricated in sections. (*From* Bedrossian E. Implant treatment planning for the edentulous patients, a graftless approach to immediate loading. St Louis (MO): Mosby, an imprint of Elsevier; 2011. Fig. 13-61B; with permission.)

without suturing. In addition, this is an excellent approach for the novice clinician to try the "All-on-4" Guided Surgery technique. Alternatively, flap or mini flap allows the clinician to do simultaneous bone grafting with implants submerged or those with minimal keratinized tissue preoperatively.

The workup for guided surgery starts with an oral examination with particular attention to be paid on the following preoperative check list[16] (**Box 13**): (1) fully healed extraction sites, (2) minimal mandibullar opening of 40 mm, (3) smile line assessment, and (4) evaluated for quantity and quality of soft tissue. A diagnostic model should be obtained verifying proper VDO and A-P tooth relationship. After clinically confirming the setup, a radiographic guide can be fabricated with at least 6 to 8 spherical

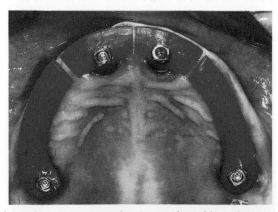

Fig. 56. Transfer the resin pattern to patient's mouth and lute the sections together with resin. (*From* Bedrossian E. Implant treatment planning for the edentulous patients, a graftless approach to immediate loading. St Louis (MO): Mosby, an imprint of Elsevier; 2011. Fig. 13-62B; with permission.)

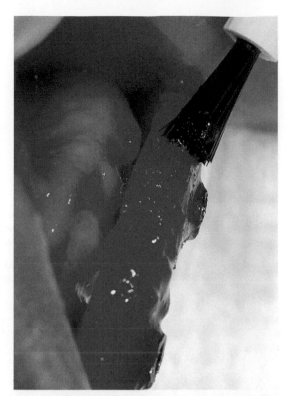

Fig. 57. Transfer the resin pattern to patient's mouth and lute the sections together with resin. (*From* Bedrossian E. Implant treatment planning for the edentulous patients, a graftless approach to immediate loading. St Louis (MO): Mosby, an imprint of Elsevier; 2011. Fig. 13-62C; with permission.)

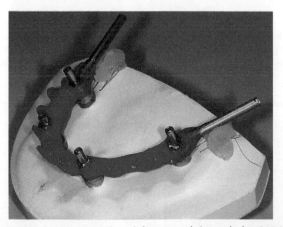

Fig. 58. This resin pattern gets scanned and framework is made by CAD/CAM technology. (*From* Bedrossian E. Implant treatment planning for the edentulous patients, a graftless approach to immediate loading. St Louis (MO): Mosby, an imprint of Elsevier; 2011. Fig. 13-64B; with permission.)

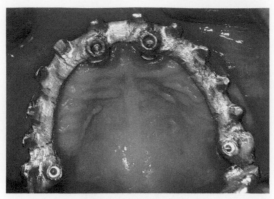

Fig. 59. Try-in framework (passive fit) in patient's mouth. (*From* Bedrossian E. Implant treatment planning for the edentulous patients, a graftless approach to immediate loading. St Louis (MO): Mosby, an imprint of Elsevier; 2011. Fig. 13-65A; with permission.)

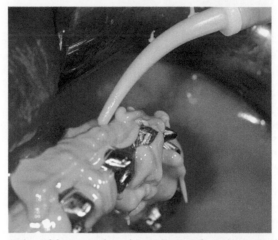

Fig. 60. Soft tissue index of framework and intaglio's surface. (*From* Bedrossian E. Implant treatment planning for the edentulous patients, a graftless approach to immediate loading. St Louis (MO): Mosby, an imprint of Elsevier; 2011. Fig. 13-67A; with permission.)

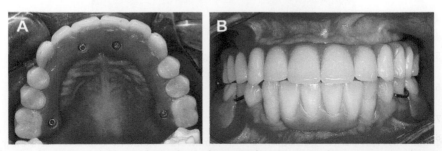

Fig. 61. (*A, B*) Final delivery of prosthesis. (*From* Bedrossian E. Implant treatment planning for the edentulous patients, a graftless approach to immediate loading. St Louis (MO): Mosby, an imprint of Elsevier; 2011. Fig. 13-69; with permission.)

Box 12	
Flow chart for guided surgery	
Flapless (Inclusion)	**Flap or Miniflap (Inclusion)**
1. Sufficient keratinized tissue	1. Minimal keratinized tissue
2. MIO >40 mm	2. Allows simultaneous bone grafting
3. Requires no preprosthetic surgery	3. MIO >40 mm
4. Partial or edentulous arch(es)	4. Partial or edentulous arch(es)
5. Decrease surgery time, bleeding, and swelling	

Data from Nobel Biocare "All-on-4" concept manual for conventional and guided surgery 2012, Zurich (Switzerland): 2012.

reference points by using either an existing denture or a new wax-up in clear acrylic (see **Fig. 62**).[16] A surgical index is created by using laboratory putty with the radiographic guide seated against a mounted model of a semi-adjustable articulator. This surgical index will ensure proper seating of the radiographic guide during scanning and later for proper alignment of the surgical prior to surgery guide.[16] NobelClinican software (Nobel Biocare AB) requires a dual scan technique for fabrication of the NobelGuide surgical guide. The first CT scan is taken with the radiographic guide along with the surgical index in the patient's mouth.[16] The second one is scanned by itself.[16] These reference points should coincide with one another to ensure a high degree of accuracy of the radiographic guide.

NobelClinician Software (Nobel Biocare AB) has the ability to perform an entire prosthetically driven implant case by virtual planning, including preoperative virtual planning of implants, abutments, immediate and final prosthesis, along with the NobelGuide

Box 13
Clinical evaluation and workup for guided surgery
1. (*Visit 1*) Clinical exam (1. fully healed extraction sites, 2. MIO > 40 mm, 3. smile line assessment, 4. evaluate soft tissue quality & quantity.)
2. (*Visit 1*) Diagnostic impression
3. (*Visit 2*) Diagnostic models (verify VDO & tooth set-up)
4. (*Laboratory procedure*) = Create a radiographic guide with 6–8 spherical points (**Fig. 62**)
5. Create a surgical index with radiographic guide or guides against counter model mounted on an articulator
6. (*Visit 3*) Dual scan technique (patient with surgical guide with surgical index and surgical guide alone)
7. Perform virtual planning (prosthetic driven approach) using software 16 (**Figs. 63** and **64**)
8. Laboratory technician fabricates (surgical guide, provisional prosthesis, and Jig)

Data from Bedrossian E. Implant treatment planning for the edentulous patients, a graftless approach to immediate loading. St Louis (MO): Mosby, an imprint of Elsevier; 2011.

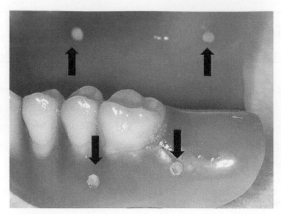

Fig. 62. Create a radiographic guide with 6 to 8 spherical points (*arrows*). (*From* Bedrossian E. Implant treatment planning for the edentulous patients, a graftless approach to immediate loading. St Louis (MO): Mosby, an imprint of Elsevier; 2011. Fig. 10-2; with permission.)

Surgical Template (NobelGuide, Nobel Biocare AB). This sagittal view demonstrates the proposed location of the anterior implant at the maxillary canine position with the prosthesis "turned on" (see **Fig. 63**).[16] The prosthesis mode can be "turned off," only viewing implant positioning.[16] After completing the virtual planning, these implants and anchor pins can be viewed to determine if collision exists; this is best seen with the bony window "turned off" (see **Fig. 64**).[16] The information is transferred to the Nobel Biocare's laboratory in Mahwah, New Jersey for surgical guide fabrication. Afterward, with the surgical guide available, the laboratory technician can then fabricate provisional prosthesis for immediate load and the jig. The purpose of the jig is to properly seat the 30° multiunit nonengaging abutments from cast to patient.

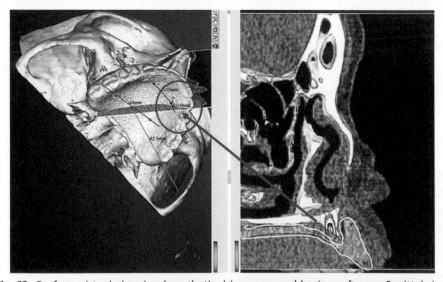

Fig. 63. Perform virtual planning (prosthetic-driven approach) using software. Sagittal view of maxillary canine with prosthesis "turned on." (*From* Bedrossian E. Implant treatment planning for the edentulous patients, a graftless approach to immediate loading. St Louis (MO): Mosby, an imprint of Elsevier; 2011. Fig. 10-15; with permission.)

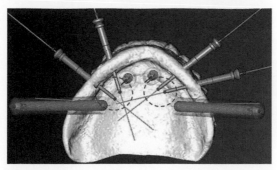

Fig. 64. Perform virtual planning (prosthetic driven approach) using software. Bony window "turned off" to view implants and anchor pins for possible collision. (*From* Bedrossian E. Implant treatment planning for the edentulous patients, a graftless approach to immediate loading. St Louis (MO): Mosby, an imprint of Elsevier; 2011. Fig. 10-23; with permission.)

"Flapless Surgical" Technique for "All-on-4" Guided Surgery: NobelGuide

The NobelGuide surgical guide is light and moisture-sensitive with deformation of the guide possible with greater than 30 minutes of exposure.[16] Disinfect the guide with approved disinfectants (ie, Betadine, Cidex, OPA, Actril, chlorhexadine, alcohol, or similar agents).[27] The NobelGuide surgical guide gets inserted in the patient's mouth (**Box 14**).[16,28] The same surgical index is required to ensure proper seating of the surgical guide.[27] Placement of an appropriate number of anchor pins on the surgical guide will provide stable retention during the procedure.[27]

The guided surgical protocol described later is for RP 4.0 × 13 mm straight implants in medium bone density (ie, NobelReplace Straight, Replace Select Straight, and NobelSpeedy Replace) for edentulous maxilla with 4 implants. Place the surgical guide in the mouth along with the surgical index in centric relations and secure the guide with anchor pins (**Figs. 65** and **66**).[16] Using the flapless approach, a tissue punch is needed to access the surgical sites (**Box 15**).[28] Place the Guided Drill Guide (RP 2.0 mm) in the

---

Box 14
Armamentarium for guided surgery

1. Surgical kits for guided surgery (2 kits) and implants
   a. Guided surgery kit
   b. Guided drill guides
2. Planning report from NobelClinician software
3. Surgical guide with disinfectant and master cast
4. Surgical index
5. Prosthetic components
6. Provisional prosthesis
7. Jig construction: for seating the 30° multiunit abutment nonengaging in the patient's mouth[a]

[a] 30° multiunit abutment nonengaging is only available in RP (trichannel) and external hex connection.
Data from Bedrossian E. Implant treatment planning for the edentulous patients, a graftless approach to immediate loading. St Louis (MO): Mosby, an imprint of Elsevier; 2011; and Nobel Biocare product catalog 2013/2014, Zurich (Switzerland): 2013.

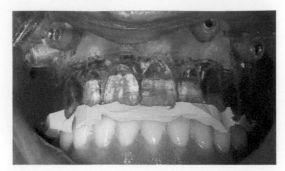

Fig. 65. Place surgical guide in mouth with surgical index in centric and secure guide with anchor pins. (*From* Bedrossian E. Implant treatment planning for the edentulous patients, a graftless approach to immediate loading. St Louis (MO): Mosby, an imprint of Elsevier; 2011. Fig. 10-60; with permission.)

first implant sleeve and start the osteotomy with the Guided Start Drill (round bur) to the built-in stop followed by a 2.0-mm Guided Twist Drill to 13 mm (**Fig. 67**).[16] Switch the Guided Drill Guide to (RP 3.2) and use the 3.2-mm Guided Twist Drill for the final osteotomy to 13 mm. The maximum recommended speed is 800 rpm for all osteotomy sites. A Guided Screw Tap Drill is preferred for dense bone regions, ensuring proper seating of implant. If needed, the Guided Counterbore RP Drill is used for counter-sinking the osteotomy to provide adequate access for the Guided Implant Mount.[16] Use the corresponding Guided Implant Mount NobelReplace to insert these implants with a handpiece at 45 Ncm maximally (**Fig. 68**).[16] For multiple implant placement, alternate insertion at different sides of the arch so further stabilization can be achieved on the surgical guide. Intimate contact of the implant mount to the surgical guide should be noted on completion of the surgical phase.[16]

Provisional Prosthesis-guided Surgery

Remove the surgical guide when all implants are inserted. The implants are torque-tested and need to be at least greater than 35 Ncm before abutment placement (**Box 16**).[16] Place the anterior abutments first and torque them down to 35 Ncm (**Fig. 69**).[16] Place the jig and tighten the impression coping open tray multiunit through

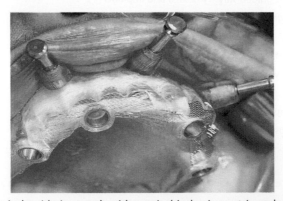

Fig. 66. Place surgical guide in mouth with surgical index in centric and secure guide with anchor pins. (*From* Bedrossian E. Implant treatment planning for the edentulous patients, a graftless approach to immediate loading. St Louis (MO): Mosby, an imprint of Elsevier; 2011. Fig. 10-62; with permission.)

Box 15
Drill sequence for guided surgery (RP) 4.0 × 13 mm NobelSpeedy replace straight implant in medium bone density

1. Place surgical guide in mouth with surgical index in centric and secure guide with anchor pins (max. 800 rpm) (see **Figs. 65** and **66**)

2. Guided tissue punch with (RP sleeve)

3. Guided start drill (round bur) to built-in stop

4. Guided drill guide (RP 2.0 mm) with 2.0-mm guided twist drill to 13 mm (max. 800 rpm) (see **Fig. 67**)

5. Guided drill guide (RP 3.2 mm) with 3.2-mm guided twist drill to 13 mm (max. 800 rpm)

6. (Optional) Guided start drill/Counterbore RP for countersinking at end of procedure for adequate access for guided implant mount (max. 800 rpm)

7. (Optional) Guided screw tap with guided drill guide (RP 4.0 mm) for dense bone regions (max. 45 Ncm)

8. Use corresponding guided implant mount NobelReplace to insert these implants with a handpiece at 45 Ncm maximally (see **Fig. 68**)

Data from Bedrossian E. Implant treatment planning for the edentulous patients, a graftless approach to immediate loading. St Louis (MO): Mosby, an imprint of Elsevier; 2011; and Nobel Biocare product catalog 2013/2014, Zurich (Switzerland): 2013.

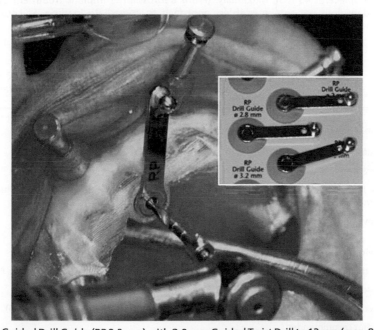

Fig. 67. Guided Drill Guide (RP 2.0 mm) with 2.0-mm Guided Twist Drill to 13 mm (max. 800 rpm). (*From* Bedrossian E. Implant treatment planning for the edentulous patients, a graftless approach to immediate loading. St Louis (MO): Mosby, an imprint of Elsevier; 2011. Fig. 10-64; with permission.)

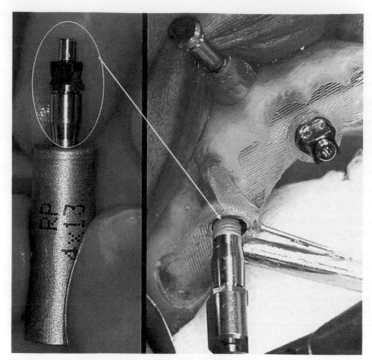

Fig. 68. Use corresponding Guided Implant Mount NobelReplace to insert these implants with a handpiece at 45 Ncm maximally. (*From* Bedrossian E. Implant treatment planning for the edentulous patients, a graftless approach to immediate loading. St Louis (MO): Mosby, an imprint of Elsevier; 2011. Fig. 10-65A; with permission.)

Box 16
Provisional prosthetic steps for guided surgery (day of surgery)

1. Torque test implants to greater than 35 Ncm

2. Place anterior abutments first and torque to 35 Ncm (see **Fig. 69**)

3. Place Jig onto the anterior abutment and the seat the posterior abutments 30° multiunit abutment nonengaging at 15 Ncm (see **Fig. 70**)

4. Remove jig (untwist the abutment holder and guide pin) (see **Fig. 71**)

5. Insert prefabricated (laboratory processed) provisional prosthesis with 3 screws at 15 Ncm (see **Fig. 72**)

6. Place the fourth temporary coping (multiunit) and lute it with fast setting acrylic (see **Fig. 73**)

7. Seal access hole

8. Bilateral group function occlusion with one tooth cantilever maximum (see **Fig. 74**)

9. Soft diet recommended

Data from Bedrossian E. Implant treatment planning for the edentulous patients, a graftless approach to immediate loading. St Louis (MO): Mosby, an imprint of Elsevier; 2011.

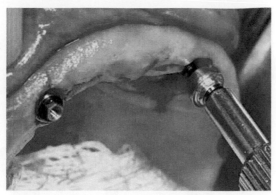

Fig. 69. Place anterior abutments first and torque to 35 Ncm. (*From* Bedrossian E. Implant treatment planning for the edentulous patients, a graftless approach to immediate loading. St Louis (MO): Mosby, an imprint of Elsevier; 2011. Fig. 10-67B; with permission.)

the guide pin with a screwdriver to the anterior site.[16] After which, tighten the abutment screw to a torque of 15 Ncm onto the 30° multiunit abutment nonengaging (**Fig. 70**).[16] The same process is performed on the contralateral side.[16] Remove the jig by untwisting the abutment holder and guide pin (**Fig. 71**).[16] Insert the prefabricated temporary prosthesis with 3 screws torqued to 15 Ncm (**Fig. 72**).[16] The fourth temporary coping (multiunit) is manually inserted into the abutment (**Fig. 73**).[10] Connect the temporary coping (multiunit) to the provisional by applying acrylic resin.[16] Adjust the occlusion to bilateral group function (**Fig. 74**).[16] A final prosthesis can be made in 4 to 6 months.

COMPLICATIONS AND REMEDY

The "All-on-4" technique has surgical and prosthetic complications. Common perio-operative complications include bleeding, swelling, bruising, pain, and possible transient parasthesia. Retraction of the flap/nerve and postoperative swelling can attribute

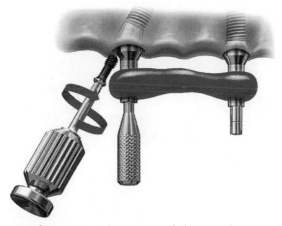

Fig. 70. Place Jig onto the anterior abutment and the seat the posterior abutments 30° multiunit abutment nonengaging at 15 Ncm. (*From* Bedrossian E. Implant treatment planning for the edentulous patients, a graftless approach to immediate loading. St Louis (MO): Mosby, an imprint of Elsevier; 2011. Fig. 10-69A; with permission.)

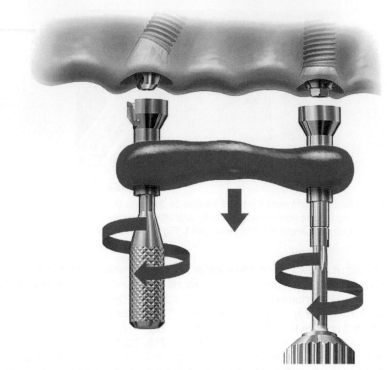

Fig. 71. Remove Jig (untwist the abutment holder and guide pin). (*From* Bedrossian E. Implant treatment planning for the edentulous patients, a graftless approach to immediate loading. St Louis (MO): Mosby, an imprint of Elsevier; 2011. Fig. 10-70B; with permission.)

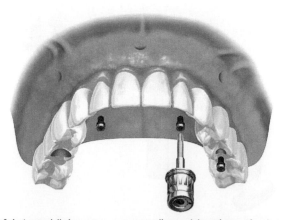

Fig. 72. Insert prefabricated (laboratory processed) provisional prosthesis with 3 screws at 15 Ncm. (*From* Bedrossian E. Implant treatment planning for the edentulous patients, a graftless approach to immediate loading. St Louis (MO): Mosby, an imprint of Elsevier; 2011. Fig. 10-71; with permission.)

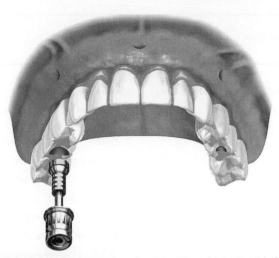

Fig. 73. Place the fourth temporary coping (multiunit) and lute it with fast setting acrylic. (*From* Bedrossian E. Implant treatment planning for the edentulous patients, a graftless approach to immediate loading. St Louis (MO): Mosby, an imprint of Elsevier; 2011. Fig. 10-72A; with permission.)

to parasthesia with resolution usually taking weeks to months. During implant installation with narrow platform implants (3.5 mm), fracture at the platform level has been reported when torque exceeds 45 Ncm(Nobel Biocare's label warning). There is one report of a fractured implant using 4.0 diameter with undisclosed reasons.[36]

Implant complications can be further classified as biological or technical after the initial postoperative period (**Box 17**).[37] Biological complication relates to the implant's hard and soft tissue architecture, although technical complication described herein is prosthetically related. In 2013, Francetti and colleagues reported poor oral hygiene as the number one cause of biological complication at 53.5%, leading to peri-implant mucositis, 30.2%, and peri-implantitis, 10.4%. Peri-implant mucositis is defined as peri-implant mucosa redness and swelling in the absence of alveolar bone loss, and peri-implantitis is the presence of peri-implant soft tissue inflammation with clinical and radiographic bone loss.[14] Strict recall maintenance, 6 months for the first 2 years

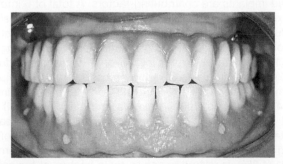

Fig. 74. Bilateral group function occlusion with one-tooth cantilever maximum. (*From* Bedrossian E. Implant treatment planning for the edentulous patients, a graftless approach to immediate loading. St Louis (MO): Mosby, an imprint of Elsevier; 2011. Fig. 10-76; with permission.)

| Box 17 | |
| Complications flow chart | |
Biological	**Technical**
Affects hard and soft tissue around implants	Relates to prosthetics
1. Peri-implant mucositis (53.5%)	1. Detachment of provisional prosthesis (10.5%)
2. Peri-implantitis (30.2%)	
3. Implant loss (8%)	2. Detachment of final prosthesis (23.2%)
	3. Fracture of provisional prosthesis (8%)
	4. Fracture of final prosthesis (7%)
	5. Others (19.8%)
	a. Screw loosening
	b. Screw fracture
	c. Loss of screw access and filling material

Data from Francetti L, Corbella S, Taschieri S, et al. Medium- and long-term complications in full-arch rehabilitations supported by upright and tilted implants. Clin Implant Dent Relat Res 2013. http://dx.doi.org/10.1111/cid.12180.

and annually thereafter, should intercept these issues with proper hygiene and oral antimicrobial rinses.[38] As for the technical side, veneer fracture in the final prosthesis is the most common with 23.2%,[37] followed by detached tooth from a provisional prosthesis at 10.5%, and last, fracture of metal framework on the final prosthesis at 7%.[37] Screw loosening and screw fracture were grouped in "Others" complications with 19.8%. Most prosthetic complications are repairable. None of these prosthetic complications affected the eventual outcome of the rehabilitation.

In 2011, Parel and Phillips[18] identified several common factors that were attributed to maxillary implant failures on immediate load for the "All-on-4" technique through their retrospective study and reported a 3.47% failure rate. Opposing natural dentition, poor bone quality (Houndsfield units <100 HU), male patient, parafunctional habits, and distally placed implants are contributing factors. A total of 6 implants are advocated for the maxilla based on these findings due to softer bone quality.

In 2013, Patzelt and colleagues,[36] performed a comprehensive systemic review for "All-on-4" concepts ever publish in the English and Germanic language looking into 3 particular areas: (1) implant survival rates for "All-on-4" technique performed in maxilla and mandible; (2) survival rates for fixed prosthesis; and (3) evaluate bone level changes at the implant level. Of the 478 articles, only 13 met their inclusion criteria. A cumulative of 4808 implants (2000 in maxilla and mandible 2804) were surveyed (**Box 18**).[36] Most implants, 55 of 74 (74%), failed within the first year of placement and were attributed to patients with certain risk factors, with most of them linked to cigarette smoking and bisphosphonate therapy. The most common prosthetic complication, 57 of 1201 (4.8%), is related to acrylic resin fracture at the anterior abutment region without mental reinforcement. Most of these cases are seen within the first 6 months. Short-face morphology and a drastic change from soft to hard diet are the 2 common denominators found by these authors.[26,31,39–45] These problems

---

Box 18
Complications and remedy

1. Implant failure = 55/74 (74%) failure with in the first year

    Cause = 1. Smoking; 2. Bisphophonate therapy

    Remedy = Removal of implant

2. Prosthesis = 57/1201 (4.8%) fracture denture in anterior abutment region

    Cause = Short face morphology with rapid change soft to hard diet

    Remedy = Repair of fracture acrylic denture

3. Permanent prosthesis = Fracture of prosthesis (only 3 cases reported)

    Cause = Parafunctional habits

    Remedy = Remake permanent prosthesis

4. Occlusal screw loosening = 3% within 6 months and 6% after 12 months

    Cause = Parafuctional habits

    Remedy = 1. Occlusal control; 2. Retightening of screw

5. Abutment screw loosening = 2 cases reported (provisional prosthesis)

    Cause = Parafunctional habits

    Remedy = 1. Retightening of the screw; 2. Night guard

6. Misfits of suprastructure = 13/16 patients

    Cause = CAD/CAM

    Remedy = Need to remake suprastructure with new impression

7. Poor oral hygiene = 1. (53.5%) Perimucositis; 2. (30.2%) Peri-implantitis

    Cause = Poor oral hygiene

    Remedy = 1. Closer recall schedule; 2. Improve hygiene; 3. Peridex; 4. Guided tissue regeneration for peri-implantitis

8. Cigarette smoke = Increases implant loss

    Cause = Cigarettes

    Remedy = Tobacco cessation program

9. Four risk factors for implant failure

    1. Diabetes, 2. Bisphosphonates, 3. Smokers, 4. Medically compromised patients

10. Opposing natural dentition = No reported case of failures

11. Marginal bone loss = No statistical difference when compared with axial implants

Data from Patzelt SB, Bahat O, Reynolds MA, et al. The All-on-Four treatment concept: a systemic review. Clin Implant Dent Relat Res 2013. http://dx.doi.org/10.1111/CID.12068.

---

were remedied by simple repairs. Only 3 failures were related to permanent prosthesis.[31,42,43] Occlusal screw loosening is another complication linked with provisional prosthesis at 3% within the first 6 months and 6% after 12 months,[41,43] in association with patients with parafunctional habits. The solution is to have occlusal control and retightening of the screws. Abutment screw loosening occurred in 2 patients with screw retightening and a night guard as remedies with parafunctional habits as the cause.[26,45] Prefabricated suprastructures had 13 of 16 radiographic misfits reported by Landazuri-Del Barrio and colleagues[31] in 2013, resulting in need of reimpression and delayed delivery of the provisional prosthesis. As stated earlier, poor oral hygiene has a direct association with implant complications, leading to peri-mucositis and or peri-implantitis, as quoted by Francetti and colleagues.[40] Hinze and colleagues[43] and Francetti and colleagues were the only 2 groups of authors that could not find an association between smoking and implant loss. In addition, no association with smoking and marginal bone loss on tilted implants was reported by Hinze.[43] Diabetes, bisphosphonates, smoking, and medically compromised patients were the only 4 common factors linked to high implant failures found by Malo and colleagues.[45] There is no reported complications of "All-on-4" prosthesis in opposing natural dentition. Most importantly, there is no statistically significant difference between maxilla and mandible, axial, or tilted implants relating to marginal bone loss.

CLINICAL DATA

Current data suggest highly successful clinical outcome is achievable for both maxillary and mandibular implants supported by fixed prosthesis in the medium (3–5 years) and long term (5–10 years), respectively, using the "All-on-4" concept.

Malo and colleagues[26] performed 968 implants on 242 patients in the maxilla and found a cumulative success rate of 98% at 5 years. These reports are compatible with literature review by Duello[46] in 2012, who found maxillary implants to have a cumulative success rate ranging from 92.5% to 100% in a 1- to 7-year span (**Table 1**).[46] As for marginal bone loss, Malo recorded an average of 1.52 mm below abutment-implant interface (SD = 0.3 mm) at 3 years, and 5-year marginal bone level at 1.95 mm (SD = 0.4 mm).[26]

Krekmanov, Aparicio, Calandriello and Tomatis and their colleagues were unable to demonstrate any significant differences between traditional vertical splinted implants and a combination of axial and tilted splinted implants at the marginal bone level.[3,6,11,12,47] Bellini and Romero[10] compared tilted and nontilted implants and concurred with the concept that cantilever reduction will help reduce stress at the marginal bone level.

Literature review by Duello[45] also showed mandibular implants with 1 to 10 years have a cumulative success rate of 93.8% to 100% (**Table 2**).[46] Malo and colleagues[45]

Table 1
Maxillary studies of cumulative implant survival of investigated protocol

Author	No. of Tilted Implants	Follow-up	Cumulative Survival (%)
Krekmanov et al,[3] 2002	40	5 y	95.7
Aparicio et al,[6] 2001	42	7 y	95.2
Fortin et al,[5] 2002	90	5 y	92.2
Calandrillo & Tomatis,[12] 2005	27	3 y	96.3
Capelli et al,[48] 2007	82	Up to 40 mo	97.59
Testori et al,[11] 2008	82	Up to 36 mo	97.1
Agliardi et al,[49] 2009	84	Up to 36 mo	100
Hinze et al,[43] 2010	38	1 y	94.6
Babbash et al,[50] 2011	272	Up to 18 mo	99.5

Maxillary implants have a cumulative success rate from 92.5% to 100% in a 1- to 7-year span.
From Duello GV. An evidence-based protocol for immediate rehabilitation of the edentulous patient. J Evid Based Dent Pract 2012;12(3 Suppl):172–81. Table 1; with permission.

Table 2 Mandibular studies of cumulative implant survival rate of investigated protocol			
Author	No. of Tilted Implants	Follow-up	Cumulative Survival Rate (%)
Krekmanov et al,[3] 2000	36	5 y	100
Malo et al,[15] 2003	88	3 y	98.9
Malo et al,[51] 2006	18	1 y	98.9
Capelli et al,[48] 2007	48	Up to 52 mo	97.59
Francetti et al,[40] 2008	124	Up to 48 mo	100
Malo et al,[45] 2011	980	10 y	93.8
Babbush et al,[50] 2010	436	Up to 18 mo	100

Mandibular implants with 1 to 10 years have a cumulative success rate of 93.8% to 100%.
From Duello GV. An evidence-based protocol for immediate rehabilitation of the edentulous patient. J Evid Based Dent Pract 2012;12(3 Suppl):172–81. Table 2; with permission.

in 2011 demonstrated a similar implant-related cumulative success rate at 98.1% in 245 patients with 980 implants.

In 2011, Butera and colleagues[7] reported an overall survival rate of 99.6% for immediate extraction and placement of 875 mandibular implants into 217 jaws in a 3-year clinical study.

Similarly, full-arch fixed prosthesis using the "All-on-4" design has a high degree of predictability in the medium and long term. Current data reveal a cumulative success rate of 99.2% for the mandible in 10 years and 100% in the maxilla for 5 years.[26,45]

SUMMARY

Multiple studies by various independent authors have shown the "All-on-4" technique has similar success rates as compared with the well-studied traditional vertical implants owing to the biomechanics. The "All-on-4" can be a viable option the clinician can offer to their edentulous patients who seek full arch rehabilitation even with planned extraction cases. Atrophic jaws that normally would require traditional bone grafting before implant placement will increase treatment time, costs, and morbidity associated with these grafting procedures. Furthermore, the ability to reduce length of treatment will have a positive psyche so patients can return back to normal form and function.

ACKNOWLEDGMENTS

The authors want to extend a very special thanks to Ms Franine Tidona (Chief, Library Service at Brooklyn Campus) for her tireless and unconditional efforts to help gather numerous articles for us.

REFERENCES

1. Branemark PI, Hannsson BO, Adell R, et al. Osseointegrated implant in treatment of the edentulous jaw. Experience from a 10-year period. Scand J Plast Reconstr Surg Suppl 1977;12:1–132.
2. Mattsson T, Konsell P, Gynther G, et al. Implant treatment without bone grafting in severely resorbed edentulous maxillae. J Oral Maxillofac Surg 1999;57:281–7.
3. Krekmanov L, Khan M, Rangert B, et al. Tilting of posterior mandibular and maxillary implants for improved prosthesis support. Int J Oral Maxillofac Implants 2000;15:405–14.

4. Malo P, Rangert B, Nobre M. "All-on-4" immediate-function concept with Brane-mark system implants for completely edentulous maxilla: a 1 year retrospective clinical study. Clin Implant Dent Relat Res 2005;7(Suppl 1):88–94.

5. Fortin Y, Sullivan RM, Rangert B. The Marius implant bridge: surgical and prosthetic rehabilitation for the completely edentulous upper jaw with moderate to severe resorption: a 5-year retrospective clinical study. Clin Implant Dent Relat Res 2002;4(2):69–77.

6. Aparicio C, Perales P, Ranget B. Tilted implants as an alternative to maxillary sinus grafting: A clinical, radiological and periotest study. Clin Implant Dent Relat Res 2001;3(1):39–49.

7. Butera C, Galindo DF, Jensen O. Mandibular all-on-four therapy using angled implants: a three-year clinical study of 857 implants in 219 jaws. Dent Clin North Am 2011;55:795–811.

8. Tada S, Strengolu R, Kitamura E, et al. Influence of implant design and bone quality on stress/strain distribution in bone around implants: a 3-dimensional finite element analysis. Int J Oral Maxillofac Implants 2003;18:357–68.

9. Rangert B, Sullivan RM, Jemt T. load factor control for implants in the posterior partially edentulous segment. Int J Oral Maxillofac Implants 1987;12:360–70.

10. Bellini CM, Romero D. Comparison of tilted versus nontilted implant-supported prosthetic design for the restoration of the edentulous mandible: a biomechanical study. Int J Oral Maxillofac Implants 2000;24(3):511–7.

11. Testori T, Del Fabbro M, Capellini M, et al. Immediate occlusal loading and tilted implants for the rehabilitation of the atrophic edentulous maxilla: 1-year interim results of a multicenter prospective study. Clin Oral Implants Res 2008;19:227–32.

12. Calandriello R, Tomatis M. Simplified treatment of the atrophic posterior maxilla via immediate/early function and tilted implants: a prospective 1-year clinical study. Clin Implant Dent Relat Res 2000;7:1–12.

13. Malo P, Lopes I, Nobre M. Chapter 27: the All-on-4 concept. In: Babbush C, Hahn J, Krauser J, et al, editors. Dental implants, the arts and science. 2nd edition. Maryland Heights (MO): Saunders an imprint of Elsevier; 2011. p. 435–7.

14. Corbella S, Del Fabbro M, Taschieri S, et al. Clinical evaluation of an implant maintenance protocol for the prevention of the peri-implant disease in patients treated with immediately loaded full arch rehabilitation. Int J Dent Hyg 2011;9:216–22.

15. Malo P, Rangert B, Nobre M. "All-on-4" immediate function concept with Brane-mark System Implants for completely edentulous mandibles: a retrospective clinical study. Clin Implant Dent Relat Res 2003;5(Suppl 1):2–9.

16. Bedrossian E. Implant treatment planning for the edentulous patients, a graftless approach to immediate loading. St Louis (MO): Mosby, an imprint of Elsevier; 2011.

17. Pomares C. A retrospective clinical study of edentulous patients rehabilitated according to the "all-on-four" or the "all-on-six" immediately function concept. Eur J Oral Implantol 2009;2(1):55–60.

18. Parel S, Phillips W. A risk assessment treatment planning protocol for the four implant immediate loaded maxilla: a preliminary findings. J Prosthet Dent 2011;106:359–66.

19. Parel S. Chapter 23: the evolution of the angled implants. In: Babbush C, Hahn J, Krauser J, et al, editors. Dental implants, the arts and science. 2nd edition. Maryland Heights (MO): Saunders an imprint of Elsevier; 2011. p. 370–88.

20. Bedrossian E. Chapter 15: graftless solution for atrophic maxilla. In: Babbush C, Hahn J, Krauser J, et al, editors. Dental implants, the arts and science. 2nd edition. Maryland Heights (MO): Saunders an imprint of Elsevier; 2011. p. 251–9.

21. Jensen OT, Adams MW. All-on-4 treatment of highly atrophic mandible with mandibular V-4: report of 2 cases. J Oral Maxillofac Surg 2009;67:1503–9.
22. Jensen OT, Adams M, Cottam J, et al. The All-on-4: shelf. J Oral Maxillofac Surg 2010;68:2520–7.
23. Jensen OT, Adams M, Cottam J, et al. The All on 4 shelf: mandible. J Oral Maxillofac Surg 2011;69:175–81.
24. Jensen OT, Cottam J, Ringeman J, et al. Trans-sinus dental implants, bone morphogenic protein 2, and immediate function for all-on-4 treatment of severe maxillary atrophy. J Oral Maxillofac Surg 2012;70:141–8.
25. Nobel Biocare "All-on-4" Procedures & Products Manuel 2007.
26. Malo P, De Araujo Nobre M, Lopes A, et al. "All-on-4" immediate function concept for completely edentulous maxillae: a clinical report on the medium (3 years) and long-term (5 years) outcomes. Clin Implant Dent Relat Res 2011;14(Suppl 1): e139–50.
27. Nobel Biocare "All-on-4" Concept manual for conventional and guided surgery 2012.
28. Nobel Biocare product catalog 2013/2014.
29. Babbush C, Rosenlicht J. Chapter 14; inferior alveolar nerve lateralization and mental neurovascular distalization. In: Babbush C, Hahn J, Krauser J, et al, editors. Dental implants, the arts and science, second edition. Maryland Heights (MO): Elsevier 2011. p. 237.
30. Babbush C, Kanawarti A, Brokloft J. A new approach to the All-on-Four treatment concept using narrow platform NobelActive implants. J Oral Implantol 2013; 39(3):314–25.
31. Landazuri-Del Barrio R, Cosyn J, De Paula W, et al. A prospective study on implants installed with flapless-guided surgery using the all-on-four concept in the mandible. Clin Oral Implants Res 2013;24:428–33.
32. Brodala N. Flapless surgery and its effects on dental implants outcomes. Int J Oral Maxillofac Implants 2009;24(Suppl):118–25.
33. D'Haese J, Van De Velde T, Komiyama A, et al. Accuracy and complications using computer-designed stereolithographic surgical guides for oral rehabilitation by means of dental implants: a review of the literature. Clin Implant Dent Relat Res 2010. http://dx.doi.org/10.1111/j.1708–8208.2010.
34. Jung RE, Schneider D, Ganeles J, et al. Computer technology applications in surgical implant dentistry: a systemic review. Int J Oral Maxillofac Implants 2009; 24(Suppl):92–109.
35. Schneider D, Marquardt P, Zwahlen M, et al. A systemic review on the accuracy and the clinical outcome of computer-guided template-based implants dentistry. Clin Oral Implants Res 2009;20(Suppl 4):73–86.
36. Patzelt SB, Bahat O, Reynolds MA, et al. The All-on-Four treatment concept: a systemic review. Clin Implant Dent Relat Res 2013. http://dx.doi.org/10.1111/CID.12068.
37. Francetti L, Corbella S, Taschieri S, et al. Medium- and long-term complications in full arch rehabilitation supported by upright and tilted implants. Clin Implant Dent Relat Res 2013. http://dx.doi.org/10.1111/cid.12180.
38. De Siena F, Francetti L, Corbella S, et al. Topical application of 1% chlorhexadine gel versus 0.2% mouthwash in the treatment of peri-implant mucositis. An observational study. Int J Dent Hyg 2013;11:41–7.
39. Agliardi E, Panigatti S, Clerico M, et al. Immediate rehabilitation of the edentulous jaws with full fixed prostheses supported by four implants: interim results of a single cohort prospective study. Clin Oral Implants Res 2010;21:459–65.

40. Francetti L, Agliardi E, Testori T, et al. Immediate rehabilitation of the mandible with fixed full prosthesis supported by axial and tilted implants interim results of a single cohort prospective study. Clin Implant Dent Relat Res 2008;10: 255–63.

41. Crespin R, Vinci R, Cappare P, et al. A clinical study of edentulous patients rehabilitated according to the "all-on-4" immediate function protocol. Int J Oral Maxillofac Implants 2012;27:428–34.

42. Francetti L, Romero D, Corbella S, et al. Bone level changes around axial and tilted implants in full-arch fixed immediate restorations. Interim results of a prospective study. Clin Implant Dent Relat Res 2012;14:646–54.

43. Hinze M, Thalmair T, Bolzano W, et al. Immediate loading of fixed provisional prostheses using four implants for the rehabilitation of the edentulous arch: a prospective clinical study. Int J Oral Maxillofac Implants 2010;25:1011–8.

44. Malo P, De Araujo Nobre M, Lopes A. The use of computer-guided flapless implant surgery and four implants placed in immediate function to support a fixed denture: preliminary results after a mean follow-up period of thirteen months. J Prosthet Dent 2007;97:S26–34.

45. Malo P, De Araujo Nobre M, Lopes A, et al. A longitudinal study of the survival of All-on-4 implants in the mandible with up to 10 years of follow-up. J Am Dent Assoc 2011;142:310–20.

46. Duello GV. An evidence-based protocol for immediate rehabilitation of the edentulous patient. J Evid Based Dent Pract 2012;12(3 Suppl):172–81.

47. Aparicio C, Arevalo X, Ouzzani W, et al. A retrospective clinical and radiographic evaluation of tilted implants used in treatment of the severely resorbed edentulous maxilla. Apple Osseointegration Res 2002;3:17–21.

48. Capelli M, Zuffetti F, Testori T, et al. Immediate rehabilitation of the completely edentulous jaws with fixed prostheses supported by either upright or tilted implants: a multicenter clinical study. Int J Oral Maxillofac Implants 2007;22:639–44.

49. Agliardi EL, Francetti L, Romeo D, et al. Immediate rehabilitation of the edentulous maxilla: preliminary results of a single-cohort prospective study. Int J Oral Maxillofac Implants 2009;24:887–95.

50. Babbash C, Kutsko G, Brokloff J. The all-on-four immediate function concept with NobelActive Implants: a retrospective study. J Oral Implantol 2011;38(4):431–45.

51. Malo P, Rangert B, Nobre M, et al. A pilot study of completely edentulous rehabilitation with immediate function using a new implant design: case series. Clin Implant Dent Relat Res 2006;8:223–32.

52. Taruna M, Chittaranjan B, Sudheer N, et al. Prosthetic Perspective to All-on-4 Concept for dental implants. Journal of Clinical and Diagnostic Research 2014; 8(10):16–9.

Soft Tissue Surgery for Implants

Hussam Batal, DMD[a],*, Amir Yavari, DDS[b], Pushkar Mehra, BDS, DMD[a]

KEYWORDS

- Subepithelial connective tissue graft • Epithelial connective tissue graft
- Gingival biotype • Pouch technique • VIP connective tissue graft
- Free subepithelial connective tissue graft
- Single-incision technique for harvest of subepithelial connective tissue graft
- Two-incision technique for harvest of subepithelial connective tissue graft

KEY POINTS

- Improving the quality of soft tissue around dental implants improves the final esthetic outcome.
- Soft tissue grafts play an integral role in increasing volume and morphology of attached gingiva.
- The pouch technique is ideal for augmentation of the soft tissue at the time of immediate implant placement.
- The VIP-CT graft is ideal augmentation of horizontal and vertical soft tissue augmentation.

INTRODUCTION

There are two common reasons for implant surgery: esthetics and function. In both cases, the treatment is aimed at re-establishing the missing soft and hard tissue architecture. Implant surgery success is no longer judged by the ability to osseointegrate, but rather by the ability of the clinicians involved in delivering care to predictably provide an acceptable esthetic result that is stable long-term under functional load.

It has long been established that appropriate quality and quantity of soft tissue provides the most optimal peri-implant environment. Attached tissue around dental implants increases soft tissue stability and decreases the incidence of peri-implant mucositis. Having an adequate band and thickness of soft tissue in the esthetic zone is often needed to provide the much-needed optimal esthetic outcome that allows the final restoration to seamlessly blend with the surrounding dentition.[1]

The authors have nothing to disclose.
[a] Oral and Maxillofacial Surgery, Boston University, 100 East Newton Street, G407, Boston, MA 02118, USA; [b] Private practice, Boston, MA 02118, USA
* Corresponding author.
E-mail address: batalhs@bu.edu

Dent Clin N Am 59 (2015) 471–491
http://dx.doi.org/10.1016/j.cden.2014.10.012
0011-8532/15/$ – see front matter Published by Elsevier Inc.

GINGIVAL BIOTYPE

Esthetic outcomes in implant dentistry strongly correlate with the patient's gingival biotype. The gingival perspective depends on gingival complex, tooth morphology, contact points, hard and soft tissue considerations, periodontal bioform, and biotype. Two distinct biotypes have been described by Olsson and Lindhe[2]: thin scalloped and thick flat. There are three key areas of variation between the two biotypes and these include differences in soft tissue, bone, and teeth morphology. Determination of biotypes in a specific individual is controversial and can be quite challenging, especially because parameters used for assessment are often subjective. Thus, use of objective criteria is recommended and combining direct measurement of soft tissue thickness and tooth morphology can aid in the determination and classification.

Thin Scalloped Gingival Biotype

The bony and soft tissue architecture tends to be highly scalloped, the soft tissue is thin, and this type of tissue reacts to insult with recession (**Fig. 1**). The underlying buccal plate tends to be thin with frequent fenestration and dehiscence type of defects. The bony architecture tends to undergo extensive remodeling after extraction of teeth including increased loss of height of the buccal plate and socket dimension compared with patients with a thicker buccal plate. The teeth tend to be more triangular in shape with narrow contact areas located in the incisal one-third and the crowns at the cervical area are either flat or have a subtle convexity with a flat emergence profile.[3]

Thick Flat Gingival Biotype

The bony and soft tissue architecture tends to be flat with short interdental papillae, supported further by a dense and thick band of attached tissue (**Fig. 2**). There is dense fibrotic tissue, and this kind of soft tissue reacts to insult with pocket formation rather than recession. The underlying bony architecture is thick and rarely has dehiscences or fenestrations. The thick plate tends to undergo lesser remodeling after surgical procedures. The teeth tend to be squarer in shape with long contact areas extending to the cervical one-third. The emergence profile tends to be pronounced.

There is general consensus that the addition of soft tissue graft to the surgical implant protocol in patients with thin scalloped biotype increases gingival thickness and improves esthetic outcomes, especially at the buccal gingival margin level. It is likely to even improve longer-term soft tissue stability.[4]

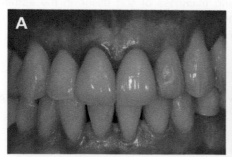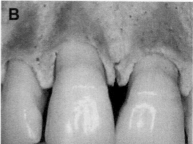

Fig. 1. (*A*) Thin scalloped gingival biotype with triangular-shaped teeth. (*B*) Thin biotype with thin buccal plate and fenestrations. Also note the scalloping of the bony architecture.

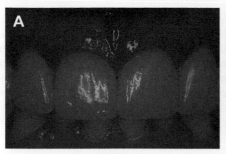
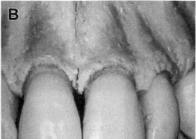

Fig. 2. (A) Thick flat gingival biotype with square-shaped teeth. (B) Thick biotype with thick buccal plate. Also note the flat bony architecture.

GENERAL PRINCIPLES OF SOFT TISSUE GRAFTING

When performing soft tissue grafting, there are general principles that increase the chances of success and decrease the incidence of complications. In general, these principles are divided into recipient site preparation and donor site management guidelines.[5] These general principles are derived from the physiologic healing process and the local and systemic conditions needed to achieve them. In brief, they are (1) creation of an adequate recipient site; (2) adequate hemostasis at the recipient site; (3) good adaptation of the graft; (4) immobilization of the graft; and (5) primary closure, when feasible (dual blood supply).

Soft tissue graft healing depends on adequate preparation and the vascularity of the recipient site.[6,7] Grafts initially survive by plasmatic diffusion and then by revascularization. Good adaptation and immobility of the graft is critical for these processes to occur effectively. Early mobility could disrupt the revascularization process and increase the chance of necrosis of the graft. Intimate adaptation to the recipient site is imperative to success and decreases the diffusion and capillary travel distance by providing early nutrition to the graft. Also, adequate hemostasis at the recipient site decreases capillary bleeding or large clot formation, both of which could impair the nutrient supply. In cases where there is decreased vascularity at the recipient site (scarring, implant abutment, root surface), use of a pedicled graft with contiguous blood supply should be considered rather than free grafts. If a pedicled graft is not feasible, care should be taken so that the recipient site and graft are wide enough to allow for peripheral circulation that supports the graft over the poorly vascularized area. When preparing the recipient site, clinicians should ensure that the surface is uniform and allows for adequate immobilization of the grafted tissue. Adequate hemostasis is mandatory to permit for adequate adaptation of the graft to the recipient bed.

Generally speaking, intact and viable periosteum is considered an ideal coverage layer. Periosteum has an excellent blood supply, is nonmovable, and allows for adequate immobilization and suturing of the graft. The graft should be of uniform thickness; this allows for better adaptation of the graft to the recipient site. The thickness of the graft plays a role in the healing process and could also determine the amount of secondary contracture of the graft. Thin and intermediate-thickness grafts have a higher percentage of survival. Contrastingly, thicker grafts yield better clinical outcomes with less secondary contracture but are more technique sensitive. Finally, whenever possible, creation of a flap at the recipient site that permits primary closure is likely to improve outcomes and decrease the possibility of graft necrosis.

TIMING OF SOFT TISSUE GRAFTING

Soft tissue grafting can be performed at a variety of timelines during implant therapy. It can be performed before bone grafting, at the same time or after bone grafting, at the time of implant placement, at the time of second-stage abutment placement, and after prosthetic crown connection. The predictability of stable and successful outcomes decreases when performed after crown connection.

TYPES OF SOFT TISSUE GRAFTS
Connective Tissue Autografts

A variety of intraoral donor sites have been described for connective tissue grafts. The most commonly used source is the hard palate. An alternative donor site is the maxillary tuberosity region. Although the greatest thickness of tissue is usually present in the maxillary tuberosity area, the maximum volume of tissue obtainable is from the palate. The amount of tissue available tends to be limited in the fully dentate patient. Types of connective tissue that are harvested from intraoral sites can be divided as either subepithelial connective tissue grafts[8] or epithelial connective tissue grafts (**Fig. 3**).

Subepithelial Connective Tissue Graft

These grafts are most commonly harvested from the palate from an area between the palatal root of the first molar and the canine tooth.[9] The soft tissue of the hard palate tissue tends to be thickest in this region. During the harvesting procedure, careful attention should be given so as not to injure the greater palatine artery.[10] According to the study by Reiser and coworkers,[10] the greater palatine artery enters the palate in the area of the greater palatine foramen and travels across the palate anteriorly in the direction of the incisive foramen (**Fig. 4**A). The greater palatine foramen is most commonly located at the junction of the horizontal and vertical shelf of the palatine bone in an area corresponding to the position between the second and third molar. The neurovascular bundle is located between 7 and 17 mm from the cementoenamel junction (CEJ) of the teeth, with an average 12 mm distance (see **Fig. 4**B). The distance

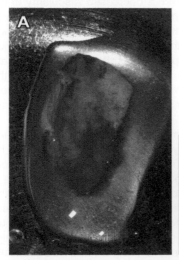
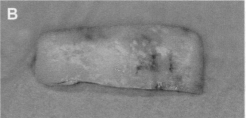

Fig. 3. (*A*) Subepithelial connective tissue graft. (*B*) Epithelial connective tissue graft.

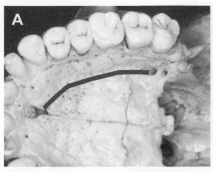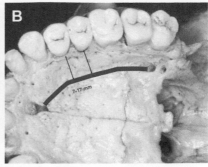

Fig. 4. (A) Course of the greater palatine artery existing the greater palatine foramen and crossing the palate in the direction of incisive canal. Crossing at the junction of the horizontal and vertical shelf of the palate. (B) The greater palatine artery is located between 7 and 17 mm from the cementoenamel junction (CEJ) of the teeth with an average distance of 12 mm.

is shorter in patients with a shallow palatal vault and longer in patients with higher palatal vault. Injury to the greater palatine artery closer to the foramen can cause extensive bleeding when compared with vasculature damage to the anterior palatal area. Limiting the dissection to 8 mm in height limits the risk of bleeding in most patients.

The palatal soft tissue is composed of three layers: (1) epithelium, (2) subepithelial connective tissue, and (3) submucosa. In the anterior palatal area, especially in the area of the rugae, the subepithelial layer is rich in fat. After harvesting of the graft, the fat layer should be removed with scissors before suturing; this minimizes subsequent mobility of the graft.[11] Moreover, it allows the graft to be uniform in size and optimize its adaptation to the host recipient bed. To maintain vitality, it is advisable to keep the harvested and prepared graft in saline or saline-soaked sponges for temporary storage.

Various techniques for harvesting of subepithelial connective tissue grafts have been described. The main variation between them is in the number and type of surface incisions.

Single-incision surgical technique

After adequate local anesthetic with vasoconstrictor has been infiltrated in the area, a horizontal incision is made 2 to 3 mm apical to the CEJ, extending from the mesial aspect of the first molar to the canine area (**Fig. 5A**). The blade is next used to start a split-thickness incision within the first horizontal incision. The direction of dissection is parallel to the palatal tissue (see **Fig. 5B**). The flap should be a least 1 mm thick to decrease the chances of sloughing and necrosis that could cause postoperative pain and discomfort. This incision also determines the thickness of the tissue that is harvested. The dissection is carried on with sharp instruments to the height of approximately 8 mm. This usually corresponds to the cutting portion of the #15 scalpel blade. A properly carried out dissection should create a rectangular pouch. Once the pouch is created, a second horizontal incision is made within the pocket all the way down to bone around 1 mm apical to the initial incision (see **Fig. 5C**). This leaves a 1-mm ledge of connective tissue, which can be sutured to the epithelial flap with an aim to increase potential for primary healing and decrease chances of dehiscence and failure.[12]

Next, an anterior incision is made inside the pouch at the most anterior aspect all the way down to bone to the desired depth (see **Fig. 5D**) and another incision is made in a

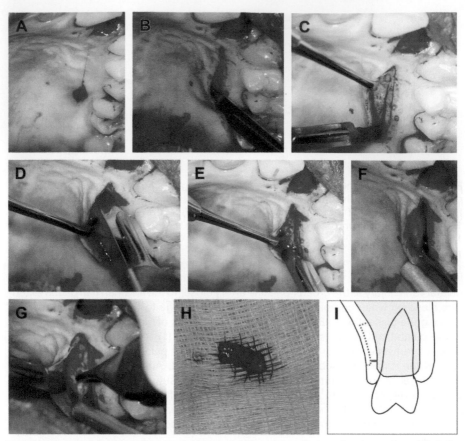

Fig. 5. (*A*) Initial horizontal split-thickness incision from first molar to canine. (*B*) Split-thickness dissection is carried to a depth of 8 to 10 mm. (*C*) Second horizontal full-thickness incision 1 mm apical to the first incision. (*D*) Anterior full-thickness incision. (*E*) Posterior full-thickness incision. (*F*) Dissection is carried in a subperiosteal fashion reflecting the graft. (*G*) A full-thickness incision is made along the apical aspect and the graft is harvested. (*H*) Sub-epithelial graft is harvested and fat is trimmed. (*I*) Diagram of the single-incision technique using stepped approach. The *dotted line* shows initial split-thickness incision. *Solid line* shows the second incision that is placed 1 mm apical to the initial incision.

similar fashion at the posterior aspect (see **Fig. 5**E). A Woodson or similar instrument, such as a periosteal elevator, is used to elevate the graft in a subperiosteal plane (see **Fig. 5**F). The partially elevated graft is held with tissue pickups and an incision made at the most apical aspect (see **Fig. 5**G) and using tissue forceps and gentle traction, the graft is harvested (see **Fig. 5**H, I). Pressure is applied to the donor site and a collagen or hemostatic dressing placed in harvest site and secured into place with overlying 4–0 resorbable sutures. One should always aim to harvest a subepithelial connective tissue graft with attached periosteum, because this makes handling easier and decreases secondary shrinkage and contraction of the graft.

Some clinicians use a modified variation of the above-mentioned single-incision technique. The initial horizontal incision (**Fig. 6**A) is a full-thickness incision to the bone. Then a split-thickness incision is started within the first incision (see **Fig. 6**B) and carried in a similar fashion to the technique described previously.

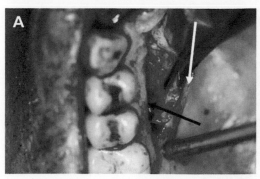 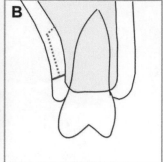

Fig. 6. (A) Initial horizontal incision is a full-thickness incision (*black arrow*), the split-thickness incision is started within the first incision (*white arrow*). (B) Diagram of the single-incision technique, *dotted line* split-thickness incision, *solid line* full-thickness incision.

Two-incision surgical technique

This technique is commonly used when an epithelial collar is desired. After adequate local anesthetic with vasoconstrictor has been infiltrated in the area, a horizontal incision is made 2 to 3 mm apical to the sulcular gingival margin, extending from the mesial aspect of the first molar to the canine area. The first incision is extended in a full-thickness fashion all the way to the bone. Then, a second horizontal incision is placed 1 to 2 mm apical to the first incision. This second incision should be a split-thickness incision to an approximate depth of 1 to 1.5 mm. Using this incision, development of a split-thickness flap is initiated with the use of a #15 blade. The direction of dissection should be parallel to the palatal tissue and associated vault (**Fig. 7**A). The flap should be a least 1 mm thick to decrease the chances of sloughing and necrosis that could cause postoperative pain and discomfort, besides failure. This incision also determines the thickness of the tissue that is harvested. The dissection is carried on with sharp instruments to the height of approximately 8 mm. This usually corresponds to the cutting portion of the #15 scalpel blade. A properly carried out dissection should create a rectangular pouch. Once the pouch is created, an anterior incision is made inside the pouch at the most anterior aspect all the way down to bone to the desired depth. Next, an incision is made in a similar fashion at the posterior aspect. A Woodson or periosteal elevator is used to elevate the graft in a subperiosteal plane. The partially elevated graft is held with tissue pickups and an incision made at the most apical aspect (see **Fig. 7**B) and the graft is harvested (see **Fig. 7**C).

Pouch technique

The pouch technique is commonly used for augmentation of soft tissue in the buccal area. It is ideal for augmentation at the time of immediate implant placement, or correction of soft tissue defects around nonsubmerged or restored implants.

A horizontal incision is made with the use of keratome knives (**Fig. 8**A, B). The incision is made at right angles to the epithelium and dissection is ideally carried in a supraperiosteal fashion to allow for dual blood supply to the graft. The pouch must have enough thickness to decrease the incidence of flap perforation, sloughing, or tearing during tunneling of the graft. This technique is extremely technique sensitive and dependent on operator variability. Thus, in the authors' opinion, it is better to develop a thicker pouch, even if the level of dissection is subperiosteal.

The dissection should be extended laterally to allow for increased blood supply to the graft (see **Fig. 8**C). The dissection should be extended beyond the mucogingival

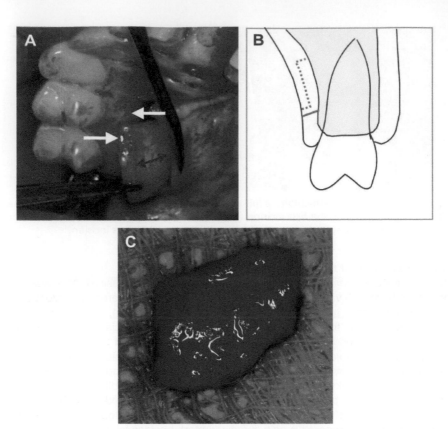

Fig. 7. (*A*) Two-incision technique, initial incision a full-thickness incision (*white arrows*). Second incision is placed 1 to 1.5 mm apical and carried in a split-thickness fashion (*gray arrow*). (*B*) Diagram of two-incision technique, *dotted line* split-thickness incision, *solid line* full-thickness incision. (*C*) Subepithelial connective tissue graft with epithelial collar.

junction because this facilitates subsequent tunneling of the graft. Once the pouch is completed, a Woodson or similar elevator is used to estimate the size of the pocket. The graft is harvested from the palate and trimmed to match the size of the created pouch (see **Fig. 8**D, E). Appropriate suture material (eg, 3–0 Vicryl suture on PS2 needle) is passed from an area beyond the mucogingival junction through the pocket and then through the connective tissue graft and back through the graft, then through the pocket out through the mucogingival junction (see **Fig. 8**F, G). The graft is then secured manually by pulling the suture with one hand and using a Woodson elevator on the other hand simultaneously to push the graft down into the pouch. Once the graft is positioned in the desired position the suture is tied to prevent the graft from getting displaced apically (see **Fig. 8**G). The graft can be further secured with a few horizontal mattress sutures (see **Fig. 8**H). Pressure is applied to the area for 5 to 10 minutes. During the dissection careful attention should be made to avoid reflection of the dental papilla or the buccal flap. This decreases the possibility of graft mobility and loss of the graft (see **Fig. 8**I).

A variation of this technique involves creation of a subperiosteal pouch with the use of a Buser or Woodson elevator but making sure the pouch extends into the

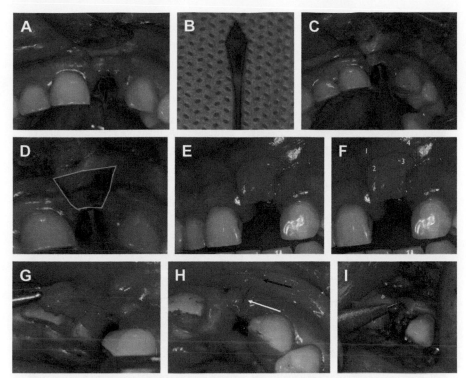

Fig. 8. (*A*) A keratome knife is used to create a pouch. (*B*) Keratome knife. (*C*) During creation of the pouch, the dissection should extend beyond the mucogingival junction. (*D*) Outline of the pouch that will be created. (*E*) A graft that corresponds to the size of the pocket is harvested. (*F*) Sequence in which the suture is passed to facilitate tunneling of the graft. (*G*) Graft with suture in place just before starting the process of tunneling the graft. (*H*) The graft is secured in place with the use of horizontal mattress suture (*white arrow*), also the suture that was used to tunnel the graft was tied and secured (*black arrow*). (*I*) During the development of the pouch attention should be made to avoid reflection of the papilla or buccal flap.

mucogingival junction. The graft is tunneled in a similar manner as in the technique described previously (**Figs. 9** and **10**).

Indications for this technique include (1) converting a thin gingival biotype into a thick biotype, (2) increasing soft tissue thickness, and (3) correction of soft tissue defects around restored implants. It cannot be used for vertical augmentation.

Free Subepithelial Connective Tissue Grafts

This technique is commonly used for augmentation of soft tissue defects at the time of implant placement or during placement of the healing abutment connection. It is commonly used for horizontal soft tissue augmentation and also less frequently for vertical augmentation.

Technique and procedure

Preparation of the recipient site depends on the timing of the soft tissue graft (**Fig. 11**A–C). A split- or full-thickness flap is reflected, and a subepithelial connective tissue graft harvested from the palate (see **Fig. 11**D, E). The graft is trimmed and

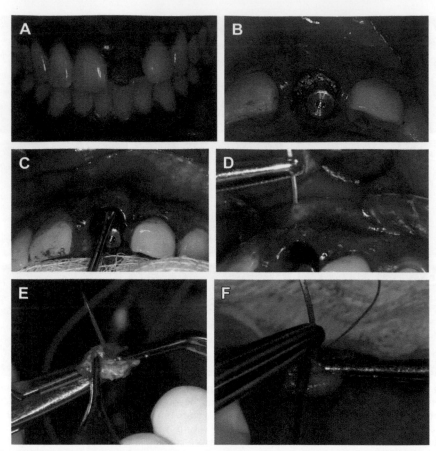

Fig. 9. (*A*) Patient with nonrestorable tooth #9, also existing long restored implant in area of tooth #8. (*B*) After extraction of tooth #9 an immediate implant is placed and gap between the implant and the buccal plate is grafted with a xenograft. (*C*) A pouch is created with the use of a Woodson elevator and the pouch is extended beyond the mucogingival junction. (*D*) A needle is passed through the mucogingival junction exiting under the gingival margin on the buccal aspect. (*E*) The suture is passed through the connective tissue graft on the inferior aspect (periosteal side). (*F*) The suture is passed again through the connective tissue graft from the superior aspect of graft. (*G*) The graft is tunneled by pulling the graft with the suture and pushing the graft with a Woodson inside the pouch. (*H*) Graft tunneled in the pouch before final suturing. (*I*) Graft in place with custom temporary healing abutment. (*J*) Healed graft before temporization. (*K*) Frontal view 1 year after implant placement with graft.

adapted to the buccal aspect of the flap. Once the graft is appropriately sized, the graft is positioned based on the desired area of augmentation and the flap is secured with a horizontal mattress resorbable suture. The suture is used to secure the graft to the buccal flap in the desired area of augmentation (see **Fig. 11**F–H).[13] The flap is sutured and this closure automatically further secures the graft in place (see **Fig. 11**I, J). An alternative option is to secure the graft to the recipient periosteal bed first, and then suture the buccal flap over so as to completely cover the connective tissue graft.

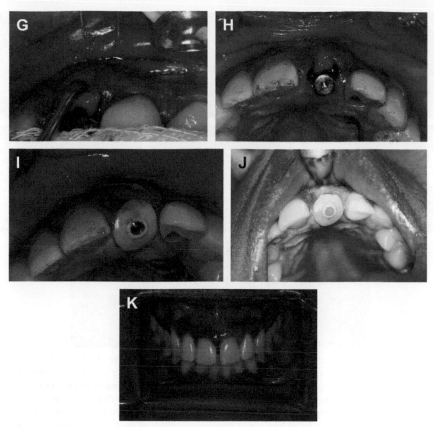

Fig. 9. (*continued*).

Vascularized Interpositional Periosteal–Connective Tissue Flap

Sclar[5] described this flap for augmentation of large soft tissue defects many years ago and since then some minor modifications have been proposed. This technique involves rotation of a pedicled subepithelial finger flap to the anterior maxillary area. The blood supply to the flap is random-pattern. One of the main advantages of the vascularized interpositional periosteal–connective tissue (VIP-CT) flap is its ability to be effective during simultaneous hard and soft tissue augmentation. The VIP-CT flap allows for superior soft tissue augmentation in vertical and horizontal directions when compared with conventional free soft tissue grafts. Practitioners can expect increased graft stability with decreased secondary shrinkage when using these flaps relative to other techniques. It is also an ideal graft to use when the tissue bed is compromised (eg, extensive scarring at recipient site with decreased blood supply to the area) and is ideal for correction of large soft tissue defects. The only downside of this flap is that it cannot be used if concomitant temporization is desired and when the implant is not submerged.

Technique and procedure

Local anesthesia with vasoconstrictor is infiltrated in a standard manner. The initial step involves preparation of the recipient site. Generally speaking, a curvilinear,

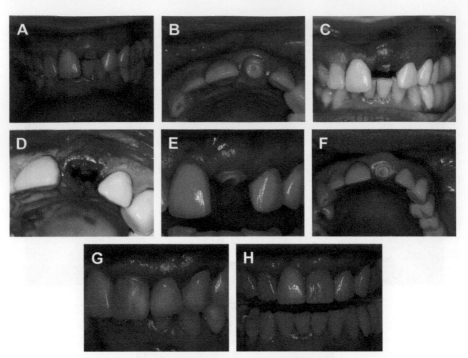

Fig. 10. (*A*) Frontal view of nonrestorable tooth #9. (*B*) Occlusal view of nonrestorable tooth #9. (*C*) Implant placed in area of tooth #9 with soft tissue graft using pouch technique with a custom temporary healing abutment. (*D*) Occlusal view of implant placed in area of tooth #9 with soft tissue graft using pouch technique before placing custom temporary healing abutment. (*E*) Frontal view after 4 months of healing; note preservation of root prominence. (*F*) Occlusal view after 4 months of healing; note preservation of root prominence. (*G*) Lateral view with temporary crown in place. (*H*) Frontal view with temporary crown in place.

papilla-sparing incision is most commonly used. In the crestal area, the incision is placed on the palatal aspect of the ridge because this allows for complete exposure of the alveolar ridge and also results in an increase in vertical soft tissue thickness at the end of the procedure (**Fig. 12**A, B). The papilla-sparing mucosal incision is next extended palatally in an exaggerated fashion, on the mesial and distal aspects of the edentulous space. A second horizontal, full-thickness, palatal incision is made approximately 3 mm below the free gingival margin and extended to connect with the distal palatal incision. Next, a split-thickness palatal incision is initiated at the first molar area and extended anteriorly in split-thickness manner to the palatal incision area (see **Fig. 12**C, D). As the dissection is carried anteriorly, the flap becomes harder to develop especially in the palatal rugae area. Maintaining a good thickness of the flap (at least 1 mm) and starting the dissection from posterior to anterior facilitates flap development. It is recommended that the split-thickness portion of the flap be developed completely at this stage (see **Fig. 12**E, F).

Next, a vertical incision is made in the distal aspect of the second premolar. The incision is carried down to bone and extended as far apically as possible without damage to the greater palatine artery. A second horizontal incision is next made at the most apical aspect of the previous vertical incision. The incision is made parallel to the previous horizontal incision extending to the mesial of the first premolar. At that point, the incision is curved toward the midpalatal area aiming for a line distal to the incisive papilla in order not to interrupt the blood supply to the flap (see **Fig. 12**G, H). A Buser or similar elevator is used to reflect in a subperiosteal plane, starting at the most distal aspect in the second premolar area and extending anteriorly to the midpalatal area. The more anterior the desired final resting position of the VIP-CT flap, the longer is the arc of rotation of the graft and more is the dissection required. For severe cases, a reverse cutback may be needed. After releasing the pedicled finger flap, it is secured to the recipient site with the use of 4–0 chromic gut sutures (see **Fig. 12**I, J). It is usually beneficial to keep the periosteal aspect of the graft facing the bone because this takes advantage of the osteoblastic potential of the flap. On occasion, when increased height of soft tissue thickness is needed, the flap can be rotated with the periosteum facing away from bone; this allows for increased augmentation of the soft tissue height. After securing the flap, a collagen or hemostatic dressing is placed in the area where the graft was harvested and the area is closed with overlying resorbable sutures (see **Fig. 12**K, L).

The buccal flap is then approximated to the palatal flap using standard suturing techniques. On occasion, primary closure might not be achieved and small areas of the pedicle may remain exposed; usually these areas epithelize over the pedicle without loss of any of the graft (see **Fig. 12**M, N). The use of removable partial denture (flipper) is not recommended given that it may put pressure on the palatal pedicle, thereby compromising its inherent blood supply. Moreover, dentists frequently encounter considerable difficulty with adjusting the denture to fit the space because of the volume of the grafted tissue on the palate. The authors prefer the use of an Essex type of retainer as opposed to a conventional denture in these cases (**Figs. 13** and **14**).

Modified Palatal Roll Technique

Abrams[14] described the original "palatal roll technique." In his technique, a split-thickness palatal flap is reflected separating the epithelium from the connective tissue. The connective tissue is reflected from the palate and rolled onto the buccal to correct a buccolingual soft tissue deficiency. In 1992, Scharf and Tarnow[15] described a modification of the original palatal roll technique. Common indications for this technique include correction of minor soft tissue defects on the buccal aspect at the time of implant placement or during connection of the healing abutment.

Technique and procedure

A #15 blade is used to make a full-thickness palatal incision extending from the crest of the ridge to the palatal area. This incision should be papilla sparing and should be of sufficient length to allow the tissue to be rolled the desired area on the buccal (see **Fig. 13**A). A similar incision is also made on the contralateral side. A partial-thickness incision connecting the two vertical incisions is made on the palatal aspect of the alveolar ridge. A partial-thickness trap door–type flap is reflected (see **Fig. 13**B). A full-thickness incision then is carried through the connective tissue down to periosteum at the apical extent of the two vertical incisions (see **Fig. 13**C). The palatal pedicle is reflected with the use of a Woodson or similar elevator. The pedicle is rolled on the buccal aspect (see **Fig. 13**D). A horizontal mattress suture is used to stabilize the graft on the buccal aspect. This technique can be effectively used for correction of minor soft tissue defects on the buccal aspect (see **Fig. 13**E). Note that this technique is harder to execute in the anterior maxillary area, especially in patients with pronounced palatal rugae. The flap is much easier to develop in the premolar area, because the palatal tissue is thicker

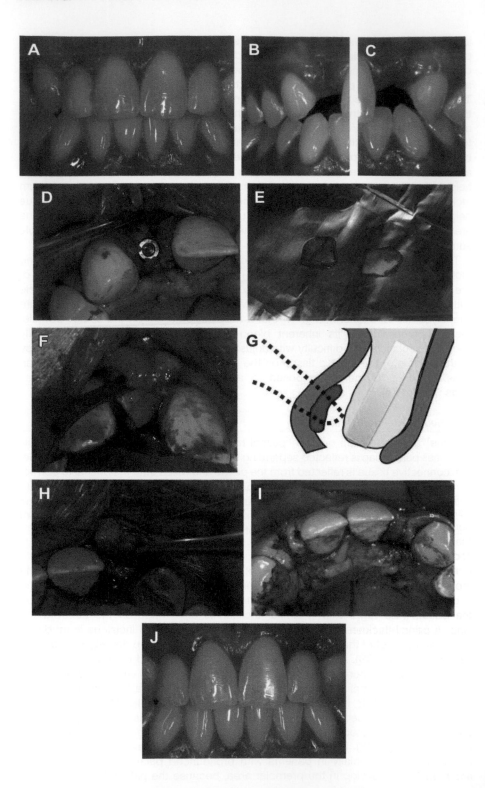

and provides better yield. A downside to this technique is decreased thickness of the palatal tissue.

The authors' prefer to use a subepithelial connective tissue graft instead of the palatal roll technique for most soft tissue deficiency cases. In their experience, the former is easier to perform, and provides for more optimal clinical results on a predictable basis. A modification of the classic palatal roll can be used at the time of exposure and connection of the healing abutment. The location of the implant should be determined with the use of a periodontal probe. The gingiva occlusal to the implant is de-epithelized with diamond bur, laser, or #15 blade (see **Fig. 14A**). Then a semicircular incision is made down to bone and the implant on the palatal aspect (see **Fig. 14B**). Then the tissue is rotated and tunneled on the buccal (see **Fig. 14C**) and secured in place with the use of a horizontal mattress suture. Finally, a healing abutment or the temporary crown is placed (see **Fig. 14D**).

Epithelialized Palatal Graft

Epithelialized palatal grafts have been widely used for correction of mucogingival defects for many years. Bjorn and coworkers[7] were the first to describe the free gingival autograft. Sullivan and colleagues[6] divided gingival grafts based on their thickness into full-thickness and split-thickness grafts. Free grafts are classified as either full-thickness or split-thickness grafts. A full-thickness graft, by definition, consists of the epithelium and the entire zone of lamina propria. Split-thickness grafts are those containing epithelium and less than the full thickness of lamina propria. Split-thickness grafts are subdivided, according to the width of lamina propria included in them, as thick, intermediate, or thin. Thin split-thickness grafts consist of epithelium and a minimal amount of lamina propria. The use of a thicker gingival graft is ideal for cases where the main purpose is to increase the zone of attached tissue. Thicker grafts are more technique sensitive but provide better outcomes. These grafts undergo less secondary graft contraction when compared with split-thickness grafts. Indications for these grafts include mucogingival defects and a requirement to increase the zone of attached or keratinized tissue.

Technique

Using a #15c blade, a desired length incision is made at the junction of the attached and nonattached tissue. At either end of the horizontal incisions, two vertical incisions are then placed. A partial-thickness flap is next developed and reflected using instruments of choice (scissors and/or blades). It is critical to dissect as close to the periosteum to remove epithelium, connective tissue, and muscle fibers; this minimizes the amount of movable tissue that is present. Performing this step carefully decreases the incidence of graft mobility and promotes healing. The dissection is next carried in a supraperiosteal fashion (**Fig. 15A, B**). The periosteum is an ideal layer to which to suture the graft. Once the flap has been developed, it can either be sutured apically or excised.

Fig. 11. (*A*) Patient with congenitally missing laterals. (*B*) After removal of bridge clefting is visible in the soft tissue. (*C*) After removal of bridge clefting is visible in the soft tissue. (*D*) Implant in place. (*E*) Supepithelial connective tissue graft harvested from the palate. (*F*) Graft positioned in the desired position. (*G*) Graft secured to the buccal flap with a horizontal mattress suture. *Dotted line* is suture, *pink* is buccal flap, *red* is subpeithelial graft, and *yellow* is bone. (*H*) The suture is tied to secure the graft to the buccal flap. (*I*) Occlusal view with graft in place on the right side and no graft on the left side. (*J*) Final crown, teeth #7 and #10.

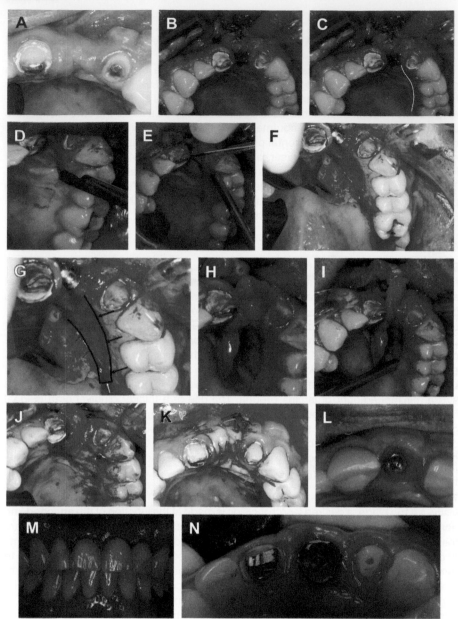

Fig. 12. (*A*) Occlusal view of edentulous space. (*B*) Papilla-sparing incision, also note the incision is extended palatally. (*C*) Full-thickness incision is extended from the distal papilla-sparing incision to mesial aspect of the first molar (*white line*). Another small 4-mm full-thickness incision is extended from the mesial papilla-sparing incision (*black line*). (*D*) A split incision is made on the palatal aspect starting from the first molar area and extending anteriorly. (*E*) The split-thickness incision is extended anteriorly and medially. (*F*) Completed palatal split-thickness incision. (*G*) Outline of the planned finger flap initial full-thickness flap around 3 mm from the CEJ of teeth (*black arrows*), then a second full incision from distal of second premolar (*white arrow*). Then a third incision parallel to the initial incision and curved medially (*gray arrows*). (*H*) Pedicled finger flap reflected. (*I*) Pedicled finger flap reflected and rotated anteriorly. (*J*) Pedicled flap rotated and secured in place. (*K*) Final suturing of the buccal and palatal flaps. (*L*) Final occlusal view showing increased tissue volume after exposure of the implant. (*M*) Final crown frontal view. (*N*) Final crown occlusal view.

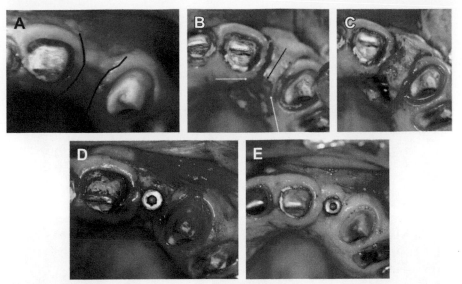

Fig. 13. (*A*) Two full-thickness papilla-sparing incisions extend far enough into the palatal aspect. (*B*) A horizontal (*black arrow*) partial-thickness incision connects the two full-thickness papilla-sparing incisions (*white arrows*). (*C*) After reflection of partial-thickness palatal flap, a full-thickness incision at the palatal apical area is made and the tissue is reflected off the palate. (*D*) The palatal tissue is rolled under the buccal gingival tissue and secured with a horizontal mattress suture. (*E*) Area after 12 weeks of healing. Note increased volume on buccal but thin tissue on the palatal aspect.

After preparation of the recipient site, attention is diverted to the harvest site. A template is used to estimate the desired size of the graft. The graft is commonly harvested from the palate, from the distal aspect of the second premolar to the mesial aspect of the canine avoiding the midline and paramidline rugae area. The graft is outlined with the use of a #15c blade. The most superior aspect of the incision is then made, staying approximately 3 mm apical to the CEJ of the teeth. The dissection is carried down to the desired depth throughout the graft length with either a #15c blade or a sharp scissors, such as the Deans scissor (see **Fig. 15C**). Once the graft has been harvested, it is trimmed to the desired shape and thinned out, if needed (see **Fig. 15D**). The graft is adapted to the recipient site and secured with several 4–0 or 5–0 resorbable sutures. The graft is initially secured at the mesial and distal corners and this ensures that the entire area is covered and that the graft is well adapted to the recipient site. Sutures are then placed in other areas to fully secure the graft. If desired, additional sling or horizontal mattress sutures can be added to further stabilize the graft. Once suturing is complete, pressure is applied to the graft for approximately 10 minutes; this aids with hemostasis, and decreases the dead space between the graft and recipient site. Biophysiologically, during this time and beyond, plasma is converted into fibrin, and this further binds the graft to the recipient site and promotes diffusion of nutrition into the graft (see **Fig. 15E, F**).

HEALING OF SOFT TISSUE GRAFTS

The subepithelial graft is ideal for reconstruction of most soft tissue defects. This graft is mostly composed of connective tissue matrix that allows for ingrowth of new

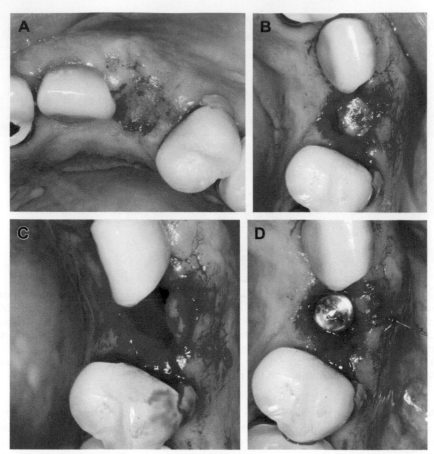

Fig. 14. (*A*) After probing the location of the implant, the epithelium is de-epithelized. (*B*) A semicircular full-thickness incision is made on the palatal aspect. (*C*) Tissue is reflected and then tunneled under the buccal flap. (*D*) The tissue is tunneled under the buccal tissue and secured in place with a horizontal mattress suture.

fibroblasts that are in addition to the fibroblasts already transported with the graft. The initial healing depends on plasmatic imbibition or diffusion during the first 24 to 48 hours. The initial hypoxic gradient between the graft and the recipient site is responsible for initiating this process. This initial plasmatic diffusion is responsible for the initial metabolite influx to the graft. Inflammatory mediators stimulate neovascularization of new capillaries from the recipient site into the graft. Anastomosis between the vessels of the recipient site and graft is established and the graft has adequate blood supply by approximately postoperative day 8. During the revascularization process, connective tissue reattachment between the graft and the recipient bed occurs. This process is completed by postoperative day 10. After final healing, the graft undergoes secondary contraction.

POSTOPERATIVE CARE

Pain management with over-the-counter medication or narcotics is recommended. Chlorhexidine 0.12% oral rinse twice a day for 10 days and warm normal saline oral

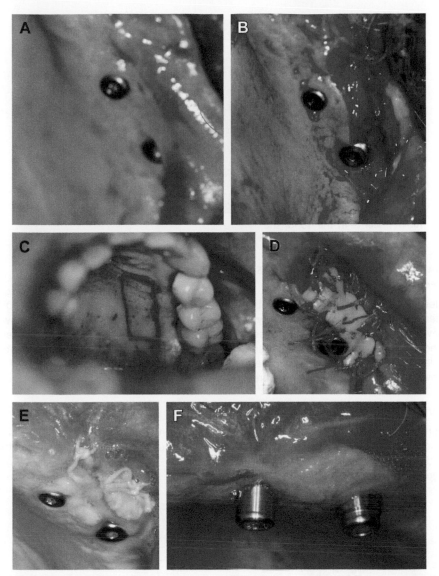

Fig. 15. (*A*) Preoperative view showing no attached tissue on the buccal aspect of the posterior implant. (*B*) Split-thickness incision is developed buccal to the implant and sutured apically. (*C*) Split-thickness epithelial graft is harvested. (*D*) Graft secured and sutured in place. (*E*) Graft at the 4-week postoperative visit. (*F*) Graft 2 years postoperative.

rinses three to five times daily are prescribed. Patients should be instructed not to use a Water-Pik or an electric toothbrush around the graft area for 4 weeks. Cold pack applications to the face over the area for 10 minutes at a time, twice an hour, for the first 6 hours and soft diet for 1 week are encouraged. Smoking should be avoided for 4 to 6 weeks.

A follow-up appointment should be scheduled 7 to 14 days after surgery to examine the progress of healing. If a periodontal dressing is placed it is usually discontinued at the same time as suture removal.

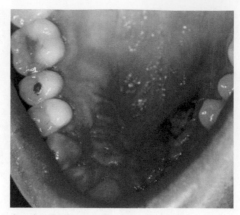

Fig. 16. Dehiscence at the donor site.

MANAGEMENT OF COMPLICATIONS
Bleeding

Bleeding could be encountered at the time of surgery or in the postoperative period. Bleeding is commonly managed with application of pressure, which usually slows down bleeding. If the source of bleeding is identified it can be cauterized or ligated. If no source is identified several sutures can be placed along the course of the greater palatine artery to compress the artery; also local with epinephrine can be injected to slow the bleeding and additional pressure applied.

Dehiscence at the Donor Site

Dehiscence at the donor site is one of the most common causes of postoperative discomfort (**Fig. 16**). Conservative management is recommended; the area granulates and completely heals over 3 to 4 weeks.

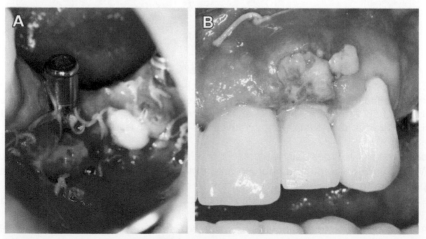

Fig. 17. (*A*) Partial loss of epithelialized connective tissue graft. (*B*) Partial loss of subepithelial connective tissue graft.

Partial or Complete Loss of the Graft

Connective tissue grafts have a high success rate, but in general partial or complete loss of the graft is possible (**Fig. 17**). Recommended management includes conservative debridement of necrotic tissue. If any tissue seems fibrinous in nature observation is recommended. One of the key factors in prevention is immobilization of the graft at the time of surgery.

REFERENCES

1. Fürhauser R, Florescu D, Benesch T, et al. Evaluation of soft tissue around single-tooth implant crowns: the pink esthetic score. Clin Oral Implants Res 2005;16(6): 639–44.
2. Olsson M, Lindhe J. Periodontal characteristics in individuals with varying form of the upper central incisors. J Clin Periodontol 1991;18(1):78–82.
3. Olsson M, Lindhe J, Marinello CP. On the relationship between crown form and clinical features of the gingiva in adolescents. J Clin Periodontol 1993;20(8): 570–7.
4. Bhat V, Shetty S. Prevalence of different gingival biotypes in individuals with varying forms of maxillary central incisors: a survey. J Dent Implants 2013;3(2): 116–21.
5. Sclar A. Soft tissue and esthetic considerations in implant therapy. Quintessence Publishing; 2003.
6. Sullivan HC, Atkins JH. Free autogenous gingival grafts. I. Principles of successful grafting. Periodontics 1968;6(3):121–9.
7. Bjorn H. Free transplantation of gingival propria. Sven Tandlak Tidskr 1963;22: 684–5.
8. Rees TD, Brasher WJ. A technique for obtaining thin split-thickness grafts in periodontal surgery. Oral Surg Oral Med Oral Pathol 1970;29(1):148–54.
9. Dibart S, Karima M. Practical Periodontal plastic surgery. Danvers (MA): Blackwell; 2006.
10. Reiser GM, Bruno JF, Mahan PE, et al. The subepithelial connective tissue graft palatal donor site: anatomic considerations for surgeons. Int J Periodontics Restorative Dent 1996;16(2):130–7.
11. Langer B, Langer L. Subepithelial connective tissue graft technique for root coverage. J Periodontol 1985;56(12):715–20.
12. Zuhr O, Hurzeler M. Plastic – esthetic periodontal and implant surgery a microsurgical approach. United Kingdom: Quintessence Publishing; 2012.
13. Palacci P. Esthetic implant dentistry, soft and hard tissue management. Quintessence Publishing; 2001.
14. Abrams L. Augmentation of the deformed residual edentulous ridge for fixed prosthesis. Comp Contin Educ Gen Dent 1980;1(3):205–13.
15. Scharf DR, Tarnow DP. Modified roll technique for localized alveolar ridge augmentation. Int J Periodontics Restorative Dent 1992;12(5):415–25.

Bone Morphogenic Protein

Application in Implant Dentistry

Dustin Bowler, DDS[a],*, Harry Dym, DDS[b,c,d,e]

KEYWORDS

- Bone morphogenic protein • Vertical and horizontal ridge augmentation
- Maxillary sinus lift • Implant site grafting and preparation

KEY POINTS

- Alveolar bone that is insufficient to support implant placement due to lack of height or width may be augmented with grafting materials including bone morphogenic protein (BMP) to create sites that are adequate for implant placement and long-term stability of an implant-supported prosthesis.
- BMP can be used alone or in concert with other bone graft materials as an alternative to invasive allograft bone-harvesting procedures.
- Patients who would otherwise not have been suitable candidates for major autologous bone grafting procedures can continue to benefit from implant reconstruction, with a less debilitating bone reconstructive procedure.

INTRODUCTION

Implant-supported prostheses are currently widely accepted as the preferred treatment, by patients and doctors alike, for the partially and completely edentulous patient. Even though implant treatment is preferred, many patients present with insufficient alveolar bone to obtain implant osseointegration. Such a lack of quality alveolar bone (**Fig. 1**), a contraindication of implant placement, is common in patients with long-standing or traumatic edentulism. Many treatments have been developed to prepare the site for implant placement and increase the likelihood of long-term implant stability.

Bone grafting, in particular the autogenous bone graft, has emerged as the treatment of choice of many dentists and oral surgeons. Autogenous bone grafts from the hip and tibia are considered to be the gold standard for large bony defects, but

The authors have nothing to disclose.

[a] Oral and Maxillofacial Surgery Training Program, The Brooklyn Hospital Center, 121 Dekalb Ave, Brooklyn, NY 11201, USA; [b] Dentistry/Oral and Maxillofacial Surgery, Residency Training Program, The Brooklyn Hospital Center, 121 Dekalb Ave, Brooklyn, NY 11201, USA; [c] Oral and Maxillofacial Surgery, Columbia University College of Dental Medicine, 630 West 168th street, NY 10032, USA; [d] Woodhull Hospital, 760 Broadway, Brooklyn, NY 11206, USA; [e] New York Harbor Healthcare System, 423 East 23rd street, New York, NY 10010, USA
* Corresponding author.
E-mail address: dustinbowler@gmail.com

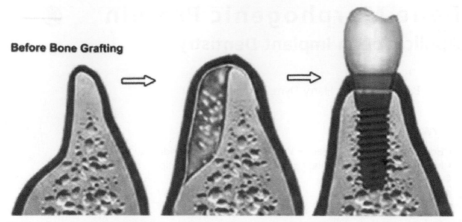

Before Bone Grafting

Fig. 1. Common alveolar buccal atrophy in need of preimplant reconstruction. (*From* Dym H, Pierse J. Advanced techniques in bone grafting procedures. Dent Clin North Am 2011; 55(3):454; with permission.)

they can be less than ideal for a large number of patients. These procedures often require general anesthesia, hospitalization, and potentially serious postoperative complications at the donor site. Elderly patients, who often are the most in need of extensive preimplant grafting, are particularly susceptible to many postoperative complications including donor site morbidity, delayed wound healing, and gait disturbances. Given the potential complications and additional surgical sites, many patients are not good candidates for such grafting procedures, and additional patients may elect not to pursue what they view as such invasive treatment.

Given the large and growing patient population requiring nonautogenous bone grafting procedures, there is clearly a need in the general population for a nonautologous graft material that can be used to augment alveolar bone prior to implant placement. Many alloplastic materials and allografts (**Table 1**) have been used. Most alloplastic materials are considered adequate but less than ideal. The ideal alloplastic material should not only be osteoconductive, but also osteoinductive (**Box 1, Table 2**).

The search for such a material has led the dental community to bone morphogenic proteins (BMPs).

Table 1 Bone substitute synopsis		
Graft Material	**Characteristics**	**Examples**
Allograft	A graft that is taken from a member of the same species as the host but is genetically dissimilar	Cadaver cortical/cancellous bone, FDBA, DFDBA
Xenograft	Graft derived from a genetically different species than the host	Bio-Oss, coralline HA, red algae
Alloplast (synthetic materials)	Fabricated graft materials	Calcium sulfate, bioactive glasses, HA, NiTi

Abbreviations: Bio-Oss, bovine bone derivative; FDBA, freeze-dried bone allografts; HA, hydroxyapatite; NiTi, nickel titanium alloy.
Data from Kao ST, Scott DD. A review of bone substitutes. Oral Maxillofac Surg Clin North Am 2007;19:514.

> **Box 1**
> **Bone formation definitions**
>
> **Osteogenesis**
>
> Osteogenesis refers to living cells, such as osteoblasts, that form new bone. The success of any bone grafting procedure depends on having enough bone-forming or osteogenic cells in the area. Iliac crest bone graft (ICBG), a type of autograft, is the only bone graft that contains enough cells to be considered osteogenic. Local bone from the primary surgical site generally contains cortical bone with much fewer cells. However, the presence of mesenchymal stem cells does not make a bone graft osteogenic. These stem cells require a signal, such as bone morphogenetic protein (BMP), to differentiate into osteoblasts.
>
> **Osteoconduction**
>
> Osteoconduction refers to the ability of some materials to serve as a scaffold onto which bone cells can attach, migrate, grow, and divide. In this way, the bone healing response is conducted through the graft site, just as a vine uses a trellis for support. Osteogenic cells generally work much better when they have a matrix or scaffold for attachment. Ceramics are strictly osteoconductive scaffolds and fall in the category of autograft extender or bone void filler.
>
> **Osteoinduction**
>
> Osteoinduction refers to the capacity of normal growth factors in the body to attract, proliferate, and differentiate primitive stem cells or immature bone cells to grow and mature, forming healthy bone tissue. Most of these signals are part of a group of protein molecules called BMPs, which are found in normal bone. Highly osteoinductive bone grafts have been evaluated as an autograft alternative in certain indications.

PROPERTIES AND HISTORY

BMPs are members of the transforming growth factor-b superfamily that were first described by Urist[1] after observing ectopic bone formation in a rodent model from implanted devitalized cadaveric bone. This family of proteins is highly osteoinductive and contains powerful stimulants of endochondral and intramembranous bone formation from pluripotent mesenchymal cells. Several types of BMPs have been isolated and cloned using recombinant DNA technology; however, the most studied has been bone morphogenic protein-2 (Rh-BMP-2). BMPs act as growth and differentiation factors and chemotactic agents. BMPs stimulate angiogenesis and migration, proliferation, and differentiation of mesenchymal stem cells into cartilage and hard tissue, forming cells in an area of bone injury.

Two major clinical studies were performed to examine the feasibility, safety, and efficacy of using Rh-BMP-2 in oral and maxillofacial applications. Boyne and colleagues[2] performed a randomized prospective controlled study utilizing Rh-BMP-2

Table 2
Bone graft material characteristics

Characteristic	Graft Material
Osteogenesis	Autograft
Osteoinduction	BMP, DFDBA, DBM
Osteoconduction	Bio-Oss, calcium phosphates, calcium sulfate, collagen, FDBA, glass ionomers HA, NiTi, BMP

Data from Kao ST, Scott DD. A review of bone substitutes. Oral Maxillofacial Surg Clin North Am 2007;19:514.

delivery via an absorbable collagen sponge (ACS) as an adjunct in maxillary sinus floor augmentation. Fiorellini and colleagues[3] performed randomized prospective controlled studies on the use of Rh-BMP-2/ACS in extraction site preservation and augmentation. Both studies demonstrated that Rh-BMP-2/ACS at 1.5 mg/cc induced significant bone formation suitable for implant placement. The bone induced by Rh-BMP-2/ACS was found to be biologically similar to native bone and capable of implant osseointegration and supporting the functional loading of a dental prosthesis.

The identification and development of Rh-BMP has led to the commercial availability of an osteoinductive alloplastic bone graft material (Infuse Bone Graft, Medtronic Spinal and Biologics, Memphis, TN, USA).

In March 2007, Infuse bone graft was approved by the US Food and Drug Administration (FDA) as an alternative to autogenous bone graft for use in sinus augmentation and localized alveolar ridge augmentation (extraction socket preservation). Infuse bone graft is also approved for use many neurosurgical and orthopedic surgical procedures, including interbody spine fusion and fresh tibial fractures.

SURGICAL PROCEDURE

Another added benefit of the Infuse graft material is the ease of use. The Rh-BMP-2/ACS (Infuse) device comes packaged as a powder and liquid with an ACS (**Fig. 2**). The carrier component or ACS is derived from highly purified bovine tendon type-1 collagen and provides the matrix for the delivery of the Rh-BMP-2. The Rh-BMP-2 comes as a powder that must first be reconstituted with dilution and then evenly expressed onto the ACS carrier (need to wait 15 minutes). At this point, if the material is to be used for postextraction socket preservation, the prepared graft is inserted into an extraction site defect and closed with a tension-free soft tissue closure. For use in maxillary sinus augmentation, the graft material is placed in the sinus cavity below the elevated sinus membrane. For augmentation of buccal wall defects and posterior mandibular height and width augmentation, it is best to secure (using small bone screws) a 0.2 mm titanium mesh to maintain the Rh-BMP-2 in place. This titanium mesh technique is not always used and should be based on the individual surgeon's preference and past experience. One of the authors (HD) also perforates the buccal plate with a small round burr before placing Rh-BMP-2/ACS. The titanium mesh material is available in sheets, which are easily custom fitted by the treating clinician, although

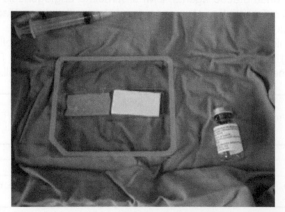

Fig. 2. Powder/liquid and absorbable collagen sponge of Infuse product. (*Courtesy of* Medtronic Spinal and Biologics, Memphis, TN, USA.)

prebent and contoured titanium mesh is now available from select vendors. Many of these treatments will be discussed further in the Clinical Case Examples section.

SAFETY, ADVERSE EFFECTS, AND COMPLICATIONS

Since the inception of the use of BMPs in treatment, there have been many studies investigating the safety, adverse effects, and possible complication of its use. The investigations are found, almost exclusively, in the neurosurgery and orthopedic literature. Although no studies are currently found in the literature specifically reporting the complications of Rh-BMP-2/ACS (Infuse) usage in oral and maxillofacial surgery procedures, the manufacturer does supply specific recommendations and warnings (**Box 2**) for use in oral and maxillofacial procedures including sinus augmentation, socket preservation, and augmentation of alveolar ridge in extractions socket defects.

The dental literature does report some adverse effects with varying severity and incidence. Edema and seroma were noted clinically following Rh-BMP-2 placement in a clinical study previously noted by Boyne and colleagues. They observed that patients in the Rh-BMP-2/ACS treatment group experienced a significantly greater amount of facial edema than those in the bone-grafted treatment group. This edema is thought not to be the result of surgical trauma or an allergic response but rather due to the activity of the Rh-BMP-2, causing an influx of fluid and cells into the treatment area related to the chemotaxis and neovascularization of the site.[4] They concluded that no other reported events were felt to be related to the Rh-BMP-2.

Rh-BMP-2 has been widely evaluated for use in neurosurgical applications including neck and spine fusion procedures. Although such use is FDA approved, recently the FDA placed a cautionary warning in usage in anterior cervical spine surgery due to increased soft tissue swelling resulting in airway restriction and compromise in patients.[5] Off-label neurosurgical usage of Rh-BMP-2/ACS (Infuse) has been reportedly linked with cancer, neurologic deficits, arachnoiditis, swelling, hematoma, infection, osteolysis, seroma, heterogenic ossification, retrograde ejaculation, and/or the need for intubation/tracheostomy.[6] Often these complications have been reported in cases in which high-doses of Rh-BMP-2 and Rh-BMP-7 were used.

The data summary published by FDA in 2002,[7] with the exception 1 study,[8] reported that the risk of cancer is the same among the control and Rh-BMP-2 group in

---

Box 2
Infuse warnings for Oral maxillofacial surgery procedures

Scar formation

Allergic reaction

Development of antibodies to:

  Rh-BMP-2/ACS

  Bovine collagen

  Human type I collagen

Ectopic bone formation

Complications in development of a fetus

Itching

Nerve or tissue damage

Possible death

24-month follow-up. A recent study[5] found that at high concentrations of Rh-BMP-2 (40 mg, AMPLIFY), there is a higher risk of cancer (3.8%) when compared with the control groups in 24 month follow-up. The same study has reported that lower dosages (4.2–4.8 mg) of Rh-BMP-2 showed no increase in the risk of cancer among trial groups, implying the risk of cancer may be dose-dependent An additional study[9] reported no statistically significant association or promotion of metastasis or tumorigenesis in review of clinical and basic science studies.

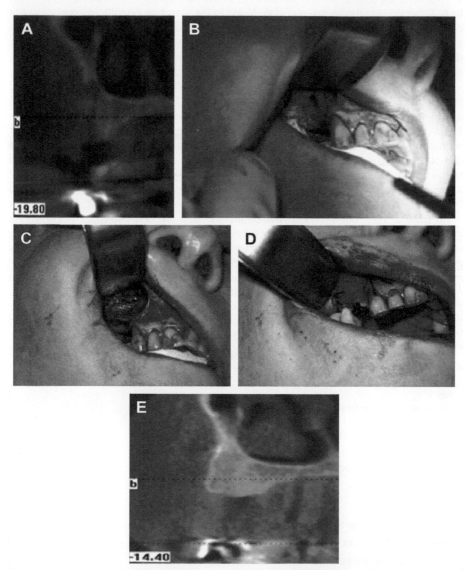

Fig. 3. (*A*) Cone beam study showing buccal wall defect in the #6 area. (*B*) Buccal alveolar defect in area of #6. (*C*) Titanium mesh secured to alveolus containing BMP-2 collagen sponge. (*D*) Primary closure obtained with buccal flap. (*E*) Buccal plate regenerated, 6 months after Infuse placement. (*From* Dym H, Pierse J. Advanced techniques in bone grafting procedures. Dent Clin North Am 2011;55(3):457; with permission.)

Please note that the concentrations that yielded differences in cancer rates were significantly more concentrated than the dosages used in oral and maxillofacial procedures. There have been no studies demonstrating increased risks of cancer using BMP-2 doses and concentrations that are within the recommendations for oral and maxillofacial reconstruction procedures. Dental practitioners need to be mindful of the contraindications with usage of Infuse and the recommended doses just as with any other medication and treatment.

CLINICAL CASE EXAMPLES
Case 1

A 78-year-old woman who had a failed implant removed in the #6 position was seen by cone beam studies to have small bone fragments with no plate of bone remaining. Infuse graft was placed with a titanium mesh technique. The patient returned 6 months later for implant placement. Excellent results were obtained without having to resort to using an autologous onlay graft or particulate allograft and membrane (**Fig. 3**).

Case 2

This case involved a 72-year-old woman with a history of failed endosseous implants in the upper left maxilla. The patient had no existing alveolar bone and was in need of a major sinus augmentation. The patient underwent a standard lateral maxillary window sinus procedure, but only the Infuse graft was used as the primary bone graft materials. The patient had excellent results and was restored with the placement of 4 endosseous implants (**Fig. 4**).

Case 3

This case involved a 16-year-old boy with an alveolar cleft that required bone grafting (**Fig. 5**). The patient and his family were given an option of autologous, allograft, or Infuse-type bone graft procedure. The patient's family wished to have the procedure done with Infuse graft. The standard exposure was performed, and Infuse was inserted. Six months later, good bone bridging was seen. Note: this was an off-label

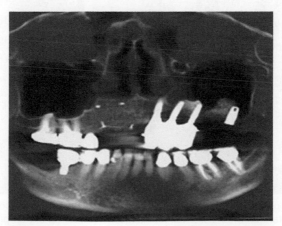

Fig. 4. Maxillary sinus grafted only with Infuse material followed by implant placement. (*From* Dym H, Pierse J. Advanced techniques in bone grafting procedures. Dent Clin North Am 2011;55(3):458; with permission.)

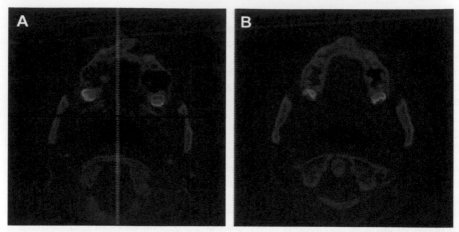

Fig. 5. (A) Preoperative axial cone beam view showing alveolar anterior bone cleft defect. (B) Six months following Infuse bone graft showing bone growth. (From Dym H, Pierse J. Advanced techniques in bone grafting procedures. Dent Clin North Am 2011;55(3):458; with permission.)

use of the product, and the patient and his family were made aware of this before its use.

Case 4

A 26-year-old woman with a history of right mandibular molar extractions required bone grafting to augment her mandibular-deficient alveolus in both vertical and horizontal dimension. The patient underwent an Infuse bone graft procedure with the use of titanium mesh. Excellent results were obtained without the need of resorting to autologous block bone graft procedure, and implants were placed into the site 6 months later (Fig. 6).

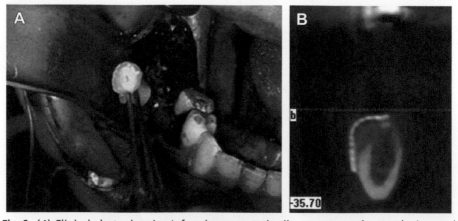

Fig. 6. (A) Clinical photo showing Infuse-impregnated collagen sponge about to be inserted underneath the titanium mesh material. (B) Six-month follow-up digital picture of atrophic posterior mandible augmented with Infuse material using mesh. (From Dym H, Pierse J. Advanced techniques in bone grafting procedures. Dent Clin North Am 2011;55(3):459; with permission.)

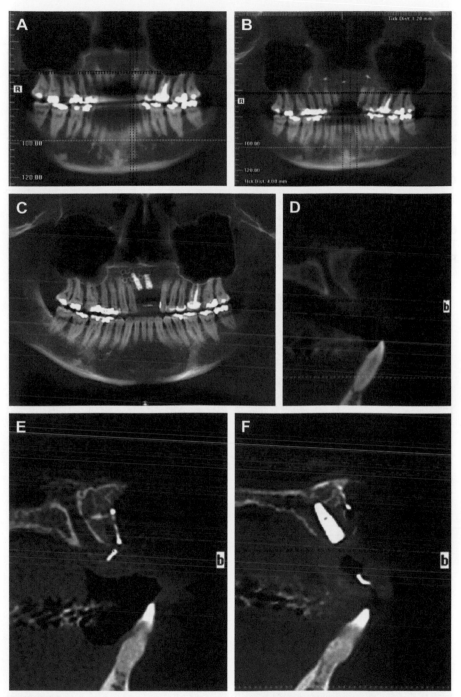

Fig. 7. (*A*) Preoperative panoramic radiograph with deficient anterior maxilla. (*B*) Panoramic radiograph status after BMP-2 and mesh placement. (*C*) Panoramic radiograph status after implant placement. (*D*) CBCT view of edentulous site anterior maxilla. (*E*) CBCT slice status after BMP-2 and mesh placement. (*F*) CBCT slice status after implant placement.

Case 5

This patient presented with post-traumatic loss of teeth in the anterior maxilla. Like many traumatic edentulous patients, the loss of alveolar bone was significant in this case. Preoperative panoramic radiograph and CBCT slices are shown below (**Fig. 7**). The anterior maxilla was grafted using Rh-BMP-2 with a titanium mesh. After 6 months healing time, the site was reopened for planned mesh retrieval and implant placement. At this time, the new bone formation had overgrown the titanium mesh to the point that removal of the mesh would compromise the bone graft. The patient was advised about the mesh and accepted the treating physician's recommendation to leave the mesh undisturbed. Implants were placed, as planned, without complication.

Case 6

This patient presented with left pneumatized maxillary sinus. Left maxillary sinus lift was performed. Rh-BMP-2 was used as a graft material to elevate the sinus floor. After 6 months of healing, the left maxillary quadrant was restored using 3 dental implants. The level of increased bone height can clearly be seen in the radiographs displayed in **Fig. 8**.

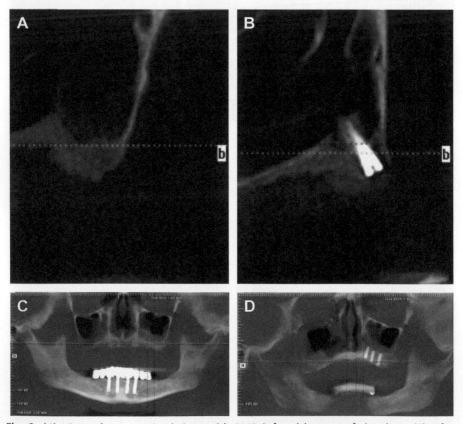

Fig. 8. (*A*) View of pneumatized sinus with BMP infused bone graft in place. (*B*) After 6 months of healing, dental implant placed at site with primary stability. (*C*) Panoramic view of pneumatized sinus with BMP infused bone graft in place in left maxillary sinus. (*D*) Postoperative panoramic film of implants placed in left maxilla.

SUMMARY

The development of alloplastic bone grafting materials infused with purified proteins or stem cells to induce osteogenesis is a significant contribution to patient care. Patients who would otherwise not have been suitable candidates for major autologous bone grafting procedures can continue to benefit from implant reconstruction, with a less debilitating bone reconstructive procedure.

REFERENCES

1. Urist MR. Bone: formation by autoinduction. Science 1965;150:893–9.
2. Boyne PJ, Lilly LC, Marx RE, et al. De novo bone induction by recombinant human morphogenetic protien-2 (rhBMP-2) in maxillary sinus floor augmentation. J Oral Maxillofac Surg 2005;63:1693–707.
3. Fiorellini JP, Howell TH, Cochran D, et al. Randomized study evaluating recombinant bone morphogenetic protein-2 for extraction socket augmentation. J Periodontol 2005;76:605–13.
4. Triplett RG, Nevins M, Marx RE, et al. Pivotal, parallel evaluation of recombinant human bone morphogenetic protein-2/absorbable collagen sponge and autogenous bone graft for maxillary sinus floor augmentation. J Oral Maxillofac Surg 2009;67:1947–60.
5. Devine JG, Dettori JR, France JC, et al. The use of rhBMP in spine surgery: is there a cancer risk? Evid Based Spine Care J 2012;3:35–41.
6. Epstein NE. Complications due to the use of BMP/INFUSE in spine surgery: the evidence continues to mount. Surg Neurol Int 2013;4(Suppl 5):S343–52.
7. Food and Drug Administration. Summary of Safety and Effectiveness Data (SSED) for P000058 Medtronic's InFUSE™ Bone Graft/LT-CAGE™ lumbar tapered fusion device. Orthopaedic and Rehabilitation Devices Advisory Panel. 2002. Available at: http://www.accessdata.fda.gov/cdrh_docs/pdf/P000058b.pdf. Accessed July, 2014.
8. Burkus JK, Gornet MF, Dickman CA, et al. Anterior lumbar interbody fusion using rhBMP-2 with tapered interbody cages. J Spinal Disord Tech 2002;15(5):337–49.
9. Thawani JP, Wang AC, Than KD, et al. Bone morphogenetic proteins and cancer: review of the literature. Neurosurgery 2010;66(2):233–46 [discussion: 246].

Implant Surface Material, Design, and Osseointegration

 CrossMark

Orrett E. Ogle, DDS[a,b,c],*

KEYWORDS

• Dental implants • Titanium surface • Implant design • Osseointegration

KEY POINTS

- The structural and functional union of the implant with living bone is greatly influenced by the surface properties of the implant.
- The success of a dental implant depends on the chemical, physical, mechanical, and topographic characteristics of its surface.
- The influence of surface topography on osseointegration has translated to shorter healing times from implant placement to restoration.

The fusion of the surface of a dental implant with the surrounding bone plays a crucial role in the longevity and the function of the implant-supported prosthesis. In fact, the most important biological event in the clinical healing phase of dental implants is cell adhesion at the interface between the host tissue and the implant. This structural and functional union of the implant with living bone is greatly influenced by the surface properties of the implant. In reality, the success of a dental implant is highly dependent on its chemical, physical, mechanical, and topographic characteristics of its surface. These different properties interact and determine the activity of the attached cells that are close to the dental implant surface.[1] The topography of the implant surface has been shown to influence the differentiation and proliferation of osteoblasts, and the up-regulation of transcription factors that are responsible for the expression of bone matrix formation genes. The influence of surface topography on osseointegration has translated to shorter healing times from implant placement to restoration.[2]

At present, the vast majority of dental implants marketed in the United States are made from commercially pure titanium (cpTi) or titanium alloys. A smaller group of

The author has nothing to disclose.
[a] Mona Dental Program, Faculty of Medical Sciences, University of the West Indies, Mona Campus, Kingston, Jamaica; [b] The Brooklyn Hospital Center, Brooklyn, NY 11201, USA; [c] Oral and Maxillofacial Surgery, Woodhull Hospital, Brooklyn, NY 11206, USA
* 4974 Golf Valley Court, Douglasville, GA 30135.
E-mail address: oeogle@aol.com

Dent Clin N Am 59 (2015) 505–520
http://dx.doi.org/10.1016/j.cden.2014.12.003
0011-8532/15/$ – see front matter © 2015 Elsevier Inc. All rights reserved.

implants are made out of a surface-coated hydroxyapatite (HA) or zirconium. Neither cpTi, its alloys, nor any of the other surface materials are fully 100% capable of directly bonding with living bone. Analysis of retrieved titanium implants showed that the bone-to-implant fusion was not entirely complete. Albrektsson and colleagues[3] reported that the percentage of bone-to-implant contact area averaged 70% to 80%. However, even 60% bone-to-implant contact was enough osseointegration for successful implants that lasted for up to 17 years. Because of this recognized imperfection in total osseointegration, modifications of the implant surfaces are continuously being made for the purpose of enhancing and also shortening the time for osseointegration with each manufacturer claiming that theirs is the best.

There are several studies that compare one implant system with another, but a great number of them are comparisons with the Branemark system (Nobel Biocare, Zurich, Switzerland). There are no well-documented series of scientific studies that show the superiority of one implant surface over the other or one product versus another. Most of the better studies only focus on one implant system and documentation of their success. A good criterion for the quality of a dental implant is that studies should document that the implant survived for at least 5 years under function in the oral cavity. In this article, relevant scientific data are presented that should allow the clinician to better understand the information coming from implant manufacturers and that should allow for better implant selection.

IMPLANT MATERIAL

cpTi, titanium alloy (with or without HA), and zirconium are the materials of choice for dental implants. Implants made from other materials should not be used unless the manufacturer can produce sound scientific evidence with good clinical trials. Laboratory studies should not be accepted as validity for the quality of a dental implant because it is not able to predict actual patient outcome and clinical longevity.

Titanium

Titanium is biologically inert and has a high resistance to corrosion because of the spontaneous formation of a film of titanium oxide (TiO_2) on its surface,[4] which separates the metal from its environment. Typically, the thickness of this oxide layer is about 3 to 10 nm.[5] It is known that the protective and stable oxides on titanium surfaces are able to provide favorable osseointegration. The stability of the oxide depends strongly on the composition structure and thickness of the film.[6] It is this oxide film that gives titanium and its alloys such good biocompatibility when used for dental implants. The passive film that forms on titanium is stable, even in a biological system as hostile as the oral cavity.

cpTi and titanium alloys are currently the materials of choice for dental implants. Unalloyed cpTi has various degrees of purity, which are graded from 1 to 4. The grading is related to the corrosion resistance, ductility, and strength. cpTi grade 1 has the highest purity, the highest corrosion resistance, formability, and lowest strength, whereas grade 4 offers the highest strength and moderate formability. Most dental implants are made from grade 4 cpTi because it is stronger than the other grades.[7]

The titanium alloy used for dental implants is specially made for dental implant applications. The specific alloy used is grade 5 titanium alloy, which has greater yield strength and fatigue properties than pure titanium. Grade 5 alloy, which is usually designated as Ti6Al4V, has a chemical composition of 6% aluminum, 4% vanadium, 0.25% (maximum) iron, 0.2% (maximum) oxygen, and 90% titanium.[8] The advantages of Ti6Al4V are its superior corrosion resistance, high fatigue strength, and low elastic modulus, which reduces stress shielding.[4]

cpTi has limited mechanical properties. In cases where good mechanical characteristics are required, as in the posterior jaw where biting forces are high, Ti6Al4V alloy is preferred.

Hydroxyapatite

HA, the mineral component of bones and teeth, is used as a coating on the implant surface in an attempt to provide titanium and its alloys with improved bonding ability to living bone. Because bone contains HA, implants coated with this material are thought to be a good biomaterial for implant surface because of its excellent biocompatibility and good mechanical properties. HA coating has been shown to give improved bone implant attachment and, being osteoconductive in nature, more bone deposition has been noted.[9] Enhancement of the osteoconductivity will increase the initial stability of the implant and shorten the treatment time.

Titanium under load-bearing conditions has good clinically biocompatibility coupled with high strength and fracture resistance but does not form a chemical bond with bone tissue. It is thought that HA coatings on titanium dental implants will accelerate surface bone apposition, thereby shortening the waiting period for dental implant restoration.

Studies have shown good primary stability of dental implants coated with HA with improved bone implant attachment.[9] However, in a meta-analysis of HA-coated implants, the survival rates reported for HA-coated implants were similar to other implants, but the success rates were significantly lower than the overall survival rates. The 10-year survival rate was 87.39% compared with the 10-year success rate of 63.84%.[10] These implants integrate fast and will survive but were only 64% clinically successful. The current HA applications of 1 μm thickness have now reduced the risk of loosening of the implant from the bone and have improved the success rate.[11] Specific indications for the selection of HA-coated implants over metallic implants are reactions to metals, the need for a greater initial bone implant interface contact, placement in type IV bone, fresh extraction sites, and newly grafted sites.[12]

Zirconium

Zirconia (Zr) is a "ceramic" compound, which is highly biocompatible and possesses the capacity to osseointegrate (**Fig. 1**).[13,14]

In its pure form, zirconium cannot be used in dentistry. It has to be manufactured, following many different steps, to be usable in dentistry. The manufacturing process of zirconium implants is very strict but varies for each implant company.[15] The companies have not provided extensive information about the surface characteristics of their implants; this represents some difficulty in the evaluation of its surface because the final product may have different chemical compositions. Regardless of the composition, however, it has been shown that the biocompatibility of zirconium is good, even if the composition of the tested materials is different.

As a biomaterial for dental implants, zirconium possesses very favorable physical properties, such as flexural strength (900–1200 MPa), hardness (1200 Vickers), as well as a favorable threshold stress intensity factor.[16] Another quality is its resistance to corrosion. Although highly unlikely, titanium can be subjected to corrosion, thus making the longevity and durability theoretically less than zirconium. The corrosion possibilities of titanium are almost entirely dependent on the iron content. At room temperature, titanium normally forms a stable oxide coating on its surface, which

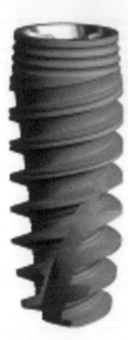

Fig. 1. Zirconium implant from Nobel Biocare. (*Courtesy of* Nobel Biocare, Zurich, Switzerland.)

limits further oxidation. This oxide coating is very adherent, and chemically stable, and is capable of spontaneously and instantaneously repairing itself if damaged by its environment. cpTi grade 4, the strongest of the grades, has the highest allowable iron content of the unalloyed grades of 0.50% maximum iron. Despite its relatively high iron content, the corrosion resistance of cpTi grade 4 is very high based on the presence of the stable, continuous, tightly adherent oxide layer, which forms spontaneously on exposure to oxygen.

Animal studies indicate similar biocompatibility and osseointegration for zirconium compared with titanium implants.[17] In a recent extensive review article, the literature suggested that zirconium implants had an inferior degree of osseointegration (removal torque tests) compared with titanium implants, but that some surface structural modifications allowed removal torque test values to come close to those obtained by titanium implants. The removal torque test values will depend more on the surface structure than on the implant material itself.[15] To date, there does not appear to be consistency in the zirconium materials used and in their long-term stability. Its major indications are a replacement for metals and improved esthetic qualities in anterior restorations. Wennerberg and Albrektsson[11] recommended proceeding slowly and with caution when considering Zr ceramic implants.

SURFACE CHARACTERISTICS

To improve the rate and quality of osseointegration, survivability, and function, manufacturers have focused on topographic changes of implant surfaces rather than alterations of chemical properties. One such significant alteration that affects the mechanical stability of the implant/tissue interface is the creation of surface irregularities that improve the mechanical interlocking between bone tissue and implant materials. Irregular surfaces improve metal shear strength and decrease implant loosening. In addition to providing better mechanical stability between bone tissue and the implant surface, roughness is also a configuration that will retain blood clots completely and stimulates the bone-healing process. Clinically, it has been known for a long time that the amount of bone-to-implant contact is an important factor in the long-term success of dental implants. This bone-to-implant contact is enhanced by implant surface roughness.[18] Controlled surface roughness now plays an important role in enhancing the osseointegration of titanium implants.

Biochemical methods of surface modifications, for example, adding rhBMP-2 or fluoride, have been tried but have had a limited effect on the level of osseointegration. The general goals of biochemical modifications are to immobilize proteins, enzymes, or peptides on biomaterials for the purpose of inducing specific cell and tissue responses, or in other words, to control the tissue-implant interface with molecules that are delivered directly to the interface.[19]

The rate and quality of osseointegration of dental implants are highly related to their composition and surface roughness. Rough-surfaced implants improve bone anchoring and biomechanical stability, and several reports have documented that the surface roughness of titanium and other implants affect the rate of osseointegration and the biomechanical fixation.[20] High roughness results in mechanical interlocking between the implant surface and the adjacent bone along with stimulation of the bone-healing process. Because of this, it has been suggested that these types of implants can be loaded earlier than machined implants. A surface roughness in the range of 1 to 10 μm will maximize the interlocking between mineralized bone and the surface of the implant.[20] Surface roughness in this range will result in greater bone-to-implant contact and higher resistance to torque removal. A theoretic approach suggested that the ideal surface should be covered with hemispherical pits approximately 1.5 μm in depth and 4 μm in diameter.[21,22] However, there is currently no consensus on the degree of surface roughness that is optimum for bone cell attachment.

Implant surface irregularities can be achieved by surface concave texturing or by surface convex texturing. Surface concave textures are achieved by either etching the material by chemical or electrochemical actions or creating mechanical indentations by sand-blasting, shot-peening, or laser-peening. Convex textured surface is formed by depositing certain types of particles on the implant surface, for example, plasma-spraying (**Fig. 2**).

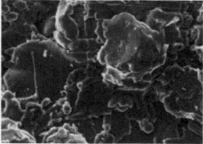

Fig. 2. Surface roughness created by Ti plasma spraying. (*From* Le Guehennec L, Soueidan A, Layrolle P, et al. Surface treatments of titanium dental implants for rapid osseointegration. Dent Mater 2007;23:847; with permission.)

Titanium

The titanium surface is modified to concave texture by the following techniques.

Sand-blasting

Blasting is a technique used to create a porous layer on the implant surface through the collision with microscopic particles. The nature of the porous layer can be altered by the size of the granule particles. Sand and grit blasting are used to modify the implant surface by using TiO_2 and alumina particles. TiO_2 particles measuring 25 μm are used to grit the blast (**Fig. 3**).

Shot-peening and laser-peening

Shot-peening (similar to sand-blasting but more controlled) is a cold working process in which the surface is bombarded with small spherical particles called shots that create small indentations or dimples on the implant surface. Laser peening involves striking the metal with high-intensity pulses of laser light beam that produces a deep and regular honeycomb pattern with small pores.

Convex textures Convex texturing is achieved by adding particles to the implant surface (see **Fig. 2**). The process is achieved by plasma deposition, which in some cases is able to create an engineered surface with features usually standing below 100 nm. The coating layers that produce the convexities are only functional and effective, however, if they adhere firmly to the metal substrate and if they are strong enough to transfer all load.

Hydroxyapatite coating

HA coating is added on the Ti implant surface to achieve better osteoconductivity (**Fig. 4**A–C). It is generally applied as spherical beads typically 20 to 80 μm in size, but HA granules ranging in size from 1 to 8 μm have also been used. A plasma spray method is used as the apatite-coating method because it gives tight adhesion between the apatite coating and Ti. Plasma-sprayed HA coatings on dental implants consist of mixtures of amorphous calcium phosphate with varying ratios of crystalline calcium phosphate and HA.

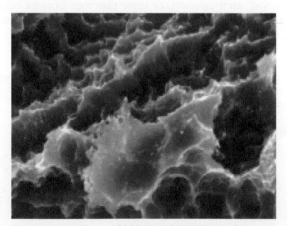

Fig. 3. Surface roughness created by sand blasting. (*From* Le Guehennec L, Soueidan A, Layrolle P, et al. Surface treatments of titanium dental implants for rapid osseointegration. Dent Mater 2007;23:844–54; with permission.)

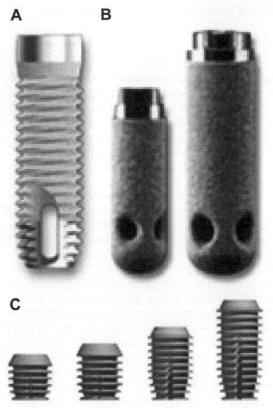

Fig. 4. (*A*) Zimmer HA-coated implant. (*B*) Zimmer HA spline reliance. (*C*) Bicon short implant system. Available in diameters from 4.5 to 6.0 mm and lengths from 5 to 11 mm. Please note that this HA-coated implant has been discontinued. (*Courtesy of* [*A, B*] Zimmer Dental, Carlsbad, CA, USA; and [*C*] Bicon Dental Implants, Boston, MA, USA.)

Titanium plasma sprayed The plasma spray process is also used to enable titanium particles to be coated onto the underlying implant surface with a uniform pattern.

Zirconium

Roughening the surfaces of Zr implants also enhances bone apposition and has a beneficial effect on interfacial shear strength; however, the mean removal torque values were higher for sand-blasted acid-etched titanium implants. The roughed Zr implants showed resistance to torque forces almost similar to machined TiO and 4-fold to 5-fold increase compared with machined Zr implants.[23]

The results from an animal study comparing bone-to-implant contact of 4 different types of titanium implant surfaces showed that adding roughness to the implant surface produced numerically superior bone-to-implant contact.[24] The results were as follows:

Machined = 41.7%
Titanium plasma spray (TPS) = 48.9%
HA coated = 57.9%
Sandblasting w/soluble particles = 68.5%.

INFLUENCE OF IMPLANT MATERIAL ON OSSEOINTEGRATION

There are no excellent scientific studies from which it can be deduced which implant design or surfaces are superior. Most of the time, implant success will depend on treatment planning, surgical skills, prosthetic design, and patient behavior rather than on the implant surface. In a retrospective analysis of 2349 implants in 677 patients to identify risk factors associated with failures of Biocon implants using a multivariant regression analysis, it was determined that implant surface was not a factor, but that failures were due to tobacco use, implant length, staging, well size, and immediate implants.[25] Osseointegration per se is not linked to any particular surface characteristics, because a great number of different surfaces achieve clinical osseointegration. However, the stronger or weaker bone responses may be related to the surface characteristics.[11]

Implant manufacturers do not fully disclose the exact compositions of their implant surfaces so it is difficult to compare the surface properties of one with the other. Most of the published studies were not standardized and they used different surfaces, cell populations, or animal models. Whatever their chemical composition may be, however, most of these surfaces have proven clinical successful with greater than 95% survival over a period of 5 years. Tracking the success rates of different implants in clinical use may be somewhat helpful in deciding on an implant system. In Finland, a national register for dental implants was initiated by their National Agency for Medicines in 1994. They systematically tracked the numbers of implants placed and the numbers removed in the period between 1994 and 2000. During the period, 43,533 implant placements and 808 removals were registered (1.9% failure). A higher proportion of removals than average were recorded for the Branemark system, 324/8075 = 4.0%; IMZ, 63/1812 = 3.5%; and Frialit, 39/1533 = 2.5%. Implant brands with a lower than the mean removal rate were ITI, 199/17,270 = 1.2%; Astra Tech, 77/7289 = 1.1%; and 3i, 11/1229 = 0.9%.[26] The reasons for removals were not stated, nor in what timeframe the implants were removed. Using these data as indicators of estimations of clinical performance of different implants, although interesting, may not be valid because implant success depends more on selecting the correct implant to match the clinical needs than the implant surface characteristics. The Branemark system being in use for the longest period of time may explain their higher removal rates.

Although surface roughness plays a crucial role in implant stability and osseointegration, some studies have indicated that in the case of a favorable bone quality (type 1 or 2 bone) the surface roughness plays only a minor role.[27] A more positive effect of the surface roughness has been observed in poor quality bone.[19] Over the years, it has been noted that the survival rate of oral implants placed into type 4 bone is markedly decreased compared with other bone qualities. Huang and colleagues[28] showed that when roughened implants were placed in type 4 bone, there was a difference in density between the bone inside and that immediately outside the threads that was statistically significant. This finding reflects a remodeling process in the immediate osteotomy site. The results suggest that the porous TiO_2 surface possesses considerable osteoconductive potential in promoting a high level of implant osseointegration in type 4 bone. Roughened implants have also been associated with higher survival rates in grafted sinuses,[29] and the consensus is that the implant-bone response is influenced by the topographic surface of the implant.

IMPLANT DESIGN

The features of the design of dental implants are one of the most critical factors that have an effect on primary stability and on the implant's ability to sustain loading after osseointegration. The overall stability of the bone-implant interface is important in maintaining the longevity of the implant. One of the most important criteria for the stability of the bone-implant interface is load transfer at the interface by using different lengths, diameters, surface materials, and thread designs. In evaluating the biomechanical features of the various implant designs, the stress transmission between the implant and the surrounding bone is of great significance in determining the success or failure of the implant. Factors that influence the load transfer at the bone-implant interface include the type of loading, material properties of the implant and prosthesis, implant geometry length, diameter as well as shape, implant surface structure, the nature of the bone-implant interface, and quality and quantity of the surrounding bone.[30]

The most important biomechanical factors that influence the load transfer at the bone-implant interface are the length, diameter, and body/thread shape. The optimum length and diameter necessary for long-term implantation success depend on the quality of the bone support. In type 1 and 2 bone, length and diameter do not seem to be significant factors for implant success. In type 3 and 4 bone, large-diameter implants are recommended and short implants should be avoided.[31] Clinical experience has shown that if the bone quality is poor, then a larger-diameter implant is needed. By increasing the implant diameter and/or by increasing the length, the peak stress values will decrease and stress distributions will be more homogenous. The parameter that mainly affects the implant stress-based performances is the diameter, irrespective of the length.[32] In a finite element analysis, Anitua and colleagues[33] reported stress values of 122.9 MPa with an implant of 2.5-mm diameter and 8.5-mm length, whereas with an implant of 5.0-mm diameter and 15-mm length, the stress value was 39.6 MPa. Increasing the diameter from 2.5 mm to 3.3 mm (30%) reduced the stress value by 31%, whereas increasing the length from 8.5 mm to 15.0 mm resulted in a reduction of only 1.7%.

A comparison of implant stability readings by Bailleri and colleagues[34] failed to demonstrate a direct relationship between implant length and primary stability. Their results indicated that a short implant could be as stable as a long implant. Primary implant stability plays a significant role in successful osseointegration.

An increase in implant diameter induces a significant reduction of stress peaks at cortical bone, whereas the variation in implant length produces its influence only on stress patterns at the cancellous bone-implant interface.[35] The highest stresses on the cortical bone are located at the crestal bone around the implant, which corresponded with the clinical finding of crestal bone loss. For the trabecular bone, the stress was concentrated in the region of the implant-trabecular bone interface, at the tip of the threads, and at the end of the implant. Under conditions of prosthetic overloading, the risks for failure are greater in cancellous bone than in cortical bone.

In addition to length and width, thread shape and thread details also play a dominant role on local stress patterns at the bone-implant interface. Thread geometry in terms of pitch, depth, and width will affect the stress distribution forces all around the implant-contacted bone. The ultimate goal of the thread design should be to avoid or minimize stress peaks under loading. In this regard, thread depths (the distance between the major and minor diameter of the thread) seemed to play a very significant role on implant stability in both trabecular and cortical bone, whereas variations of pitch (the distance from the center of the thread to the center of the next thread) and the thread face angle (the angle between a face of a thread and a plane perpendicular to the long axis of the implant) do not influence implant stability in trabecular bone.[36] Chung and colleagues[37] found that implants with a pitch distance of 0.6 mm had more crestal cortical bone loss than implants with 0.5-mm pitch. These authors concluded that as pitch decreased, the surface area increased, leading to a more favorable stress distribution. Implant with a higher number of threads is advisable in poor bone quality, areas with high occlusal forces, and in short implants. However, from a surgical point of view, the fewer the threads, the easier and faster it will be to insert the implant. Misch and colleagues[38] stated that "the deeper the threads, the wider the surface area of the implant," which is a design that is very advantageous in softer bone and higher occlusal force areas because of a higher functional surface area in contact with the bone itself. In summary, implant threads should allow for increased stability and more implant surface contact area.

IMPLANT SHAPE

Surface modifications and implant shape are independent conditions that can alter the response at the implant/bone interface. Three types of loads are generated at the interface: compressive, tensile, and shear forces. Compressive force tends to increase the bone density and thus increases its strength, whereas tensile and shear forces result in a poorer interface, with shear being the worst.[38] The type of force generated depends on the shape of the implant and on the site of placement. An ideal implant design, therefore, should provide a balance between compressive and tensile forces while minimizing the initiation of shear forces.

There is a wide variation in the shape of implants with a trend toward having implants with 3-dimensional alterations along the vertical axis (**Fig. 5**).

The advantage of having a geometric feature on the implant is that it decreases the dependence on a complex drilling and placement protocol to create the level of compression needed for initial stability. On the contrary, high forces and stresses may arise at geometric notches, which may occur when a straight contour is abandoned. Implant shapes can be straight, tapered, conical, ovoid, trapezoid, or stepped (**Fig. 6**).

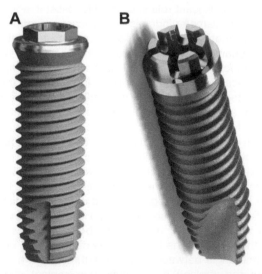

Fig. 5. (*A*) Geometric feature of Branemark system from Nobel Biocare. (*B*) Geometric feature of Zimmer system. (*Courtesy of* [*A*] Nobel Biocare, Zurich, Switzerland; and [*B*] Zimmer Dental, Carlsbad, CA, USA.)

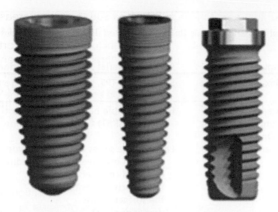

Fig. 6. Tapered and straight implants. (*Courtesy of* Nobel Biocare, Zurich, Switzerland.)

Although implant shape can affect the bone response, there are very few publications that have looked at clinical outcomes with different implant geometry, and these few studies have not clearly identified any particular implant geometry as an important factor when it relates to treatment success. To achieve high treatment success, the implant design should reduce crestal bone loss, biomechanical load, and microfractures of the bone as well as increase the primary stability of the implant.

For dense bone, type 1 and 2, design does not play a significant role and is less important. Regardless of the implant shape, higher bone quality is related to better primary stability and better long-term success. The differences between different implant designs are more pronounced in type 4 bone, mainly because of the significant decrease in primary stability in low-density bone. The goal, therefore, is to have an implant design that can result in improved primary stability in soft bone. By achieving and maintaining good stability during the remodeling of the trabecular network, more dense bone will lead to a more lasting implant.

From the early Branemark days, endosseous implants were parallel in design (see **Fig. 5**A, B), but, using finite element analysis, Rieger and colleagues[39] reported that stress is dissipated more throughout the interfacial area with tapered implants (see **Fig. 6**; **Fig. 7**). They concluded that a tapered endosseous implant with a high elastic

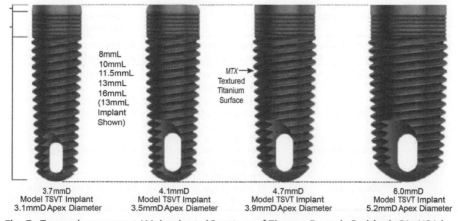

8mmL
10mmL
11.5mmL
13mmL
16mmL
(13mmL
Implant
Shown)

MTX→
Textured
Titanium
Surface

3.7mmD	4.1mmD	4.7mmD	6.0mmD
Model TSVT Implant	Model TSVT Implant	Model TSVT Implant	Model TSVT Implant
3.1mmD Apex Diameter	3.5mmD Apex Diameter	3.9mmD Apex Diameter	5.2mmD Apex Diameter

Fig. 7. Tapered screw-vent HA implant. (*Courtesy of* Zimmer Dental, Carlsbad, CA, USA.)

Table 1
Widely used dental implant systems (Indications listed are not absolute, but are simply suggestions)

Manufacturer	Implant System	Surface Material	Indication
Biocon	Max 2.5 and short	Selection of TPS. HA coated. Acid etched	Fixed, removable All bone qualities
Biohorizon	Internal/external implant systems. One piece	HA. Resorbable blast textured (RBT) titanium	All prosthetic uses All bone qualities
	Laser Lock 3.0	Laser lock (a series of precision-engineered cell-sized channels laser-machined onto the surface of the dental implant)	All prosthetic uses All bone qualities
	Single stage	RBT	All prosthetic uses
	Short	Laser lock	Removable
	Tapered	RBT	All prosthetic uses
Biomet 3i	Nanotite	Ti coated with osseotite and calcium phosphate	Extraction sockets Simultaneous grafted sites Implant placement in esthetic zone where bone preservation is critical
	Osseotite and Osseotite XP	Ti-osseotite microtextured	Fixed, removable
Dentsply	OsseoSpeed	Ti micro-roughened-fluoride-modified	All prosthetic uses All bone qualities
	XiVE	Ti-Grit-blasted	Single tooth restorations
MIS	Cl. M4. Conical Seven	Ti-sand-blasted/acid-etched	All prosthetic uses
Noble Biocare	Branemark	CP grade 4 titanium	Fixed prostheses Better for type 1 and 2 bone
	Active-tapered	CP grade 4 titanium	All prosthetic uses, extraction sites
	Noble Replace	Machined Ti	Soft to moderately hard bone
	NobelRondo Zirconia	Zr	Anterior esthetic restorations
Straumann	Roxolid SLActive	Titanium zirconium alloy	All implantology uses
	Straumann System	Ti–acid-etched	All implantology uses
Zimmer	AdVent	Titanium implant surface with HA particles and HA coating	Over dentures, single tooth Type 3, 4 bone
	Screw Vent	Titanium implant surface with HA particles and HA coating	All prosthetic uses
	Trabecular metal	Porous tantalum trabecular metal-enhanced titanium	All prosthetic uses
	One-piece	Ti alloy grade 5—microtextured	Single and multiple teeth

modulus is the most suitable shape. In a 3-dimensional finite element analysis, Huang and colleagues[40] showed that the tapered body form decreased the stresses in both cortical and trabecular bone compared with straight design. Zimmer Dental reports that their Tapered Screw-Vent HA implant (see **Fig. 7**) is now their flagship implant (Joanna Dorgan, Zimmer Dental, Carlsbad, CA, USA, personal communication, July 2014).

In an assessment of primary implant stability, O'Sullivan and colleagues[41] reported that the tapered-screw-type implant had a significantly higher initial stability in type IV bone quality compared with straight implants. There was no significant difference in initial stability values when the bone quality was satisfactory.

In good-quality bone, types 1 and 2, implant shape has very little influence on initial stability, osseointegration, and final success. The success or failure is more dependent on patient-related, procedural, and prosthetic parameters than implant shape. Tapered screw-type implants give better initial stability in poor-quality bone and distribute the occlusal force to surrounding bones more equally than straight-screw types.[42] Bone perforation is also less likely to occur because of the tapered shape.

IMPLANT SELECTION

For 90% of patients, any of the leading implant systems will give good results depending on prosthetic treatment planning, quality of surgery, and patient parameters (**Table 1**). Variations in the size and shape of implants become relevant for the exceptions, such as patients with low bone volume and poor quality bone. Determination of the size and shape to be used is a part of the diagnostic and treatment planning process used by the implant practitioner. For any implant system, it is critical that the practitioner become very familiar with the intricacies of the individual system.

As a general rule, if the practitioner is not doing many implants daily, then it is not economically advisable to have a lot of inventory on hand. It is recommended, therefore, that the dentist select an implant company that has a "presence" in the area and can get products to the office in 1 or 2 days. Most companies will be able to provide an implant to match the clinical indications. Titanium and its alloys have the widest use. In general, the widest possible implant should be used and conventional cross-sectional tomography should be the method of choice for gaining information on implant diameter for most patients. Diagnostic radiographic studies with cross-sectional imaging are significant in making implant selection for compromised implant cases. Tapered implants are now being used for many cases in which the bone narrows below the alveolar crest.

Zirconium implants (see **Fig. 1**) are indicated in anterior restorations where color is significant because of a thin gingival overlay and where the tissue could transmit an unesthetic gray hue from titanium implants. There are, however, several reports of Zr abutment fractures. The force that is expected to be loaded on the restoration must be taken into consideration.

HA-coated dental implants have been shown to improve the rate of success in patients with poor bone quality.

REFERENCES

1. Grassi S, Piattelli A, de Figueiredo LC, et al. Histologic evaluation of early human bone response to different implant surfaces. J Periodontol 2006;77(10):1736–43.
2. Cochran DL, Buser D, ten Bruggenkate CM, et al. The use of reduced healing times on ITI implants with a sandblasted and acid-etched (SLA) surface: early

results from clinical trials on ITI SLA implants. Clin Oral Implants Res 2002;13(2): 144–53.

3. Albrektsson T, Eriksson AR, Friberg B, et al. Histologic investigations on 33 retrieved Nobelpharma implants. Clin Mater 1993;12(1):1–9.

4. Jacobs JJ, Gilbert JL, Urban RM. Current concepts review: corrosion of metal orthopaedic implants. J Bone Joint Surg Am 1998;80A:268–82.

5. Neoh KG, Hu X, Zheng D, et al. Balancing osteoblast functions and bacterial adhesion on functionalized titanium surfaces. Biomaterials 2012;33:2813–22.

6. Zhu X, Chen J, Scheideler L, et al. Effects of topography and composition of titanium surface oxides on osteoblast responses. Biomaterials 2004;25:4087–103.

7. Steinemann S. Titanium - The material of choice? Periodontol 2000 1998;17(1):7–21.

8. ASM Material Data Sheet. Available at: http://asm.matweb.com/search/SpecificMaterial.asp?bassnum=MTP642. Accessed February 2014.

9. Strnad Z, Strnad J, Povysil C, et al. Effect of plasma-sprayed hydroxyapatite coating on the osteoconductivity of commercially pure titanium implants. Int J Oral Maxillofac Implants 2000;15(4):483–90.

10. Zhou W, Liu Z, Xu S, et al. Long-term survivability of hydroxyapatite-coated implants: a meta-analysis. Oral Surg 2011;4(1):2–7.

11. Wennerberg A, Albrektsson T. On implant surfaces: a review of the current knowledge and opinions. Int J Oral Maxillofac Implants 2010;25(1):63–74.

12. Anusavice K. Dental implants. In: Anusavice k, editor. Philips science of dental materials. 11th edition. St Louis (MO): Saunders -Elsevier; 2005. Chapter 23 (Kindle book. Hard copy not available).

13. Delgado-Ruiz RA, Calvo-Guirado JL, Abboud M, et al. Histologic and histomorphometric behavior of microgrooved zirconia dental implants with immediate loading. Clin Implant Dent Relat Res 2013. Available at: http://www.ncbi.nlm.nih.gov/m/pubmed/23560416/. Accessed February 2014.

14. Koch FP, Weng D, Krämer S, et al. Osseointegration of one-piece zirconia implants compared with a titanium implant of identical design: a histomorphometric study in the dog. Clin Oral Implants Res 2010;21(3):350–6.

15. Assal P. The osseointegration of zirconia dental implants. Schweiz Monatsschr Zahnmed 2013;123(7–8):644–54.

16. Andreiotelli M, Wenz HJ, Kohal RJ. Are ceramic implants a viable alternative to titanium implants? A systematic literature review. Clin Oral Implants Res 2009; 20(9 Suppl 4):32–47.

17. Moller B, Terheyden H, Acil Y, et al. A comparison of biocompatibility and osseointegration of ceramic and titanium implants: an in vivo and in vitro study. Int J Oral Maxillofac Surg 2012;41(5):638–45.

18. Soskolne W, Cohen S, Sennerby L, et al. The effect of titanium surface roughness on the adhesion of monocytes and their secretion of TNF-α and PGE 2. Clin Oral Implants Res 2002;13:86–93.

19. Garg H, Bedi G, Garg A. Implant surface modifications: a review. J Clinic Dental Research 2012;6(2):319–24.

20. Wennerberg A, Hallgren C, Johansson C, et al. A histomorphometric evaluation of screw-shaped implants each prepared with two surface roughnesses. Clin Oral Implants Res 1998;9:11–9.

21. Le Guéhennec L, Soueidan A, Layrolle P, et al. Surface treatments of titanium dental implants for rapid osseointegration. Dent Mater 2007;2(3):844–54.

22. Hansson S, Norton M. The relation between surface roughness and interfacial shear strength for bone-anchored implants. A mathematical model. J Biomech 1999;32:829–36.

23. Gahlert M, Gudehus T, Eichhorn S, et al. Biomechanical and histomorphometric comparison between zirconia implants with varying surface textures and a titanium implant in the maxilla of miniature pigs. Clin Oral Implants Res 2007;18: 662–8.

24. Novaes AB Jr, Souza SL, de Oliveria PT, et al. Histomorphometric analysis of the bone-implant contact obtained with 4 different implant surface treatments placed side by side in the dog mandible. Int J Oral Maxillofac Implants 2002;17(3): 377–83.

25. Chuang SK, Wei LJ, Douglass CW, et al. Risk factors for dental implant failure: a strategy for the analysis of clustered failure-time observations. J Dent Res 2002; 81:572–7.

26. Jokstad A, Braegger U, Brunski JB, et al. Quality of dental implants. Int Dent J 2003;53(Suppl 6):607–41.

27. Nawab Al B, Pangen U, Duschner H, et al. Turned, machined vs double etched dental implants in vivo. Clin Implant Dent Relat Res 2007;9(2):71–8.

28. Huang YH, Xiropaidis AV, Albabdar RG, et al. Bone formation at titanium porous oxide (TiUnite) oral implants in type IV bone. Clin Oral Implants Res 2005;16: 105–11.

29. Marchetti C, Pieri F, Trasarti S, et al. Impact of implant surface and grafting protocol on clinical outcomes of endosseous implants. Int J Oral Maxillofac Implants 2007;22:399–407.

30. Weinstein AM, Klawitter JJ, Anand SC, et al. Stress analysis of porous rooted dental implants. Implantologist 1997;1(2):104–9.

31. Holmgren EP, Seckingpr RJ, Kilgren LM, et al. Evaluating parameters of osseointegrated dental implants using finite element analysis – a two-dimensional comparative study examining the effects of implant diameter, implant shape, and load direction. J Oral Implantol 1998;4(2):80–8.

32. Baggi L, Di Girolamo M, Vairo G, et al. Comparative evaluation of osseointegrated dental implants based on platform-switching concept: influence of diameter, length, thread shape, and in-bone positioning depth on stress-based performance. Comput Math Methods Med 2013;2013:250929. Available at: http://www.ncbi.nlm.nih.gov/pmc/articles/PMC3703879/. Accessed February 2014.

33. Anitua A, Tapia R, Luzuriaga F, et al. Influence of implant length, diameter, and geometry on stress distribution: a finite element analysis. Int J Periodontics Restorative Dent 2010;30(1):89–95.

34. Bailleri P, Cozzolino A, Ghelli L, et al. Stability measurements of osseointegrated implants using Osstell in partially edentulous jaws after 1 year of loading. Clin Implant Dent Relat Res 2002;4(3):128–32.

35. Baggi L, Cappelloni I, Di Girolamo M, et al. The influence of implant diameter and length on stress distribution of osseointegrated implants related to crestal bone geometry: a three-dimensional finite element analysis. J Prosthet Dent 2008; 100(6):422–31.

36. Ausiello P, Franciosa P, Martorelli M, et al. Effects of thread features in osseointegrated titanium implants using a statistics-based finite element method. Dent Mater 2012;28:919–27.

37. Chung SH, Heo SJ, Koak JY, et al. Effects of implant geometry and surface treatment on osseointegration after functional loading: a dog study. J Oral Rehabil 2008;35:229–36.

38. Misch CE, Strong T, Bidez MW. Scientific rationale for dental implant design. In: Misch CE, editor. Contemporary implant dentistry. 3rd edition. St Louis (MO): Mosby; 2008. p. 200–29.

39. Rieger MR, Mayberry M, Brose MO. Finite element analysis of six endosseous implants. J Prosthet Dent 1990;63(6):671–6.

40. Huang HL, Chang CH, Hsu JT, et al. Comparison of implant body designs and threaded designs of dental implants: a 3-dimensional finite element analysis. Int J Oral Maxillofac Implants 2007;22(4):551–62.

41. O'Sullivan D, Sennerby L, Meredith N. Measurements comparing the initial stability of five designs of dental implants: a human cadaver study. Clin Implant Dent Relat Res 2000;2:85–92.

42. Glauser R, Sennerby L, Meredith N, et al. Resonance frequency analysis of implants subjected to immediate or early functional occlusal loading. Successful vs. failing implants. Clin Oral Implants Res 2004;15:428–34.

Index

Note: Page numbers of article titles are in **boldface** type.

Dent Clin N Am 59 (2015) 521–527
http://dx.doi.org/10.1016/S0011-8532(15)00009-9
0011-8532/15/$ – see front matter © 2015 Elsevier Inc. All rights reserved.

dental.theclinics.com

Printed and bound by CPI Group (UK) Ltd, Croydon, CR0 4YY

07/10/2024

01040499-0010